Also by Susan Powter
Stop the Insanity!
The Pocket Powter

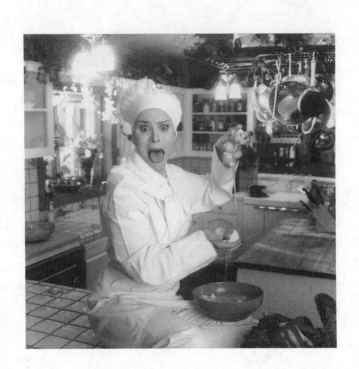

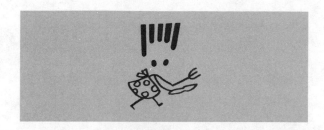

FOOD

by

Susan Powter

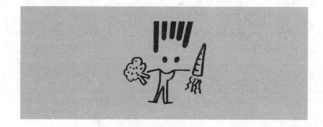

SIMON & SCHUSTER
NEW YORK LONDON TORONTO
SYDNEY TOKYO SINGAPORE

SIMON & SCHUSTER
Rockefeller Center
1230 Avenue of the Americas
New York, NY 10020

SIMON & SCHUSTER and colophon are registered trademarks of Simon & Schuster Inc.

Designed by Karolina Harris

Manufactured in the United States of America

10 9 8 7 6 5 4 3 2 1

Library of Congress Cataloging-in-Publication Data is available.

ISBN 0-671-89225-8

I first met Suzi the mom,
The most honest, wonderful mother I've met.
Then I met Suzi the friend,
The most honest, wonderful friend I've met.
Then I met Suzi the computer wizard, the organizer, the best researcher,
The most honest, wonderful person I've met.
I love meeting Suzi.
I thank her.

Deanne
Lights the candles,
Places the flowers,
Creates the beauty, the peace, the beautiful smells, and checks the ingredients.
She puts it all together with such grace.
I thank her.

Rusty
Believes, believes, believes,
Loves, loves, loves,
Works, works, works.
Without her there would be nothing.
I thank her.

Sally
Sprinkles in some organization,
Adds a dash of structure,
Fixes, mends, pieces it all together to make it whole,
With the beauty and strength of an angel.
I thank her.

Bob and Debl, who showed me what I missed in college.
Long hours sitting at a table covered in papers,
Throwing around ideas and working to the point of delirium,
Lots and lots of bad food, big fun, and organization like you've never seen.
The biggest term paper I've ever done could not have been done without their
   help.
I thank them.

Rita and Manny
Invited Rusty and me into their celebration.
We had the most wonderful, warm, tasty beyond tasty business meeting I've ever
    had.
The great-tasting, low-fat recipes that you will be preparing in your kitchens come
    from Rita to you with hard work, dedication, and love.
What a pleasure the Stern family is . . .
I thank you all.

To the thousands and thousands of women I've met over the last few years who
have asked the questions, written, phoned, networked the solutions, and made it
very clear what you want. Food, food, food, food, food, food. . . .

This book is for you, about you, and dedicated to you and your families.

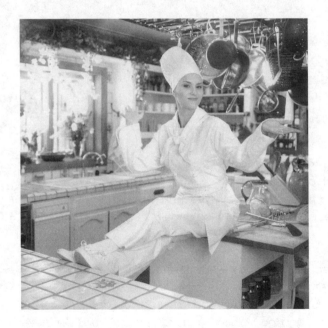

CONTENTS

Stage 3

THE FOOD CONNECTION

Food = joy.

Food = guilt.

Food = anger.

Food = pain.

Food = nurturing.

Food = friendship.

Food = hatred.

Food = the way you look and feel.

Other than genetics and environmental considerations, what determines the way you look and feel more than what you arc eating?

Food = everything you can imagine.

What is food?

It's the reward at the end of a good dental visit. When you are hurt and angry, food is warmer and more soothing than a fire on a cold winter night.

It's tasting the taste you've been craving all day, as satisfying as finally getting to a toilet when you've been dying to go.

It's the lollipop you get at the end of a shopping trip with Mommy that lets you know you've been the good little girl you try so hard to be.

It's the beating you're looking for, that food club you use when you're bingeing and hating yourself.

It's the strongest love/hate relationship I've ever had. Talk about something you can't live with and you can't live without! Food!!

Our connection with food reaches as far back as the cave and is as current as the therapist's couch.

Food is your fuel, the stuff that feeds you and keeps you going. But let's forget about that for a while, because we are jumping right into the psychology of it all. The emotion. The why, how, and what we can do to gain more control of and have a better understanding of this powerful influence in our lives. Can't you hear the tabloids now? "Susan Powter: From fitness to psychology—who does she think she is?" Well, if it's food we are talking about, and it is, then why not break it down, understand it, get the answers to the questions we all have—get it all out on the table, pardon the pun, and figure it out?????

Hi! My name is Susan Powter, and do I have a food connection story to tell you.

There has been quite a bit of psychological confusion in my life. You've probably heard about the Prince situation—such confusion there never was!!!!!

I've spent years trying to do the adult thing, grow up, heal what has to be healed—maturing. I've worked it. From forgiving the nuns who did everything in their power to turn me into a good Catholic girl with the side of a ruler, to not blaming Mom and Dad for their codependent, enabling, chemically imbalanced way of bringing us up. And other than a few sharp words blasted all over national TV, I've looked right past the industries that starved and humiliated me (the diet and fitness industries) and breezed with maturity beyond the brother who ran to the tabloids saying I was never 260 pounds (what was I, 258?) while the rest of the family stood by and watched with embarrassment and sadness.

I've slowly and painfully worked through a relationship with my ex-husband, the Prince, who was a catalyst, shall we say, for one of the biggest food connections in my life—gaining a hell of a lot of weight (133 pounds, but who's counting?) after the breakup of our marriage. Notice I say one of the biggest food connections. I've got a food connection story to tell you that will break your heart; it's the most important food connection in my life because it involves one of the people I love most in the world, my son. But one moment please . . . a round of applause for me, for being such an adult and referring to my ex-husband as a catalyst. Did you hear that: Nic the catalyst!! Growing up in the public eye, wouldn't you say—the end of an era. Bravo!

Before I was such an adult, I blamed the nuns, my parents, and of course the Prince every time I found myself shoving food in my mouth, gaining weight, and hating the way I looked and felt. But the further I get into this food thing, the more I realize how emotionally connected I am to food and how deeply rooted food is in the lives of millions of women. The thousands and thousands of letters, phone calls, conversations in grocery stores, airports, and everywhere else I go with the women I've met—you—over the last few years have made it all very clear.

Oh, the stories we have to tell! The solutions we've figured out to some of the problems. The brilliant, brilliant ways we've discovered to make the changes in our lives that have turned food from the enemy into a friend. That's what this book is about. Food—I've used it for everything it's worth, and still do, even in my newfound maturity. Listen to this:

Recently a reporter wrote an article about me that was about as mean-spirited as you get. It wasn't what the article said that hurt me. It's hard to find a reporter who doesn't screw up what you say and go for the sensationalism:

EX-FAT WOMAN'S BROTHER SAYS . . .

FITNESS GURU SAYS DIETS DON'T WORK—WHAT DOES SHE KNOW?

FROM FLAB TO FIT, EX-FATTY SAYS YOU CAN . . .

LEAN AND MEAN SELLING MACHINE . . .

FITNESS TERRORIST . . .

(That was one of the latest catchy headlines that I saw. Have you ever??)

I've seen them all. After a while you have to wonder how some of those reporters can sleep at night. This particular article was so pathetically written and the facts so wrong that it was hard to take seriously. This experience was different for me, however, because I spent a lot of time and energy with this reporter. I'd let her into my life, included her—yep, I'm sad to say it was a woman, but I'm convinced she was really a beer-guzzling redneck in drag. (Yeah, I know a lot of those beer-guzzling rednecks who dress up like women.)

This reporter followed me around for weeks. I included her in conversations with people I love, ate meals with her, shared my honest and unguarded feelings with her. I let her in, and she beat me to a pulp. She didn't understand anything we, my staff and I, were doing. It's as if she was blind, deaf, and dumb. She saw nothing we've done, only anger. My anger. (Did I mention that she was a beer-guzzling red-neck in drag?) She missed the compassion, the love, the hard work, the intelligence, the respect that my staff and I have for the message we work so very hard to get to as many women as humanly possible.

The words she wrote, what she said in her article, didn't hurt me (did I mention it was the biggest piece of crap ever written?). What hurt me, made me angry, frustrated, and sadder than sad was that I had handed her the ammunition. I opened up to this beer-guzzling red-neck, and I felt like the biggest jerk around. I gotta say it knocked me down for a day. Twenty-four hours of one of those close-the-curtains, don't-pick-up-the-phone-no-matter-how-many-times-it-rings, watch-the-worst-TV-programs-on-the-air, and-only-get-up-to-go-to-the-bathroom-and-eat-and-eat-and-eat kind of days. That's exactly how I handled it. How's that for maturity?

So there I was, moping in my jammies. Eating and moping and eating and moping some more. Closing in on evening, food wrappers everywhere, I stopped eating long enough to think about how I felt. You know what? I felt wonderful. Warm. Protected. Cozy. Snug. Lying there under the blankies, pillows and food everywhere, bad TV blasting, with the tenth bagel with jelly going down slowly—it felt great!!

Food. Connected in a big way to one of the rituals I'd been doing for years. Ritual? Sure! Can we say that yet without being burned at the stake? If not, light the match, because that's exactly what it was—a ritual. A ritual of self-pity, maybe, but think about it: What's our connection with food anyway? Nothing but one big ritual after another.

The holiday rituals:

Thanksgiving

Christmas

Hanukkah

Valentine's Day

Halloween

The good behavior rituals:

From the day I can remember, knowing that if I could keep still long enough, I'd get something sweet at the end of it all.

The love ritual:

My love ritual started with my grandmother Gilly. Her name was Ell (isn't that a beautiful name?), but we called her Gilly. Don't ask me why. Gilly would come over once a week with the biggest Cadbury chocolate bars you've ever seen, one for each of us. Those were the days when Cadbury was made in England, not New Jersey or wherever it's made now. The days when chocolate was real chocky, not some chemical concoction. We're talking the thickest, the sweetest, the best chocolate you've ever tasted. My grandmother's once weekly chocolate bar was love at its best. Grandma and chocolate—what could be better!

Love. Romance!

The romance ritual:

The romantic dinner . . . believing a romantic dinner could fix it all. My romantic dinners with the Prince didn't fix anything. Lord knows the Prince and I tried. How many times during the slow, painful breakup of our marriage did I try to have a "romantic dinner" with my husband??

You know what it's like: Organize the children, get the baby-sitter, spend time getting all dolled up, put on his favorite perfume, light the candles, have the wine and the favorite food ready, and set the stage.

The stage for reconnection? Romance? A little sex maybe, after weeks of not having time for each other.

There it all was—the tastes, smells, textures of the foods we loved most, candles, wine, all mushed together with the disappointment I felt when it didn't work. No night of passion and love. No reconciliation. No marriage saver. And then guess where it ended up? Right in:

The self-destruct ritual:

This is a big one for most of us. The self-destruct ritual that could last weeks, months, sometimes years. Powerful, no doubt about it.

Eating six bags of cookies " 'cause I'm gonna show you."

Soothing the breaking heart.

Fooling myself into believing that's what I wanted to do, and damn it, I was going to do what I wanted.

Yeah . . . My goal was to get fatter and fatter in the name of freedom of choice!

Stand up and die is what that was all about. Who cared that the person I was trying to punish by eating tons of food still had a twenty-eight-inch waist and a girlfriend? I had all the cakes and cookies anyone could dream of to keep me going.

More food, more food, more food. Soothe the pain, cushion the blow.

My self-destruct ritual usually blended nicely with the old boredom ritual.

Eating because there's nothing else to do? Bored with life, bored with it all? Tired of being sick and tired, fed up?

What is food connected to?

What isn't it connected to?

Love

Romance

Self-destruction

Boredom

Pleasure

Sadness

Desperation

Fear

Suffocation

Comfort

I've connected all this stuff with food since the day I can remember. I've done it all—I'm sure you have, too—but it was my last lie-in-bed-all-day-and-eat episode that really got me thinking.

Free from guilt (sure—now that I pig out on high-volume, low-fat food, and now that my body is lean, strong, and healthy and functions at a more efficient level, and now that I have a life, a day of eating and moping isn't the end of the world for me), I could have a look at it, take it in, and think about how it felt. Free to lie there, eat, think, eat, walk down memory lane. And here's what I came up with.

Food, my connections.

The lamb and mint sauce dinners I was raised on—very Australian, you know.

The bowls of sugary cereal I devoured.

The hot chocolate milk—a source of warmth and comfort. (Forget about the saturated fat and sugar that went right along with that fairy-tale soother.)

Dieting ever since I can remember. The minute I started to hate the way I looked or felt, I took away food—starvation—only to begin the obsessing that goes hand in hand with dieting: about the tastes, textures, and comfort of certain foods, high fat and greasy at the top of the list.

Food, the Prince, and my new fast-growing family.

Priding myself as a new wife on cooking huge dinners for the Prince, his friends, and his family. Really believing that he was eating the food, appreciating his wife, seeing my value and loving me. (The next book may be about my believing my "value" was in a dinner I was preparing for my husband. That's a whole other subject and something we should chat about, but for now let's stick with food.)

The Prince came home one day with one of his friends. My, or should I say our, older son was almost a year old, and I was as pregnant as can be.

The men went out to lift some weights, and I started preparing the meal that I knew they would need when they finished. Boy, did I put some effort into that lunch. Tasty, filling, pleasing to the eye, and ready the minute they walked in the door. I was so proud of the food I'd prepared, how tidy the kitchen was, and the atmosphere I'd created—well-dressed and clean baby quietly playing, food ready, table set, kitchen smelling like "Little House on the Prairie." That was my job, and I'd done it well.

The Prince and his friend came in, sat down, ate like animals, and ran out the door without saying, "Thank you. It tasted good. Boy, it's nice to come home to a good meal and a nice home." Nothing but a quick kiss from the Prince before he ran out the door with his friend. It broke my heart.

Now I know this is the kind of stuff in the past that's been all too quickly, and quite stupidly, attributed to the sensitivity of a very pregnant woman, but enough of that. I had worked hard on that meal, and I was hurt and mad at the Prince, I hated his friend for life, and I spent days feeling worthless and lost in my newfound role of cook without appreciation. Just an example of walking down memory lane with the food connections in my life.

These are the things I'm thinking about during my eleventh-hour, curtain-drawn, eating-and-moping-because-that-reporter-was-such-a-pig session.

It's amazing how free you really are when guilt isn't invited. So many food connections, so little time, and we haven't even talked about the biggest food connection in my life. The one I promised would break your heart is yet to come. It's about my son—excuse me, our son (who else would I use as the shining star of food allergies but my/our son?)—whose health problems were misdiagnosed by doctors for the first eight months of his life, while my marriage was breaking up and while I was pregnant with our second baby!! A fun time in the Prince and Princess's household for sure.

After much fussing and fighting with physicians, more pain and anguish than you can imagine (unless, of course, you are a mom who has had a very, very sick baby, then you understand the kind of terror that is involved), it turned out that our son's problem was food—that word, see how it's plagued my life?—allergies. (I'm obviously just throwing you a bone on this one, teasing you just a little. The details follow when we get into the food, health, allergy connection.)

I changed my/our son's diet and mine—my breast milk was loaded with the foods he was severely allergic to—and the change in his diet literally saved his life.

And if you think the food/family connection ends there, you're wrong. My mother and food. A big connection: growing up watching my mother starve herself to be thin and beautiful. She was, until she died at the age of fifty-two. I was sure it was the cancer that would eventually kill her, but the radiation therapy burned her esophagus so badly, she couldn't eat a thing. Seems to me she died of starvation.

Food.

Gaining and losing 133 pounds when the picket fence finally exploded. Getting well, taking back control in my life, and talking about it.

> Talking on TV
> On radio
> In seminars all over the country
> In books

Food and fat, food and getting lean, food and disease (it's a thought), food and the quality of our lives. Food and the energy you may or may not have. Food, food, food. I'm in it in a big way, and I've got to write about it, because everywhere I go, you guys have been asking about it.

So . . . let's talk.

Here's what you have in your hands. You have your food book, a book that the women of America and I wrote. A state fair bake-off in print. You have the program: high volume, low fat. The answers to the questions:

> Dairy?
> Meat?
> Saturated?
> Unsaturated?
> Oil?
> Kids?
> Husbands?
> Restaurants?
> Proteins?
> Carbs?
> Steamed, baked, or grilled?
> Fish or fowl?
> Healthy, unhealthy?

You're gonna get a couple of things in your food book. (I don't mean that literally. Can you imagine if you'd just paid for the book and you were going to get two things. A bargain?)

You're gonna get the answers to your questions.

Recipes by the ton.

Discussion, suggestions, solutions for some things you may or may not ever have thought about.

You're getting networking and support from some of the brightest minds around: the women of America.

Discussion, sharing, solutions, honesty, food, food, food. Investigation by Susan Powter, Food P.I.

What could be better?

The end result: a food book that will help you make your breakfast, lunch, dinner, snacking, what-the-heck-do-I-feed-the-kids? decisions easier, more understandable, and based on *your* life-style, *your* tastes, *your* physical considerations, *your* goals. You'll be the expert. You will be able to make your own decisions about what's going into your body, and you will regain some of the control in your life by increasing your awareness, making the choices you choose to make, and changing your life.

If you want to increase the quality of life, get leaner, stronger, and healthier, change the way you look and feel, food has a whole hell of a lot to do with all of these things. It's in your hands. Nothing complicated, nothing difficult: the connection. The food connection.

Just before we jump into it all, I have to tell you what's going on around me.

I'm on an airplane flying to Atlanta, and dinner has just been served. People are eating because it's dinnertime. I often wonder why people on airplanes eat anything that's put in front of them. It's as if denial sets in the minute the smiling flight attendant places the tray in front of us. I mean, airplane food? Does it get gaggier than that?

The cabin smells like grease and flesh, because that's what they're serving: greasy steak, salad, creamed veggies, all dressed up to look pretty.

This guy next to me is about forty-five, well dressed, decent-looking, if you like an aging Ken doll look. He has a slight paunch around the middle but can still pass for "ex-jock in middle-age shape." He looks a little tired, but other than that he's an average Joe. He's just poured his creamy white dressing all over a salad that looks limp and slightly brown in its little plastic salad bowl.

He's buttering his white bread roll with his little plastic knife. (I hope he doesn't look at this screen and read what Susan Powter, Food P.I., is writing about him, but I've gotta take the chance. In this business of investigating, it's nothing but chances, slow, jazzy music, and lots of smoky rooms.) He's biting into the buttered roll, soaking up some of the greasy gravy with it, and biting again, digging into the steak, about to dive into the creamy veggies. And when he finishes all that, I'm sure he'll be going right to the slice of chocolate cake that's sitting to the left of the entree plate.

Now remember where we are. On an airplane. This is airplane food we're talking about.

I'm sharing this with you for a reason. There is a strong connection between what's happening on this flight at this very moment and what happened on another flight I was on just three flights ago. My plane (sounds like I own it, doesn't it?) had to make an emergency landing in Nebraska. A man on that flight was having a heart attack. Can you imagine anything worse than having a heart attack forty thousand feet in the air? My heart (pardon the pun) went out to this guy—big heart attack, lots of pain—it was not a good thing. We landed, the ambulance met the plane, the guy was carried off not looking so good, and off we went to Denver, the original destination.

The meal served on the flight that night? Steak, creamed veggies, salad with creamy dressing, bread, butter, and beverage of your choice.

Now, I am not and never will be a self-righteous low-fat person; that's not my style. You guys who have Stopped the Insanity in your lives know that this whole thing is about choice, control, and this information working for your life-style, your tastes, your physical considerations. But let's just spend a moment here outside of judgment, free from low-fat anything. Isn't this a little scary? Don't you think it's kind of nuts? Everyone diving into a high-saturated-fat, gross, chemical meal right after this guy was wheeled out—and not making the connection? You don't have to be a low-fat vegan to have this scenario make you think.

Think about how you are feeling.

The size of your thighs.

Your energy level.

Disease.

Any connection to the foods we are eating? Come on. Couldn't be!!

Well, there is. It's time to wake up, A.M.A.; get our heads out of the sand, dietitians and nutritionists; go to hell, diet industry (sorry, that slipped in; my fingers were guided by some higher power to type that). No matter how much the "experts" want to confuse and cloud some of these issues, what we eat very much affects our lives in more ways than you can imagine.

So what's the solution?

Never eat plane food again?

Don't eat anything that comes on a little plastic plate with little plastic knives and forks?

Starve for the duration of the flight and wait to eat some of that wonderful airport terminal food?

Don't travel?

Don't ever eat steak?

HELLLLLLLLLLLL . . . P!! (Didn't think I was going to add the P, did ya?)

Well, that's exactly what this book is about. Airplane food, traveling, restaurants, home, kids, husbands, office, thighs, stomachs, cancer, heart disease, energy, control, emotional connections, food, food, food, food—how it affects us, what's right, wrong, good, bad, or indifferent. You see, while eating steak on a plane doesn't guarantee a heart attack, the connection between the steak, the creamy veggies, the butter on the white bread, the wine, and the chocolate cake—oh, I left out the nuts as an appetizer with the first cocktail (some private dick I am)—and the oblivion to the food and how-we-look-and-feel connection that most of us live our whole lives in—that's what we need to spend a little time on.

Do you want to be lean? How about some extra energy? How about any energy at all? Health—is that a consideration in your life? Are you dealing with a degenerative disease, heart condition, or a fatigue syndrome of some kind? Emotionally dependent on sweet things? There is a lot of ground to cover and a whole lot of people to talk to and hear from.

Let's go through some of the facts together, free of judgment and fear. Cast them out of your lives (sound like a revival, or what?) while you're reading this book. You and I can get the info, cover some good ground, see how food really affects our lives and the way we look and feel, and then you can decide what works for you. You figure out what you want and the best way to get it. Right back to that freedom-of-choice theme.

So while this guy next to me finishes his dinner, I'm going to begin my food book and work like hell to get you the information you need that's gonna make a huge difference in your life.

Food by Susan Powter . . . here we go again.

Stage 1

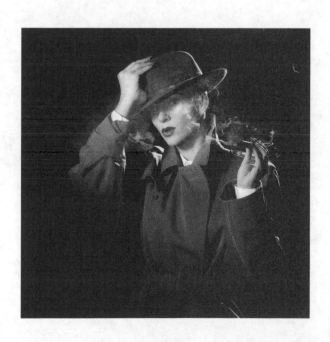

CHAPTER 1

FAT

*T*he Average Joe is finishing up his dinner, and I'm on to Fat. What else am I gonna start a food book with?

Fat by Susan Powter, Food P.I.

Nothing wrong with it. Let me begin by saying fat is:

> An important element in the human body.
>
> Necessary in our lives.
>
> Something all of us need and should have enough of.

HOLD ON!

CALL THE NEWSPAPER!

ANTI-FAT ADVOCATE, CONSUMER FAT DETECTIVE, SCREAMER AND YELLER OF THE EAT-LESS-FAT IN THE 90'S, SUSAN POWTER, HAS LOST HER MIND.

Now I'm gonna ask ya . . . who can you trust anymore? Run back to the bookstore, get your money back . . . there's no point in trying to make the change.

The bottom has fallen out.

Where can we turn?

A moment of calm, please. No need to call the tabloids just yet. Hear me out, there's more to this than meets the eye.

True, there is nothing wrong with fat. Our bodies need fat. Your vital organs wouldn't have any cushioning without it (something I wished I'd known about at 260 pounds). Apparently I was free and clear, protected as you get from the old kidney punch. Isn't my heart as vital an organ as they come? That extra 133 pounds didn't stop it from breaking. I guess the extra weight comes in handy only if you get kicked in the chest. Isn't that what the Prince did? Oh, enough of that, you get my point. The vital organs, your liver, kidney, heart, all of them need the cushioning and protection that fat gives them. Don't ask what would happen if we didn't have any fat on our bodies and the temperature suddenly dropped.

Freezing would mean exactly that, freezing. Fat helps regulate your body temperature in extreme weather conditions. (Something that's definitely necessary in Texas in the summertime. Did my 260 help or hurt? Was I being regulated or suffocating under all that extra fat?) Let's just say that if a cold spell had whipped down from the Antarctic, I would have been ready for it. Pretty necessary, this fat stuff, wouldn't you say? Well, get ready for more good fat news because it doesn't end with temperature regulation and cushioning. Fat is also a carrier for some very important vitamins. Those famous fat-soluble vitamins, A, D, E, and K, wouldn't get far without fat.

And if it's fuel you ever find yourself talking about with friends, it'll be fat, too, because fat is oxidized in your body to get you the heat/energy you need to function. It's one of the big three fuels: carbs, proteins, and you guessed it—fat. And if you think that's all fat does, you're in for a big surprise, because fat can also save our lives; it's a built-in safety mechanism against famine. Thank God for fat. Otherwise, most of us would be dead from all the dieting we've done—voluntary famine, I like to call it, much to the displeasure of the diet industry (sorry, guys; gotta call it what it is!). When you go into famine, voluntary or involuntary, your body uses its storage of fat to survive until you:

> (a) Get an airlift of food.
> (b) Get off your diet.

Either one. All your body knows is that it isn't getting any fuel, and it still has to function.

Fat: the amazing fuel, protector, built-in survival device. Unbelievable.

If you want to make sure your prostaglandins are functioning properly (and I'm sure we all do even though we don't have a clue what they are), you must have fat, because these guys regulate many functions of all the tissues in your body. This is a big job, and it's not gonna happen without fat.

Cholesterol and fat have been synonymous with the killer heart disease for

years, but you know what? Your body needs both. Fat helps regulate cholesterol. They work together, balancing your sex hormones, your menstrual
cycle, and keeping it all the way it needs to be. Your body needs fat to function properly and to be healthy. So what's the big deal, pardon the pun? Why
the fuss about fat? If it's balanced, cushioned, temp-controlled, and choles-
terol-regulating you want, aren't we then saying that at 260 I was a physical
specimen, as insulated as they come and hormonally and sexually balanced
as they get?

Nope, because I was suffering from and living with the consequences of
one very big problem. You might be familiar with the same thing. Millions
and millions are: WAY, WAY, WAY, WAY, WAY, WAY, WAY TOO MUCH FAT.

LOADS AND LOADS OF EXTRA FAT THAT IS KILLING US.

THE CONDITION: OVERFAT.

And you can't talk food without talking fat, because that's it, that's the connection, that's where it's coming from.

Here's the deal:

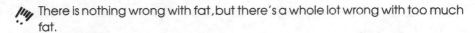 There is nothing wrong with fat, but there's a whole lot wrong with too much
fat.

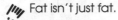 Fat isn't just fat.

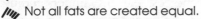 Not all fats are created equal.

The big fat picture has been presented by the experts in such a confusing
way that now nobody knows what's going on. It's time to get the skinny (pardon the hell out of that pun) on fat. You and I need to understand the big
picture if we are going to start making different decisions and choices about
this stuff. We need the real story, no holds barred. We need to know:

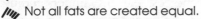 What our bodies need or don't need.

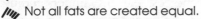 What's hurting us.

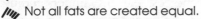 What's making us all so fat.

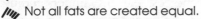 What we can do about it.

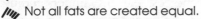 How we can make the changes necessary that will help us get rid of some
of this stuff hanging from our bodies.

We need to get rid of all the garbage that's out there, the confusion and the
wrong info. We need to get on with it so we can solve the problem of being
overfat and feeling horrible.

I went on my very own fat search, which isn't hard to do these days because everywhere you look, everything you read, and everything you hear is about fat, fat, fat, fat, fat.

It has even become a political issue. The other night on tele I watched one of this country's most outspoken, very, very fat commentators stand behind a table full of high-fat foods—steak, sausage, movie theater popcorn, oils, etc.—and suggest that it's the liberals in this country who are trying to take away our "pleasure" foods by labeling them high-fat and dangerous.

The things that "bring us pleasure" are being turned into weapons.

The liberals are taking the all-American foods such as hamburgers and hot dogs and hurting the American image by suggesting that they have anything to do with heart disease—poor boy, just a tad confused!

Fat isn't about fun. Too much fat is about being uncomfortable and unhealthy, and about killing ourselves. Just ask anyone who's having a heart attack how much fun he or she is having. Too much fat in our daily diets has nothing to do with the American flag or our country's image other than the fact that we look a little foolish with this voluntary destruction, this suicide called overfat, unfit, and unhealthy. Too much fat going into our bodies means having too much fat on our bodies, and that doesn't look or feel good, and it ain't healthy.

Cutting back on unnecessary fat isn't about falling for a political trap, it's about using common sense, having more choices, learning, understanding, and making different decisions. It's about having more control and not being controlled by anyone.

Whatever your politics, whether we agree or disagree, standing behind a table of fat making statements like that was just plain pathetic.

This particular very fat commentator can keep eating his steak, lard, the high high-fat diet. Keep chowing down on your movie theater popcorn, buddy. That'll take care of itself. It already is. Give a fool enough rope . . . you guys know the rest. It's not him I'm concerned with, it's you.

It's not getting the facts on something that's killing us. This is what's happening out there. These are the facts—not my political opinion. Let's have a look and decide what we want to do about it. Hey, let's increase our options with facts instead of following just one more opinion without thinking and closing more doors on our health, shall we?

Obesity was recognized as a health problem in 1863 with the publication of "Letter on Corpulence" by British cabinet maker William Banting. It contained the first slimming diet, The Banting System.

Here's what's going on. There is way, way, way too much fat in the American diet. We are eating tons of it, and it's killing us, making us get fat, feel bad, look bad—sapping our lives. So I tracked down some of the best fat experts out there. Read the books, articles, taped the TV shows, watched, called, got the transcripts, and surprise, surprise—guess what I found out? It's not as complicated as it appears to be.

Fat is good. Fat is important to the human body. Fat is necessary, but:

- We are eating three to four times the fat we need daily in our diets—and that, my friends, is a very, very conservative figure.

- In order for our bodies to have the cushioning, protection, and balance they need, we must have about a tablespoon of dietary fat a day.

- The average American is taking in six to eight tablespoons of fat a day.

- Since 1919 our daily fat percentage has gone from 27 percent to 40 percent.

- According to *Consumer Reports,* the nation's eating and drinking habits have been implicated in six of the ten leading causes of death—heart disease, cancer, stroke, diabetes, atherosclerosis, chronic liver disease—as well as several non-fat-related but potentially disabling disorders, such as osteoporosis and diverticulosis.

- Today, 40 percent of Americans are overweight.

- Twenty-five percent of American adults are clinically obese.

- One-fourth of U.S. children are 20 percent or more above their ideal weight.

So that's what the research says, but if you're overweight, you know what all these horrifying facts mean to you: How uncomfortable has the extra fat you're eating made you? What's it doing to your life? Yesterday Peggy told me that she couldn't get in and out of her car easily anymore because of the three hundred pounds she was carrying around. Debby said that the extra thirty pounds she has put on in the last couple of months has her running from mirrors, tired, tired, tired, and wearing tents for clothes because "nothing fits, and I'm depressed and feeling miserable."

You, me, millions of us have huge chunks of life taken from us because of the extra, unhealthy amount of fat on our bodies.

Traveling? How about not being able to fit comfortably into an airplane seat?

Are you adjusting your life because of the fat on your body? Whether it's forty extra pounds or three hundred, what we are talking about here is fat, too much of it, how it affects our lives, and where it's coming from.

That's what we have to take a moment for and research together. We just have to spend the time on some of the details of this fat stuff and sort it all out. Getting as lean as you want to be isn't difficult, but I'll tell you something

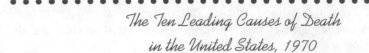

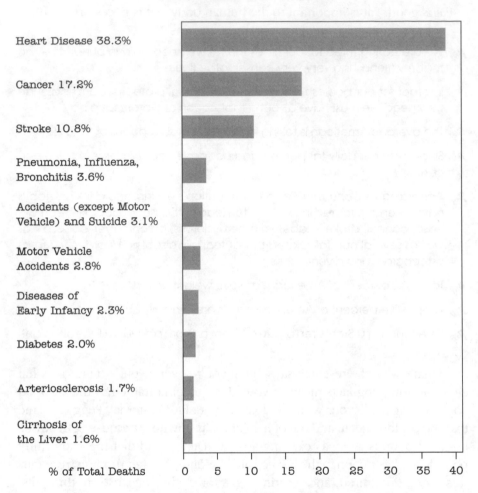

The Ten Leading Causes of Death
in the United States, 1970

Heart Disease 38.3%

Cancer 17.2%

Stroke 10.8%

Pneumonia, Influenza,
Bronchitis 3.6%

Accidents (except Motor
Vehicle) and Suicide 3.1%

Motor Vehicle
Accidents 2.8%

Diseases of
Early Infancy 2.3%

Diabetes 2.0%

Arteriosclerosis 1.7%

Cirrhosis of
the Liver 1.6%

% of Total Deaths   0   5   10   15   20   25   30   35   40

Source: *Maximum Life Span* by Roy Walford, M.D., W.W. Norton and Co., New York, London, 1983.

Heart disease, cancer, and stroke—the three big ones . . . all connected to the amount
of fat we eat.

. . . it's about a lot more than just the greatest low-fat recipes on earth (you've
already got them in your hot little hands), and it's about a whole lot more
than someone telling you what to eat and when.

It's about your understanding completely, once and for all, down to the bottom line, the facts about fat. So come on, come on, come on, let's clear it up.

The confusion is out there; it's real, and we're deep in it together. It's not too difficult to figure out why most of us choose to live with our heads in the sand when it comes to fat. All the numbers, the saturated, the unsaturated (just wait till you find out about the hydrogenated) . . . the good, the bad, the ugly. Mr. Average Joe and his airplane meal are looking better and better by the second, don't you think?

No.

No more. It's time to stop running (start walking/running to burn some fat off—always a good thing to do, a little exercise here and there—but I'm talking about that special kind of "running," as in not looking at what's right in front of our face).

Consider the buying of this book a commitment to the truth, the tangible cash exchange acknowledgment that you are going to get down to the nitty-gritty of what's high, what's low, what's good, what's bad, and what the hell we're supposed to be eating.

It's perfectly understandable why we are all so confused, with all the lying labeling guys out there and the trillions of magazine articles telling us something different every time we flip the page. The behaviorists scream the need for self love every time we binge, binge, binge on fat. Who knows what's going on anymore?

Hey, I was doing a show the other day, and this lady, we'll call her Ms. Fitness, knew all about wellness. Fifteen percent body fat. Fit as a fiddle. Sure, she knew it all until she watched a little videotape I'd done in the grocery store that talked about fish.

• • • • • • • • • • • • • • •

Light Tuna	3% fat
Cod	8%
Scallops	7%
Halibut	19%
Swordfish	30%
Salmon	40%
Orange Roughy	50%

• • • • • • • • • • • • • • •

"SALMON!! SALMON," she gasped from the audience.

"I've been eating tons of salmon!

"I thought it was good for me.

"I thought it was low-fat!!"

Gasp, gasp, gasp.

We'll get to fish and the truth behind it soon (how about that orange roughy?) and all the wonderful ways you and I can get to the truth, but you see what I'm getting at here? You and I are not so dumb. Ms. Fitness was confused, just like the rest of us. You ought to hear what I hear when it comes to confusion, food, low-fat . . .

I, like you, never thought I'd eat in a restaurant again when I went low-fat. But a lady in the airport said to me the other day, "I can order great-tasting food in restaurants and not walk out feeling like I'm going to die." How about the wonderful woman who almost exploded with excitement when she told me that her favorite thing in the world to eat was chips and hot sauce by the case, and guess what? She knows how she can do that and not get fat now that she's got the ABC's of low-fat living!!

You, me, and the rest of the world need to understand all there is to know about this stuff so that we can eat, eat, eat, eat, and look and feel good, good, good, good.

Between the confusing info that's been floating around in the last couple of years and the enormous changes that have taken place, what we thought was good is no more.

Protein should come from where?

Best source of calcium is?

What do I feed the children?

I'm supposed to eat what, when, how much? . . .

You and I don't need a roundtable discussion to figure out that we have a mess going on, but you know what? We also don't need much to sort it out.

Here's what we need: just a little info, presented by the best . . . Dr. John McDougall, right here, right now. According to Doc John, the connection to fat and all this stuff we are finding out about is very, very clear.

"Hundreds of international checks and balances give us a very clear picture of the connection between a high-fat diet, obesity, and disease."

The Finns, as in Finland, have the highest level of saturated fat in their diets, and they also have the highest rate of heart disease in the world. Congratulations, Finland. Let's award them the Heart and Arteries of Stone Award, but let's not be too judgmental or hasty to criticize, because who do you think is right behind them in second place? Get the Sash and Arteries of Stone Award ready for the runner-up: the United States of America. Yep, the greatest, smartest, most advanced country in the world is in second place in heart disease. Why?

Americans have a diet that is slightly less rich in saturated fat than the first-place heart-disease award winner, and that puts us in second place. Japan, which has a diet very low in saturated fat, has the lowest levels of blood cholesterol and cardiovascular disease of any developed nation. Do you see the interesting little connection here? This is one contest you'd want to lose because it means they are living and we are dying.

It seems pretty clear to me:

 Diets high in saturated fat—loads of heart disease.

 Diets low in saturated fat—less heart disease.

No coincidence and simple, simple, simple to see the connection.

> All I really wanted was to feel better, but as I put more and more into this new life-style, the smaller I am getting. The best part is that I am doing all of this without starving.
>
> —*Rae-Jean, Buffalo, Oklahoma*

It's not difficult to take this one step further and right out of the health arena, back to where the interest lies: the stuff that is covering your body. Let's talk. Is any of this information connected to being overfat?

How about that daily fat intake contributing to obesity or just that "extra twenty pounds that you can't seem to get rid of"? Above and beyond all the confusion, heart disease, and the horrible stats on our eating habits, what about fat and the way we look?

Just a thought. Fat. Could how much we are eating be connected at all to the problem of being overweight? I think we all know the answer to that question. I'm just interested why the "diet" experts out there don't seem to know: the doctors, the dietitians, the nutritionists, the behaviorists, and all the other people who insist on making it two different subjects—health and the fat connection, my thighs and the fat connection. Sure there are some people in this world who can eat a lot of fat and not get fat, but we hate them and could care less about them. But for most of us? You eat a lot of fat and you get fat. Pretty basic stuff.

Our daily fat intake is higher than our sedentary life-styles can burn off, get rid of. If that's not one of the biggest reasons obesity is out of control in this country, then I'll eat my hat. There are other things involved, but don't you think it's safe to say that cutting back on your daily fat intake would be a hell of a good place to start if you want to get lean?

*If you're trying to get rid of the stuff hanging from your underarms.

*If you're trying to thin that thick waist.

*Forget about the pinch. What about that wad of fat on your hips?

It's hard to cut back when you don't have a clue how. That's the way I felt when I started putting this stuff together and wanted desperately to change the direction my body was heading—from 190 to 210 pounds . . . 230 . . . 255. I tried, but I kept bumping into more and more information that got me more and more mixed up.

Do you think for a second that I ever thought I was going to be able to understand saturated fat and what it all meant to my body? Get out of here!

Solid at room temperature—what are you talking about? Like never, ever melts, no matter what?

Please!

You may be at the "eliminate anything white and creamy" beginning stages of going low-fat (a great beginning, I might add), having no clue at all why you'd even need or want to know about saturated fat.

You may be thinking to yourself: Forget about it—just give me something that I'm supposed to eat, and I'll get on with it.

No, no, no, fellow fat detective. You do need to know, because once you get this info down (by the end of this chapter), you'll realize, first, that you are as smart as anyone (very empowering indeed); second, that once you get it (the facts on fat), it's with you forever; and last but never least, nobody will be able to rip you off, put you on some stupid eating plan that sets you up for failure, or suck you into anything that's going to leave you fatter for the rest of your life. How's that for a reason to educate yourself, change your way of thinking, and take the time to understand this stuff before we run into the kitchen and try some new low-fat recipes?

I avoided learning about it all for the longest time. I lost a bit of body fat—moving slowly but surely, burning that extra one hundred-plus off, using a low-fat recipe here and there, sometimes living on the same thing for a week and a half because I had no clue what else to eat, and running as far and as fast from the fat details in my life as I'd run from parts of my past.

Was there a turning point? A moment of change? (I'm asking and thinking about the answer as I write. Is that normal?) Sure. There was a turning point.

TURNING POINT . . .

Grocery shopping, using the fat formula and being able to use easy, easy math (something I never in my life thought I'd use) to figure out how much fat was in something.

TURNING POINT . . .

Reading a label and understanding the word "hydrogenated"—understanding what it meant to my hips.

TURNING POINT . . .

Getting a clue about cholesterol and what it meant to me and my body. Getting a little "heady" at this point, thinking medical school—what could be so hard about it?

EDUCATE . . .
EMPOWER . . .
INCREASE CHOICES . . .

Okay, are you with me? I promise it won't take too long. Let's go.

SATURATED FAT 101

I'm sure you've heard it: "solid at room temperature." That's the way this stuff has been described in every article I've ever read that attempts to help us understand what saturated fat is. Solid at room temperature? Room temperature is different in Alaska in the winter than it is in Arizona in August. Does that mean that saturated fat is solid no matter what? Always solid? Can never be anything but solid? Who knows. That definition never meant anything to me until I went underground and investigated this stuff.

> Saturated fat
> The bad stuff
> The cloggy stuff
> The stuff that is somehow connected with cholesterol
> Solid and sticky

I asked, and those are the definitions I got.

Here's the scoop on saturated fat. All fats are made up of three components:

> Saturated fat
> Polyunsaturated fat
> Monounsaturated fat

Which one it is depends on the proportion of the different components. Here it is, right from the mouth of the *Wellness Encyclopedia:*

WELLNESS ENCYCLOPEDIA: *Most fats in foods are triglycerides, which consist of three fatty acids attached to a glycerol molecule [whatever that means]. These fatty acids vary in length and in degree of saturation by hydrogen atoms.*

ME: ***Now this I understand. There's a connection here between the "degree of saturation," hydrogen atoms, and saturated fat. I'm getting there.***

WELLNESS ENCYCLOPEDIA: *Fats containing mainly saturated fatty acids are described as highly saturated.*

ME: ***O.K., I'm with you now. This makes some sense. The more saturated, the more saturated. Simple.***

WELLNESS ENCYCLOPEDIA: *Saturated fatty acids are loaded with all the hydrogen atoms they can carry.*

ME: ***So, saturated fatty acids are full of hydrogen. Fat Fat. Fat. Solid. Solid. Solid. It's making sense.***

WELLNESS ENCYCLOPEDIA: *Saturated fat raises blood cholesterol because your body takes it in and converts it into cholesterol.*

Thank you, *Wellness Encyclopedia,* for finally clearing this saturated fat and cholesterol thing up in one very well stated sentence. There it is. When you are talking about raising your blood cholesterol level, and everybody is these days, you are talking about two things: saturated fat and cholesterol. Separate and together, because eating cholesterol raises blood cholesterol, and eating saturated fat (converted by your liver into cholesterol) also does the trick. Do you see it? Doesn't that make a lot of sense? You eat saturated fat, and it's converted by the liver into cholesterol and is sent through your body to do whatever your body does with cholesterol.

Are you ready for some empowerment? Ready to see how information turns into something that can absolutely change the way your body looks and feels? Think about this:

I bet you're making the big effort and eating foods that have NO CHOLESTEROL written all over them, aren't you? So you're in the grocery store, and you see something that has NO CHOLESTEROL on the label . . .

CHOLESTEROL FREE

NO CHOLESTEROL IN SIGHT

NEVER DID, NEVER WILL, COULDN'T HAVE CHOLESTEROL IN IT IF
   IT TRIED

. . . but when you turn it over and read the label, you see a saturated fat listed in the ingredients. No cholesterol, but what does the saturated fat in it tell you (now that you have just this tiny bit of info)? That your body will take this saturated fat in the food you're eating and turn it into cholesterol, because that's what our body does with saturated fat.

The companies that are stamping NO CHOLESTEROL in big red letters all over the foods they manufacture know full well that a lot of this stuff is loaded with saturated fat—which does what in the body?

GOTCHA, BOYS. A food can contain no cholesterol but tons of saturated fat. That's how you guys get away with your "healthier because it has no cholesterol added" claim. "Heart healthy," my butt—not if it has saturated fat in it. Shame on you.

Don't you see what's happening? The controversy. A place I always seem to end up. It's the same thing. Hidden fats in foods everywhere. Not just the old "98% fat free" that doesn't really mean 98 percent fat free. We're talking about "no cholesterol" not necessarily meaning no cholesterol. No cholesterol added, maybe, but once you put it in your mouth, the tons of saturated fat in the NO CHOLESTEROL food you're buying on faith, believing that the food manufacturer you've trusted for years would never, ever do anything to hurt you or your family—bammo, you have cholesterol city, unless you know what you know now.

BOYS . . . YOU CAN'T DO THAT TO US ANYMORE. We've got your number. We are getting saturated-fat smarter by the second. I happen to have some labels handy that scream "no cholesterol." Want to check them out with me?

Don't you think that knowing this, changing the amount of cholesterol and saturated fat you're eating, and being able to figure it all out are going to make a difference in your life?

Corn Oil Squeeze Spread

MADE FROM PURE CORN OIL

ZERO CHOLESTEROL

NUTRITION INFORMATION PER SERVING

SERVING SIZE	1 TBSP.	(14 grams)	FAT	10 grams
SERVINGS PER POUND	32		POLYUNSATURATED	5 grams
CALORIES	90		SATURATED	1 gram
PROTEIN		0 grams	CHOLESTEROL	0 mgs
CARBOHYDRATE		0 grams	SODIUM	95 mgs

Corn Oil Squeeze Spread—this one should be good.

"Zero Cholesterol" splashed across the front . . . zero cholesterol as in "healthy for you"? As in "good for your heart"? Think again. Turn this little goodie over and check out the nutritional information. What do you see? Sure enough, no cholesterol, but right above that zero are 10 grams of fat and one gram of that is saturated. Remember, once your liver gets ahold of that saturated fat it turns right into Mr. C.

• •

*Sugar*Free*
*Chocolate*Wafers*

CHOLESTEROL FREE
BAKED WITH 100% VEGETABLE SHORTENING

NUTRITION INFORMATION PER SERVING

SERVING SIZE	1 WAFER	SODIUM	15 mgs
SERVINGS PER PACKAGE	4	FAT	4 grams
CALORIES	60	POLYUNSATURATED	*
PROTEIN	1 gram	SATURATED	1 gram
CARBOHYDRATE	8 grams	CHOLESTEROL	0 mgs

*CONTAINS LESS THAN 1/2 GRAM PER SERVING

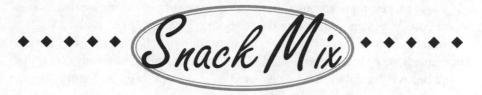

Traditional Flavor Baked Snacks
NO CHOLESTEROL

NUTRITION FACTS

SERVING SIZE ½ CUP		(32 grams)	POLYUNSATURATED FAT		0.5 grams
SERVINGS PER CONTAINER ABOUT		8	MONOUNSATURATED FAT		2.5 grams
AMOUNT PER SERVING:			CHOLESTEROL	0 mgs	0%
CALORIES		150	SODIUM	430 mgs	18%
CALORIES FROM FAT		60	TOTAL CARBOHYDRATE	21 grams	7%
% DAILY VALUE*			DIETARY FIBER	1 gram	5%
TOTAL FAT	7 grams	10%	SUGARS		2 grams
SATURATED FAT	1 gram	6%	PROTEIN		3 grams

Neapolitan
Non-Dairy Dessert

100% MILK FREE
NO LACTOSE   NO CHOLESTEROL

NUTRITION FACTS

SERVING SIZE ½ CUP		(65 grams)	CALORIES		140
SERVINGS		8	FAT CALORIES		65
AMOUNT/SERVING		%DV*	AMOUNT/SERVING		%DV*
TOTAL FAT	7 grams	11%	TOTAL CARBOHYDRATE	18 grams	6%
SATURATED FAT	1.5 grams	8%	FIBER	0 grams	0%
CHOLESTEROL	0 mgs	0%	SUGARS	12 grams	
SODIUM	70 mgs	3%	PROTEIN	1 gram	

Sugar-free Chocolate Wafers, Snack Mix, Neapolitan Dessert . . . same story. They may not be "lying" when they say No Cholesterol . . . but telling you the real truth? I don't think so! Read, read, read your labels.

It will make an enormous difference inside and out. More for the money than you ever imagined, and you're only into Chapter One.

Well, well, well. Now you know. It may scream "cholesterol free" at you, but unless you turn it around and check out the saturated fat in it, you just can't believe that label. It was designed to make you buy, no matter what it does to your, and your family's, health.

START HERE START NOW

Fettucine Alfredo is loaded with fat—twenty-eight grams of it. But wait . . . don't throw out the pasta. Change the sauce to marinara, and you've eaten only ten grams of fat. Better yet, use low-fat marinara and you've eaten only three grams of fat. WOW!

Bargain? Easy? Fun? The best thing you've ever done for yourself? Sure. But don't get too huggy kissy and trusting just yet, because first we have to talk about the "no cholesterol" saturated-fat labeling lie of all time. Half the mystery solved: We've made the connection between cholesterol and saturated fat. But when you're talking about saturated fat, where do you find this solid-at-any-room-temperature, loaded-with-hydrogen Mr. Saturated Fat?

Animals, animals, animals. Animal products, as in meats, poultry, fish, and dairy products. That's where it comes from. It is a very rare plant indeed that contains saturated fat—avocados, olives, coconuts, nuts, seeds, and cocoa products (such as chocolate, guys), four or five things out of a katrillion. Other than that, you won't find saturated fat in the plant world.

Gosh. We hear statistics on heart disease everywhere. We all are so cholesterol aware—a tad confused, but aware—and saturated fat is talked about so much lately that you'd think this news just hit the wire. Did the American Medical Association, the American Heart Association, the Surgeon General just figure this out?

Sorry. No chance. You can take this saturated fat, high cholesterol, and heart disease connection as far back as President Dwight D. Eisenhower. Yep. The good president had a heart attack, and his doctor, Paul Dudley White, published a report connecting the almost pure vegetarian diet and the astounding lack of heart disease—as in the lack of saturated fat from animal products, as in "astounding lack of heart disease." Forget about the vegetarian connection, because as you'll soon know, there are plenty of vegans out there who are getting plenty of saturated fat . . . in coconut and avocados, by the ton. We'll talk.

What we are focusing on here is the connection, the one big connection to something we've all been scratching our heads about. Fat. Heart disease.

Not feeling well. Bad health. Fat. Fat. Fat. What is it? Asking the question sends you right back to the 70's.

> Bad fashions
>
> Disco

And a massive seven-country study by Dr. Ancel Keys of the University of Minnesota School of Public Health, analyzing the correlation between the amount of saturated fat and cholesterol and the death rate from heart disease.

Finland, Greece, Italy, Japan, the Netherlands, the United States, and Yugoslavia, all talking fat, and guess what they found.

Saturated fat, cholesterol, animals . . .

Said in any language, BIG CONNECTION.

O.K., O.K., so you know. There is a connection. Let's say for one crazy moment that you picked this book up to understand the connection between heart disease and fat. Your next question would be how much is healthy, and what am I supposed to be getting in my daily intake? What's good for me and what's bad for me? How do I know where, when, and how to make sure that I get enough saturated fat in my diet to keep me healthy?

That's ten questions, not one, but the point is . . . CHART TIME, GIRLS AND BOYS. If you want to know what it is you need to be healthy, all you have to do is check out this chart that comes straight from the expert's mouth. Mr. Prevent-heart-disease himself, Mr. Saturated-fat-and-everything-you-ever-wanted-to-know-about-it, Mr. Explain-this-complicated-stuff-so-we-all-can-understand-it—Dr. Dean Ornish.

Let's do women first, shall we?

You have four listings:

> Ideal Body Weight
>
> Inactive
>
> Moderately Active
>
> Very Active

Kinda like the calorie consumption chart, this saturated fat intake seems to have a whole lot to do with how much you weigh and how active you are.

Fuel.

How much of what kind is connected to your life-style.

The gasoline in the car.

The coal in the fire. We just keep coming right back to these simple concepts . . . love, love, love, love this.

Saturated Fat Intake: Women

Ideal Body Weight	Inactive	Moderately Active	Very Active
90	4	5	5
100	5	5	5
110	5	6	6
120	6	6	6
130	6	7	7
140	7	7	7
150	7	8	8
160	7	8	9
170	8	9	9
180	8	9	9
190	9	9	10
200	9	10	11
210	9	11	11
220	10	11	12

Source: *Reversing Heart Disease* by Dr. Dean Ornish, Ballantine Books, New York, 1991.

Find the figure in the left-hand column that most closely corresponds to your desirable weight. Then move across the chart to the vertical column that corresponds to your physical activity level. At the point where your ideal weight and activity level intersect, you will find the maximum amount of saturated fat (in grams) that you should consume each day.

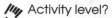 Ideal Body Weight?

Say, 120. 110 is too thin on my frame. 114–113 is the low end and the good end, but let's again go easy with the easy math, shall we?

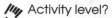 Activity level?

I'd say very active.
With the kids.
The job.
The schedule.
The working out—four to five times a week, a high-intensity level.
Very active.

The instructions at the bottom of the good doctor's chart pretty much explain what it is you need to do to get your number.

I'll do mine.

I'm supposed to have six. Six what? Six grams of saturated fat per day. O.K.

Easy enough to do. Make sure I'm as healthy as a horse. Couldn't be any easier to figure out. Now do yours. Make sure you know what you need daily, and there it is. You never have to worry about getting enough (anyone you know concerned about not getting enough?) saturated fat in your daily intake to be healthy.

Memorizing every bit of information out there isn't the solution. If you can do that, go on a game show and win a fortune or do something with your talent for trivia. Most of us just want to know what to watch for and what to eat instead of the big high saturated fat foods.

Men . . . do the same thing.

Notice how much time I spent on that one! Throw 'em a bone, include their chart, and tell them to follow our lead. I'm liking this way of doing things. Just joking, guys. It's just that we are talking among ourselves, the ladies, and

● ●

Saturated Fat Intake: Men

Ideal Body Weight	Inactive	Moderately Active	Very Active
90	5	5	5
100	5	6	6
110	6	6	7
120	6	7	7
130	7	7	8
140	7	8	8
150	8	8	9
160	8	9	9
170	9	9	10
180	9	10	11
190	10	11	11
200	10	11	12
210	11	12	12
220	11	12	13

Source: *Reversing Heart Disease* by Dr. Dean Ornish, Ballantine Books, New York, 1991.

Find the figure in the left-hand column that most closely corresponds to your desirable weight. Then move across the chart to the vertical column that corresponds to your physical activity level. At the point where your ideal weight and activity level intersect, you will find the maximum amount of saturated fat (in grams) that you should consume each day.

● ●

we need to get through this saturated fat stuff fast, because although our heart health is very, very important—health, sure, who wants to have a heart attack? Stroke couldn't be too much fun. And even though we don't see them, clogged arteries aren't something that anyone wants to strive for—it's the stuff hanging all over our bodies that we want to get rid of. Education is nice, and learning is important, but we're talking about getting lean here. As far as your butt, thighs, stomach, arms, and everything else are concerned, fat is fat is fat is fat . . . but for now, if it's tips, guides, or saturated fat suggestions you're looking for—if you want the red light alert signs for saturated fat—that's easy.

So you guys do your chart, we're moving on.

SATURATED FAT LOOKOUT

Meat. I'm not picking on the flesh manufacturers here. It's just plain fact that when it comes to saturated fat—you and I being overfat and our bodies not looking good—meat is up there as one of the big contributors. Have a look and see for yourself:

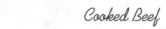

Cooked Beef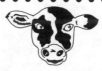

4 OZ	Calories	Fat (g)	Saturated Fat (g)	Cholesterol (mg)
Beef Frankfurter	360	32	14	70
Brisket, Trimmed	275	14	7	106
Chuck Roast	443	35	15	118
Corned Beef	287	22	7	112
Ground Beef, Lean	306	20	8	89
Ground Beef, Regular	333	21	9	115
Pastrami	399	33	12	106
Prime Rib	320	22	9	94
Rib Eye	337	24	10	95
Salami	299	24	10	74
Sirloin	238	10	4	102
T-bone Steak	245	12	5	91
Tenderloin	240	13	4	98
Top Loin	387	29	12	91

Adapted from University of California, Berkeley, ed. *The Wellness Encyclopedia*, Houghton Mifflin Company, New York, 1991.

Here we are at the old beef chart, talking about total daily fat intake and, specifically, saturated fat. Have a look at a few things with me, would you?

Frankfurter . . . total fat grams: 32

Fat formula city.

$32 \times 9 = 288$

Divide that by total calories, 360, and you have 80 percent fat PER SERVING.

You see, here it is. You're hanging out at the ballpark (yeah, something I do often) or you're at the kid's birthday party. You haven't eaten all day because there wasn't time, and you have a couple of bites of a hot dog. It's the only thing around, and what the heck—what harm could it do?

Eighty percent fat per serving worth of harm. For that much fat you could eat more low-fat, high-volume food than you could ever imagine. Forget about imagining, here's what you could have:

Ground beef. Plain old regular ground beef—burgers, tacos, meat loaf.

21 fat grams $x 9 = 189$.

189 divided by total calories, 333, equals 57 percent fat per serving.

So you have a choice. You can have your burger, the bun, the lettuce, the pickle, the tomato, the onions (or any combination) and put the 57 percent fat ground beef in the middle, making your meal a very high fat meal, or you can fill the middle with something that is lower in fat and eat twenty-five of them.

Listen, I know what you're thinking:

What goes in the middle?

Give up my beef?

My husband won't stand for this.

The kids will boycott.

What could be better than beef?

Don't panic. I've got a suggestion for you. Get your hands on a low-fat veggie burger. (If they don't sell them in your grocery store, talk to the store manager and get him to order them.)

Here's what you do. You grill, barbecue, smoke, whatever you want to do with your burger. Slap on some low-fat cheese, pile high all the fixings—lettuce, tomato, onion, relish, pickles, sauerkraut—lying the whole time to the family—and feed it to them.

What have you saved? Well, we've already figured out that regular ground beef is 57 percent fat . . . so let's do the fat formula on a low-fat veggie burger (remember to read the labels because some veggie burgers aren't low fat).

1 fat gram $x 9 = 9$

9 divided by 97 (total calories) = 9 percent fat per serving

That's 48 percent less fat per serving! And look at the saturated fat . . . zero as in "No" saturated fat in the veggie burger and 9 grams in the regular ground beef.

Eat the veggie burger . . . your thighs will get thinner, you'll be giving your heart a chance, and the family will love it!

Do the fat formula on the rest of your chart. See where the fat is and decide what you want.

• •

Chicken. Interesting fact here. Chicken may be lower in fat than beef. Chicken is animal. And animal is cholesterol. So lowering your daily fat with chicken is possible. Cutting back on cholesterol with chicken. Different story.

• •

Cooked Poultry

(4 OZ Roasted)	Calories	Fat (g)	Saturated Fat (g)	Cholesterol (mg)
Chicken				
Dark Meat, with skin	289	18	5	104
Dark Meat, without skin	234	11	3	106
Light Meat, with skin	254	12	3	96
Light Meat, without skin	198	5	1	97
Turkey				
Dark Meat, with skin	253	13	4	102
Dark Meat, without skin	214	8	3	97
Light Meat, with skin	225	9	3	87
Light Meat, without skin	179	4	1	79
Goose				
With skin	349	25	8	104
Duck				
With skin	385	32	11	96

Adapted from University of California, Berkeley, ed. *The Wellness Encyclopedia,* Houghton Mifflin, New York, 1991.

Let's have a look at Mr. Poultry and see how it stacks up in the fat department. If you look at the chart, the first thing you will notice is that just by eliminating the skin you can cut way, way, way back on your total fat intake.

Dark meat chicken with skin has 18 grams of fat per serving.

18 fat grams x 9 = 162

162 divided by total calories 289 = 56 percent fat per serving . . . not good, a bit high wouldn't you say?

Compared to light meat without skin:

5 fat grams x 9 = 45

45 divided by 195 = 23 percent fat per serving . . . much better in the total fat category, but let's look at the cholesterol column. Boy, is that a different story.

The piece of dark meat chicken with skin has 104 mg of cholesterol! That's more than the same size of sirloin steak. (Didn't you think chicken was healthier for you!)

Even the light meat without skin has 97 mg of cholesterol, just 5 mg less than the steak. . . . Maybe this stuff is better for cutting down on total fat, but cutting down on cholesterol . . . Mr. Chicky and his cousins don't seem to be doing your cholesterol intake any favors. . . .

• •

Fish. Fish you know about already. Ms. Fitness helped us with that one by realizing in front of a live television audience that she didn't quite know as much as she thought she did about low-fat eating. Everybody's eating fish because we know beef is high fat. Chicken is saving the day because it's lower in total fat. And fish is almost saintly in its presentation of a healthy, wonderful low-fat alternative. It is smashingly easy to prepare, something you can't go wrong with—unless, of course, you're chowing down on orange roughy (and millions are) or salmon. Light tuna or halibut—fab.

Cooked Fish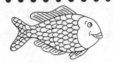

4 OZ	Calories	Fat (g)	Saturated Fat (g)	Cholesterol (mg)
Carp	185	8	2	96
Caviar, 2 tbsp	80	6	1	188
Clams, cooked	169	2	0	77
Cod	120	1	0	63
Crab, Alaskan King	111	2	0	61
Crayfish	130	1	0	203
Haddock	128	1	0	86
Halibut	160	3	0	47
Lobster	112	1	0	82
Mackerel	299	21	5	83
Mussels	197	5	1	64
Oysters	157	6	1	125
Perch	134	1	0	131
Pike	129	1	0	57
Salmon, pink, canned	159	7	2	45
Salmon, fresh	247	13	2	99
Sardines, canned in oil	238	13	3	162
Scallops, cooked	128	1	0	61
Shrimp, breaded and fried	277	14	2	202
Snapper	146	2	0	54
Squid	200	8	2	297
Swordfish	177	6	2	57
Trout, Rainbow	173	5	1	83
Tuna, light, canned in oil	226	9	2	21
Tuna, light, canned in water	150	2	0	21

Adapted from University of California, Berkeley, ed. *The Wellness Encyclopedia*, Houghton Mifflin Company, New York, 1991.

But again and again and again we see that it's about getting the info we need in order to know what the hell is going on and what's going in so that we end up having the body we want, the energy level we need to live our lives, and the prevention against heart disease, cancer, obesity, and all the other things connected to a high-fat life-style.

Dairy. If it's chart checking and saturated fat talking that we're doing, then we can't go far without chatting about dairy.

Saturated fat and dairy products? Sure.

> Dairy = animal product.
>
> Cows' milk is an animal product.
>
> Animal product = saturated fat.

I never did understand those vegetarians who looked down their noses at the beef eaters while they were eating their cheese. From a health standpoint (because this is not an animal rights book), what's the difference? Both products come from an animal, and both are loaded with saturated fat. I never understood the attitude that I've heard from so many vegetarians about the beef eaters of the world, while they eat their cheese burritos with sour cream on top. YO, seems to be something wrong with this picture, but who am I??

Well, now that you have all the numbers, you can pretty much make up your mind about how much saturated fat you want to take in daily and which source you're going to be getting it from. Nothing complicated about it, is there? If you feel you're lacking and need more saturated fat than you're getting, that's easy.

Eat it.

If you feel you're getting way, way too much, don't eat it.

Yeah, we need a nutritionist to figure this out. Sure, I'm gonna pay someone to give me this. I'm going to spend my life believing that they are smarter than I am because they know it!!

God forbid you don't get enough of whatever it is and shrivel up and die. I don't think that's gonna happen with most of us. Not getting enough saturated fat in our diet? Come on, I have plenty of other things to worry about. It's easy, it's obvious, and you can make your own decisions about it.

I am eating healthier and losing weight . . . and I try to eat a meatless dinner once or twice a week.

—*Kelli, Washington, D.C.*

So I'm in Texas figuring all this out, feeling kind of full of myself because I knew enough to know if there was an animal product in something, it had

Milk

Milk (8 fl oz)	Calories	Fat (g)	Fat Calories	Saturated Fat (g)
WHOLE (3% fat)	150	8	48%	5
LOW-FAT (2% fat)	120	5	38%	4
LOW-FAT (1% fat)	100	3	27%	2
SKIM (non-fat)	80	trace	5%	trace
BUTTERMILK (1% fat)	100	2	18%	1
DRY (non-fat, reconstituted)	80	trace	5%	trace
EVAPORATED (canned, made from whole milk, undiluted)	340	20	53%	17
LACTAID (lactase treated, 1% fat)	100	2	18%	2
GOAT'S MILK (whole)	168	10	54%	6

No surprise here that we're looking at high fat. Dairy is high fat, unless of course you go for the low-fat versions such as skim, 1%, or 2%. But if you stop for a second and take a look at your basic 2% milk, what you'll see is that it's 38 percent total fat. Confused? Sure you are—why wouldn't you be? How do they do that? Here it is: They, the dairy boys, measure the percentage of total weight and a lot of other things that we don't care about when they come up with their figures. We, on the other hand, are asking HOW MUCH FAT IS IN THIS SERVING? PLEASE, PLEASE, PLEASE, TELL US.

When you do the fat formula on the facts . . . well, let's do it.

$5 \times 9 = 45$

45 divided by total calories, 120, equals 38 percent.

See, just like they say here on this chart, but you're not gonna see that on your milk package, because what you see is only what those dairy boys want you to see—2%, 2%, 2%—and you buy it, thinking that's how much total fat you're taking in when you drink your milk.

Information—it's so interesting when you get down to the facts. Evaporated milk—who ever thought about how high in fat evaporated milk is? Fifty-three percent—it sits right next to the old goat's milk. YUCK-O. Why would you ever drink goat's milk? High fat and gross tasting.

• •

Cheese

	Calories	Fat (g)	Fat Calories	Saturated Fat (g)
American, 1 oz	105	9	77%	4
Blue, 1 oz	100	8	72%	5
Camembert or Brie, 1 oz	85	7	74%	4-5
Cheddar, 1 oz	115	9	70%	6
Cottage, creamed, ½ cup	108	5	42%	3
Cottage, low-fat, ½ cup	104	2	17%	1
Cream, 1 oz	100	10	90%	6
Feta, 1 oz	75	6	72%	4
Mozzarella, part skim, 1 oz	80	5	56%	3
Mozzarella, whole milk, 1 oz	80	6	68%	4
Muenster, 1 oz	105	9	77%	5
Neufchatel, 1 oz	74	7	85%	4
Parmesan, 1 oz	130	9	62%	5
Provolone, 1 oz	100	8	72%	5
Ricotta, part skim, ½ cup	170	10	53%	6
Ricotta, whole milk, ½ cup	216	16	66%	10
Swiss, 1 oz	105	8	67%	5

Never did I ever think I'd hear this come out of my mouth: EAT COTTAGE CHEESE. Talk about the old diet mentality. Cottage cheese, salad, and hamburger without the bun. How many of those plates have you eaten in your life?

It makes me nauseous to even think about the old cottage cheese diet plate, but when you run down this list, what's your choice?

One ounce of American cheese? Sure, it's only 105 calories, and 77 percent of those 105 calories are fat.

GET OUT OF TOWN WITH YOUR 77 PERCENT FAT.

Now I gotta stop here and talk volume for one minute.

> High volume, low fat
> High volume, low fat
> High volume, low fat

How many times have I said that in the last couple of years??? This is it. Right here is what I've been talking, talking, talking about.

> High volume?
> One slice, what are you—nuts??
> High volume—105 calories??

How long is that gonna last you, with your schedule? Like half a morning??

Low fat? We don't even need to talk about how high fat 77 percent of a slice of anything is.

The way to have the body and life of your dreams is to go the opposite way. Low fat and high volume. Why?

Low fat so it doesn't end up all over your body.

Low fat in the food you're eating so you can eat more food without getting the . . . you guessed it.

More food with less fat so you'll have the fuel your body needs to get through the day.

Fuel your body needs, without all the extra damn fat, and you'll have the energy you have to have to live. Energy to live so that you can decide how you want to live, what you want your life to be. And it all starts with cottage cheese?? You know what I mean. Lower-fat choices versus the high, high-fat-without-enough-food-to-get-you-through-the-day, one-slice-of-anything kind of foods.

• •

Yogurt

8 oz	Calories	Fat (g)	Saturated Fat (g)	Fat %
WHOLE MILK	139	7	5	45
plain				
LOW-FAT				
plain	143	4	2	25
flavored—coffee/vanilla	193	3	2	14
NON-FAT				
plain	126	0	U	0
flavored—fruit				
w/low-cal sweetener	115	0	0	0

Yogurt—the low-fat option.

Women living on nothing but a yogurt for lunch—I've seen it over and over again. Check out this chart.

• •

saturated fat in it. Knew beyond a shadow of a doubt that when and if I took in that saturated fat exactly what my liver was going to do with it: convert it into cholesterol city, which I also knew that my body needed. Then I found out that my body, your body, everybody's body make all they need, so any extra was just that—extra.

I knew this as I was eating my low-fat, no-cholesterol pretzels;

making my soups with my vegetarian soup mix;

snacking on my low-fat chip dip.

But hydrogenated? Ever heard of it? I know you've seen it because it's everywhere.

Lots and lots of snacky foods. Hydrogenated oil is in more foods than you can ever imagine.

What is it? And why am I talking about it now instead of talking about unsaturated fat? Wouldn't the logical progression be to go from saturated to unsaturated fat?

No. And you'll soon see why.

Let's start with why. Why is hydrogenated oil in everything we pick up these days? Like:

> Almost 90 percent of all breakfast cereals.
> You gotta look out for the
>> fruit loopy
>> pebbly
>> granola
>> 100% natural cereals.
> The granola bars
>> fruit roll-up things
>> box o' rice mixes
>> help-a-hamburger-along mixes
>> instant soups
>> tortillas
>> all margarines.
>
> The chippy things
>> the salty snacky things
>> the cheesy things.
>
> The things that go with the chippy,
> dippy things.
>> the french onion dip
>> the ranch dip
>> the avocado dip.
>
> Almost every frozen dinner
>> pizzas
>> lasagnas
>> egg rolls
>> fish sticks.
>
> The ready-to-bake biscuits
>> rolls
>> croissants.

The desserts
the frozen pies
cakes
cupcakes.
The make-you-slim shakes and the
make-you-slimmer snack bars.
And on and on and on . . . read the labels!

Why? I'll tell you why:

Shelf life.

Texture.

Lack of spoilage.

O.K., so what? Sounds fine, doesn't it? What's the matter with making sure our food doesn't rot in the warehouses before we even get a chance to get to the store?

Technology is good. Technology is what moves this country forward. Hold up the American flag, and let's sing a round of "The Star-Spangled Banner," shall we? Yes, yes, yes, I'd love to, because "The Star-Spangled Banner" is a beautiful song, and if you want pride and patriotism, count me in; however, technology, schmology, it ain't about that.

Hydrogenation is about taking an unsaturated fat, adding some hydrogen to it and making it a saturated fat, and using it in more packaged goods, spreads, dressings, and every other kind of food you can imagine. We eat it while having no idea that it's:

(a) A fat.

(b) A saturated fat.

- Pretzels good for you? Not if they have hydrogenated oil in them.

- Instant potato products? Potatoes are low-fat, but not if they have hydrogenated oil in them.

- Rice dishes? Not if they have hydrogenated oil in them.

- Pasta dinners? Not if they have hydrogenated oil in them.

- Stuffings, breading, pastries? Well, you know the rest . . .

Look for yourself. Go to your pantry and check it out. When you do, you'll see a couple of different kinds of hydrogenated oils listed. Don't be confused.

When you see "partially hydrogenated," it means just that: partially hydro-genated.

> Kinda saturated?
> Not fully?
> On its way?
> Could be cloggier?
> Will only last for forty years on the shelf instead of eighty?

Just another detail. The bottom line on this hydrogenation stuff is that it's a good way for the food manufacturers to use a cheaper product (why do you think margarine is so much cheaper than butter? Turn it into a despoiler and feed it to us) and sell the hell out of it. It costs them less, it lasts forever on the shelf, and as long as we are confused enough to eat this stuff without having a clue as to what we are eating, it works. The minute you question, decide that you might not want to be eating an unsaturated fat that the food company has turned into a saturated fat (which is worse for your health) in your packaged foods, then you can pick the brand of whatever it is you're eating that is made without the hydrogenated oils. You'll see things change.

Once the companies know you know about this convenient little way of feeding the American public more saturated fat (don't you think heart disease rates are high enough with the meat and milk we are eating, now that the snack foods are loaded with saturated fats? Has anyone told these guys that the amount of saturated fat is killing us by the millions? They know this and still they are adding hydrogenated/saturated fat to our food?), they'll be busted. Busted by the American women again!

It has taken a while for the Surgeon General, the American Dietetic Asso-ciation, and the American Medical Association to jump on board. They ex-panded their consciousness in the 60's and 70's—yeah, I've heard that before. It's the what-you're-eating-connected-to-how-you're-feeling train. The truth is, they had trouble seeing the train before it ran over them. Getting to the station and standing on the platform was a big deal for these "protectors of the people's health." Getting on the train was too much to ask.

According to our friend Dr. John, there has been an enormous change and consumer demand for information over the last few years.

"We first had to figure out that modern medicine doesn't work. We've been battered and beaten by modern medicine for so long while they tried to find the cure. There have been too few results, and the prob-lems keep getting worse and worse. Before we knew any better we thought science was better than God, and years later we realize that we

The Mounting Consensus
With each passing year more and more expert organizations publicly affirmed the role of saturated fat and cholesterol in heart disease.

1980	U.S. DEPT. OF AGRICULTURE/ DEPT. OF HEALTH AND HUMAN SERVICES;
1979	SURGEON GENERAL OF THE U.S.;
1977	FOOD AND AGRICULTURAL ORGANIZATION/ WORLD HEALTH ORGANIZATION; QUEBEC DEPT. OF SOCIAL AFFAIRS;
1976	NEW ZEALAND ROYAL SOCIETY; ROYAL COLLEGE OF PHYSICIANS OF LONDON/ BRITISH CARDIAC SOCIETY;
1975	AUSTRALIAN ACADEMY OF SCIENCE; FEDERAL REPUBLIC OF GERMANY REPORT; CALIFORNIA SOCIETY OF PEDIATRIC CARDIOLOGY/ CALIFORNIA HEART ASSOCIATION;
1974	NATIONAL HEART FOUNDATION OF AUSTRALIA; UNITED KINGDOM DEPT. OF HEALTH AND SOCIAL SECURITY;
1973	INTERNATIONAL SOCIETY OF CARDIOLOGY; NATIONAL ADVISORY COUNCIL ON NUTRITION OF THE NETHERLANDS; REPORT OF THE 1969 WHITE HOUSE CONFERENCE ON FOOD, NUTRITION AND HEALTH;
1972	AMERICAN HEALTH FOUNDATION; AMERICAN MEDICAL ASSOCIATION/ NATIONAL ACADEMY OF SCIENCES FOOD AND NUTRITION BOARD;
1971	NATIONAL HEART FOUNDATION OF NEW ZEALAND; TASK FORCE ON ARTERIOSCLEROSIS/NATIONAL HEART, LUNG, AND BLOOD INSTITUTE (U.S.);
1970	INTER-SOCIETY COMMISSION ON HEART DISEASE RESOURCES (U.S.)
1968	SCANDINAVIAN GOVERNMENT MEDICAL BOARDS (FINLAND, SWEDEN, AND NORWAY);
1961	AMERICAN HEART ASSOCIATION; NATIONAL HEALTH EDUCATION COMMITTEE (U.S.)

Source: *Jack Sprat's Legacy,* Patricia Hausman, Richard Marek Publishers, New York, 1981.

AHHHHHHHHH, just happen to have a chart.

1961: the American Heart Association and the National Education Committee jumped on board the connect-cholesterol-to-heart-disease train. The Surgeon General of the United States jumped on in '79. Stood on the platform eighteen years.

It took a while for the Department of Agriculture. Well, you don't wonder why, do you? Who do you think the beef and the dairy boys are? We don't think for a second that they didn't fight every step of the way against connecting the number one killer in our country to the foods they were pumping millions and millions of dollars into advertising. It's interesting to look at this chart and see who jumped on board and when. That's a whole lot of people in a whole lot of countries saying that the connection is there.

are not going to be saved by medicine. We can and must save ourselves."

Easy to see why I love this guy so much, isn't it? Statements like that make my heart sing. You and I can save ourselves by getting the information and making the changes in our life-styles that can literally save our lives. I love this guy as much now as I did when my son was eight months old and Dr. McDougall's book gave me the answers to my questions, helped me see things differently, and helped me make the connection between food and my son's health. The longest relationship I've ever had. Doc John McDougall and I together for fifteen years—bliss. We'll invite you to our fiftieth anniversary. You'll come, we'll eat, we'll all be healthy—it will be big fun.

The availability of information. The fence sitters who are stepping over and making a stand because the consumer is demanding—that's what happening here.

The fact that it's cool now to know a little about food, herbs, holistic healing, makes it easier for all of us to make these changes. Getting sick and over-fat has worked in our favor because now, based on overwhelming evidence, it's time to take a look and make a few changes.

When I asked the doctor what we could do to help people get the information they need to improve the quality of their lives, he said, "Education, education, education." Education and understanding fat. Saturated fat and now hydrogenated oil. Not so difficult. But can it be this easy?

You're probably ready to blast into your lower-saturated-fat, hydrogenated-aware life. Think you've got it down? After all, it's understandable, and you're capable of applying this to your life.

Fat. Finished.

Graduated from the fat detective school?

Understanding more than you ever thought you'd understand? Most of the confusion out of the way? It begins and ends with saturated fat, hydrogenated fat, heart disease, obesity—you've got the whole connection, right?

Wrong. Not so fast, fat detectives. If you think saturated fat was the biggest and hydrogenated the best kept secret—no, no, no, no. I've got more fat for you. Saturated may have the worst reputation in town, but there's more to fat than just saturated. How about unsaturated? Ever heard of it? Understand it any better than you understood saturated just a few short minutes ago? This, my friends, is interesting. The confusion about this unsaturated mess is beyond belief. Come on, grab your magnifying glasses and come with me into the land of mono- and polyunsaturated fats.

> I have learned not to be conned by labels (I was actually eating those little lunch-and-munch things!) and can even eat a baked potato with just a touch of salt now, instead of globs of butter (a miracle for me—but now I actually TASTE the potato!).
> —*Helen, Memphis, Tennessee*

UNSATURATED FAT

Brothers in crime, that's what this unsaturated fat amounts to. There are two of them: Mr. Monounsaturated and Mr. Polyunsaturated.

Liquid? Solid?

Good or bad for you?

Married? Unmarried?

What do they look like, these boys?

Questions you might be asking at this very moment about our friend/foe, unsaturated fat.

Nothing but liquid. If Cousin Saturated is solid at room temperature, any room temperature, and it is, then these guys can only be described as liquid at room temperature.

Remember now, all fats are a combo of saturated, polyunsaturated, and monounsaturated. It's the saturation by hydrogen atoms that determines what they are; it's the variations that determine the properties of different fats. (Some doctor said that, not me. Couldn't you tell? It doesn't scream *me*, does it?)

So depending on the number of missing hydrogen atoms, you either have monounsaturated fat, as in:

Olive

Peanut

Canola

Avocado

or you have polyunsaturated:

Corn

Safflower

Sesame

So here's the difference between saturated and unsaturated.

> Liquid as opposed to solid.
> Less hydrogen here or there.
> And you've got a different name.

Since the day I figured out that fat had something to do with my being fat, the lists and lists of poly or mono or saturated fats have clogged my brain and confused me no end. I still can't tell you which is which.

Why shouldn't we just concentrate on fat being fat, and who cares if it blocks your arteries and puts fat in you, or goes right to your fat cells and puts fat on you? What's the difference and why so complicated? That's what I was thinking. Then it dawned on me. It took a couple of hits on the head with a hammer, but I got it.

Aren't you under the impression that one is good for you and one is bad? Doesn't one increase blood cholesterol and another decrease—as in make better?

Aren't we supposed to be eating one and avoiding the other like the plague?

Isn't that what you're walking around believing but not understanding?

Doesn't corn oil do something that peanut oil doesn't?

Or is it olive oil that is so good for you and reverses something inside your bloodstream? Wait a minute. Safflower—something in safflower oil is good for something in your body?

When you make that salad dressing, which one do you use?

This is exactly where I was when the hammer hit me on the head. So I picked up my cigar, put on my topcoat, and went out on the streets to ask, ask, ask the questions.

Dean Ornish pretty much sums it up in his book, *Reversing Heart Disease:*

"Several studies have shown that *replacing* oils high in saturated fats (like coconut oil) with oils high in monounsaturated fat (like olive oil) or oils high in polyunsaturated fat (such as safflower oil) will, in fact, lower cholesterol levels. This is because olive oil and safflower oil contain less saturated fat, not because they contain more monounsaturated or polyunsaturated fat. In other words, olive oil and safflower oil are not 'good' for you; they are less 'bad' for you."

Hey, hey, hey, what are you saying? Saturated fat in olive oil? I thought it was unsaturated, meaning no saturated fat? You see, I thought that unsaturated fats were O.K. because they weren't saturated. All I had to do was look beyond the nose on my face (there's a little expression my mother always, always used to use; inner child having a fit, pardon me for one moment) to find out that all oil, let me repeat, ALL OIL contains saturated fat.

Surprised me just a bit. Did you know that? Did you, like me, think that unsaturated meant no saturated fat, none as in "un," and that saturated meant saturated? And so the good/bad rep, right? Didn't you think that?

That's not what it means. Unsaturated oil has saturated fat in it. Look and see for yourself.

Interesting stuff! Check out the saturated fat in coconut oil. My God, that's high.

Butterfat is a close second.

Beef fat . . . well, we could have figured that.

Safflower oil—1.3 grams of fat. Wait a minute. I thought that was supposed to be the "good for you" kind of oil?

Canola is low. That's good. But Ornish is right (he's probably relieved that I've confirmed his facts for him!). Some more than others, but we're talking saturated fat in all oils, and when you put that together with all oils being 100 percent fat, it isn't looking good for oils.

According to the brilliant doctor, adding any oil to your food will raise your blood cholesterol level, because all oils contain some saturated fat.

Look. Olive oil contains 1.9 grams of saturated fat per tablespoon. That's 14 percent saturated fat. That's not *no* saturated fat, that's 14 percent saturated fat.

Safflower oil has 1.3 grams of saturated fat per tablespoon. HEY, BOYS IN THE AMA AND DIETITIANS OF THIS COUNTRY, that's 1.3 grams of saturated fat any way you look at it.

"One tablespoon of any oil contains almost fourteen grams of total fat."

Forget about the cousin and the brothers right now. Did you hear that right from the expert's mouth? That's a hell of a lot of fat per tablespoon. Talk about low volume, high fat!! One teaspoon and all that fat—for what?

Don't you think one tablespoon of anything that high in fat is going to contribute to a weight problem?

Separating saturated fat from unsaturated fat is important if all you are interested in is cholesterol levels and clogged arteries. (But apparently there isn't that much of a separation. Saturated fat is in all oil, and saturated fat is

• •

TYPE OF FAT	SATURATED (g)	MONOUNSATURATED (g)	POLYUNSATURATED (g)
Beef Fat	**7.1**	6.0	0.5
Butterfat	**9.0**	4.1	0.6
Canola (Puritan) Oil	**0.8**	8.4	4.4
Chicken Fat	4.2	6.4	3.0
Coconut Oil	**11.7**	0.8	0.2
Corn Oil	1.7	3.4	7.9
Cottonseed Oil	3.6	2.6	6.9
Crisco	3.8	6.0	3.8
Lard	5.6	6.4	1.6
Olive Oil	**1.9**	9.8	1.2
Peanut Oil	2.6	6.2	4.1
Safflower Oil	**1.3**	1.7	10.0
Soybean Oil	2.0	3.1	7.8
Sunflower Oil	1.4	2.8	8.7

(Fat content is for 1 tablespoon of oil)

Source: *Reversing Heart Disease*, Dr. Dean Ornish, Ballantine Books, New York, 1991.

In case your doctor thinks you've gone out of your mind when you tell him/her that all oil has saturated fat in it, show him/her this chart.

Start with the statement that all oil is 100 percent fat.

Go to the saturated fat.

Then ask, Which oil is "heart healthy" and why?

How do they figure that out?

• •

connected to heart disease. So I'm still confused about where the good and the bad rep comes in, but forget about this for a minute.)

Why are we doing this? What's the point? How could anything this important get so screwed up? Why shouldn't we just look at fat and cut back on it if we want to get leaner and healthier? Healthier was never my motivation, but can't you see starting to care just a little bit about it as you learn more and more about the connection between your health and the way your body looks? What you're eating may be causing the exhaustion in your life, your butt widening, your heart trouble, your high blood cholesterol level, your triglyceride level.

You probably didn't know the connection between all that extra upper body weight you've put on and the bad HDL and LDL level you just got from your doctor.

You know you're unhealthy because you don't feel good. You know you don't look good because you have mirrors in your house.

I raised a question that I haven't answered yet. Why all the confusion? It seems very simple to me. I have a theory: I think they want us to be confused. You see, when you are overwhelmed with contradictory information, sometimes you give up. That's what happened to me. It keeps us buying their products, it keeps us feeling as if we aren't capable of figuring it out.

Not solving the problem, getting caught up in the symptoms, spending energy on the details when the bottom line seems to be total fat—that's what most of us are doing. If you want to make it easy, do what I did. At 260 pounds I couldn't have been bothered with all the confusion, so I looked at fat as fat and cut it way, way, way back. Down to 15 percent of my daily intake.

Saturated = animals, except for a couple of plant things that I couldn't remember for years.

I cut way, way, way back on animal products. I found ways to think beyond grilled chicken and started getting creative with my plate of food, no matter where I was. There's nothing wrong with combining a couple of different entrees in a restaurant to make a meal without the foods that were high in fat. You can take the baked potato from one dish and combine it with the corn from another, throw in braised chicken from another, have a little extra pasta salad, and, what the hell, go for the sorbet for dessert. Tell them to name the plate after you. The Peggy, Jackie, Bonnie plate. Fat is easy to cut out of your life. Cut the animal stuff. Read the labels: When you see coconut oil, run for the hills; palm oil, anything that smells of the tropics, forget it. That's how I cut my daily fat intake from 50 percent to 15 percent.

≈ Polyunsaturated and monounsaturated? Simple, cut back on the oil, all oils.

≈ Hydrogenated? Easier: Check the labels. Pick the brand that doesn't include it . . . eat their pretzels.

What do you think will happen when you do that? Where's the fat gonna come from if we don't eat it? You know the end of my story (if you don't, flip to my before and after pictures in *Stop the Insanity!*, they say it all, as far as I'm concerned). I may remember which oil is a poly or a mono, saturated or unsaturated, when I've had a good eight hours of sleep and a big breakfast and no stress and I've been reading about it all for a few days, but ask me when I am tired, haven't thought about it for a while, am trying like hell to keep up with life, and I'll get it wrong every time. I still get it wrong every time unless I refer back to the experts, such as Ornish and McDougall. Why bother memorizing all the stats? I don't know about you, but it seems to me that there is a much simpler solution.

> My children now ask how much fat is in something, and at the grocery store we all read labels and do our calculation!
>
> —*Laura, Troutdale, Oregon*

Start with the famous, the easy to use, the golden FAT FORMULA.

After I started talking about the fat formula (surprised to find out that I didn't invent it?) I've heard . . .

"Love your formula."

"Your formula changed my life."

"That formula of yours really made sense to me."

"What's that formula that you made up?"

As much as I'd like to take full credit for the fat formula—and I would quickly if there was a way to get away with it—I can't. It's the AMA, the American Heart Association, the dietitians and nutritionists came up with the thing. The problem is that they forgot to tell us how the hell to use it. What it means. How we are supposed to apply it to our lives. And what to do if we are mathematically brain dead, as I am, and still want to know how much fat is in the food we are eating. So, as I just said to one of the biggest names in nutrition when he said I was "doing good work," it's all your stuff, I'm just the mouthpiece. Charming, don't you think?

Discovering the fat formula changed my life. Shopping was never the same after I figured out how to use it. So simple. So informative. So easy to use. We'll do it together, and then you'll know. You'll have the power of the golden fat formula.

Here's what you do to get the magic:

Turn around every canned, packaged, labeled anything you put into your mouth and get the number of fat grams.

Take the number of fat grams x 9 = "whatever."

Take "whatever" and divide that by the total calories. That will answer the question that's on everyone's mind: How much fat is in the total serving of food that I'm about to put into my mouth and onto my hips? That's what you want to know. Is it 10 percent fat or 80 percent? That's the deal—how much of it is fat??

So, fine. You do. And you get your answers. Then what are you supposed to do with it? You've done your formula and you've got your answers.

// The bread is 10 percent fat.

// Lettuce—so little it's not worth mentioning.

// Tomato—so little it's not worth mentioning.

// Mayo—100 percent.

// Lunch meat—that ham may say 98 percent fat free, but once you do the formula, you may find out it's 67 percent fat.

So what then? Does it all add up? One item at a time giving you the number that's "right," "healthy"? Do you do this with every meal and add up all the numbers at the end of the day?

Have no fear, simple math and common sense are here. This is what I do, based on the American Heart Association's standards, of course:

According to the American Heart Association, 30 percent of our daily intake should be fat. That means 30 percent of our total calories is fat, and the rest is carbs and protein and all the wonderful minerals and vitamins that we need to stay healthy.

That, my friends, is a load of junk.

You can go much, much lower, all the way down to 10 percent (Dean Ornish's results haven't been too shabby). You can go to the high end, the AHA's 30 percent daily recommendation, or you can take in anything in between.

Guess who should decide what your daily fat intake is? You.

// Based on how overfat you are and how much fat you want to lose.

// Based on your heart.

// Based on what your HDL and LDL and triglycerides all add up to.

// Based on how healthy, well, and lean you want to be.

I keep mine at 15 percent of my daily intake because I don't want to get fat. And here's how you do it—10 percent, 15 percent, 20 percent, or 30 percent, whatever you want in your life.

// Don't add it all up because it takes too much time.

// Forget about gram counting all day long.

Who wants to spend any more time on this stuff than you have to? There's plenty more to do with your time than count food grams all day long.

Here it is: The simplest way on earth to make sure that you stay within your daily fat intake.

- Pick a number, any number—say, 20 percent. Do the fat formula on every food you've ever had in your cupboard or fridge or in your favorite restaurant, and get to know its fat percentage.

- Snack foods—check out how much fat per serving.

- Lunch meats—fat per serving is?

- Cakes, cookies, frozen whatever you've been eating—do that fat formula.

- See how much fat is in the food you're eating.

- If it's a higher percentage than the 20 percent you've decided on, then don't eat it.

- Think about this. If everything you eat is 20 percent fat or under, how can you exceed your 20 percent total daily fat intake? You can't.

Another way of saying the same thing is if you don't eat anything that's over 20 percent fat, why would you bother calculating it? You wouldn't because you know that nothing you've eaten is above 20 percent fat.

If you don't want to do it my way, the simple-minded way, then here's what you can do:

Say you are eating a meal and one ingredient is 20 percent fat, another is 45 percent, one is 10 percent fat, and the last is 23 percent.

- Don't add up your percentages here. Write down all the fat grams in each food you're eating and the calories right beside them. All day long. Everything you put into your mouth.

- Then, at the end of the day, do the fat formula on the totals.

Saturated fat, understood.

Unsaturated, down.

Fat formula, done.

Daily percentage, piece of cake (pardon that high-fat reference).

What more can we say about fat? More involved than you could have ever imagined?? Yep. See how easy it was to keep us all in the dark? It's easy to hide behind all this info—twist and turn it around so that we're so confused.

Are you begging me to stop yet? Fat making you tired? Sick to death of finding out information that's making you madder and madder by the minute? Don't worry, you'll be out of your mind by the time you get past this section of the fat discussion. Bear with me for one more part of the whole big fat story.

• •

20 Percent Daily Menu

	Calories	Fat Grams
BREAKFAST		
Bell pepper egg white omelette	99	1
English muffin w/1 tbsp strawberry jam	182	1
Coffee (black)	4	0
MORNING SNACK		
Apple	81	.5
LUNCH		
Tuna sandwich	404	19
(water-packed light tuna with mayo on cracked wheat bread)		
Dill pickle	12	trace
Low-fat baked tortilla chips without oil (1 oz)	110	1
AFTERNOON SNACK		
Vanilla frozen yogurt (8 oz)	359	13
DINNER		
Shrimp kabobs	301	4
(½ lb shrimp, bell pepper, onions, barbecue sauce)		
served over ½ cup steamed brown rice	108	1
Corn on the cob	59	.5
Angel food cake with ½ cup strawberries	159	.1

Total calories: 1,878
Total fat grams: 41
Total fat percentage: 20

When you look down at the bottom of this daily eating plan, you have your basic-20-percent-of-your-daily-intake-kind-of-fat day. Good day, anyone talking low fat would say. And all you have to do to find the big fat contributors is look at your lunch sandwich, with its mayo, and check your afternoon snack, regular yogurt—the biggest, fattest contributors by far.

Twenty percent daily fat is very low fat. It will get you lean, lean, lean, and doesn't seem too difficult to do. Check it out. Great breakfast. Not such a great morning snack (fruit, so what?).

Lunch. Fine.

Dinner, YUMMMMMMMMM.

Now here's what I'd do.

I'd blow off the mayo and the yogurt and add tons more food to my day. Low-, low-, low-fat food, that is. More for the money, more for less fat, just more food, that's always been my motto (that's how I got to be 260). Still live by the more food motto, just without the fat.

The fat's in the mayo. If you took it out and added curry and non-fat mayo, you could have six-plus, almost seven tuna sandwiches for the same amount of fat. Now let's get to the frozen yogurt. In place of your regular eight-ounce frozen yogurt, you could have the equivalent in fat of 285 non-fat frozen yogurts.

• •

• •

30 Percent Daily Menu

	Calories	Fat Grams
BREAKFAST		
Oatmeal (1 cup cooked)	145	2.5
Banana	104	.5
Whole wheat toast with 1 tbsp butter	161	13
MID-MORNING SNACK		
½ cinnamon raisin bagel with 1 oz cream cheese	256	11
LUNCH		
Bean burrito (2)	447	14
Steamed brown rice (1 cup)	216	2
Low-fat baked tortilla chips with oil (2 oz)	220	2
Salsa (¼ cup)	11	trace
AFTERNOON SNACK		
6 gingersnaps	180	4
DINNER		
Cubed beef Sirloin (3½ oz) with Cream of		
Mushroom Soup over 1 cup cooked linguini	564	26
Steamed broccoli and carrots topped with		
2 tbsp Parmesan cheese	112	4
Pound cake with ½ cup strawberries	139	6

Total calories:	2,555
Total fat grams:	85
Total fat percentage:	30

Well, well, well—seems to me that there's something to be said for this high-volume, low-fat eating, and we haven't even begun, because we're not at the really high-fat daily intake yet.

Thirty percent of our daily intake is the standard. What do we have to do to this in order to eat higher volume and lower fat, and how much more could we eat?

Take off the tablespoon of butter, and you can have fourteen pieces of whole wheat toast.

The cream cheese—remember, we are talking one stupid ounce—goes, and you can have five bagels.

Two bean burritos—still bean burritos. Just take out the lard and get yourself some non-fat refried beans, and you can have fifteen bean burritos for lunch. How about it? Think you'd be full? Worried about getting enough food? Understanding a little better now high volume, low fat, and the reason for it?

Hey, the main course for dinner tells us one thing. Switch the beef in your stroganoff with chicken, change your whole milk cream of mushroom soup to low-fat cream of mushroom soup, and you have yourself six servings for the same amount of fat.

Dessert. Pound cake with strawberries. All you gotta do with this is have angel food cake with strawberries, and you can have eight servings instead of one.

This is the most fun ever for me. You can see why. It's a great way to make a point. I would never suggest that you actually go out and eat seven tuna sandwiches, 285 ounces of non-fat yogurt, fifteen non-fat refried burritos, or eight pieces of angel food cake, because that's too much food for anyone to eat. Calories are not what we need to be counting anymore, because you've cut back on the fattest ones—fat calories— and you've gotta move to burn up the rest of the calories, for sure. But if it's fat for fat we're talking about, and a great example of more food for less fat that we're talk- ing about, what could be better than this?

Come on, let's get to the next example, the 60 percent menu. I'm dying to . . .

● ●

60 Percent Daily Menu

	Calories	Fat Grams
BREAKFAST		
Fried egg (1 egg fried in butter)	92	6
Bacon (2 slices)	73	6
Croissant with 1 pat butter	333	24
Coffee with cream (1 tbsp Half & Half)	25	2
MID-MORNING SNACK		
Glazed doughnut	242	14
Coffee with cream (1 tbsp Half & Half)	25	2
LUNCH		
Fried chicken (2 pieces dark)	431	27
Biscuit with butter	378	25
French fries	235	12
AFTERNOON SNACK		
Potato chips (1 small bag)	304	20
DINNER		
Barbecued brisket (3.5%)	367	30
Baked potato with sour cream, butter, chives, and cheese	542	34
Coleslaw salad (1 cup)	178	13
Cheesecake	295	21

Total calories:	3,520
Total fat grams:	236
Total fat percentage:	60

One fried egg with margarine equals eight scrambled egg whites without the yolk or margarine.

Croissant with butter. You want more food? How about eight English muffins with jam instead? How's that for breakfast?

Chicken, chicken, chicken—preparation says it all, right here.

For your two pieces of fried chicken (dark meat), you can have eighteen servings of skinless roasted chicken breasts. With that much chicken you could

continued

Have a sandwich.
Cook a stew.
Cut it in cubes and stir-fry it.
Host a chicken party.

My point is you have to eat a lot of fat to have a daily fat intake of 60 percent or even 30 percent fat. I know because I did, and that's why I put on 133 pounds. I ate it. You have to work hard to get heart disease, you have to work hard to get fat. It doesn't just happen, it isn't coming from nowhere, and you could be eating twice, three times, four times the amount of food and not get the fat.

• •

The really big subject, the one we've been referring to right along with saturated fat, is cholesterol!!

It's a subject you certainly can't tackle yourself. You need a degree in something to understand this, don't you? Surely it requires a brilliant mind. And the consequences of attempting to explain this big, big subject without those things would be . . .

Devastating?

Potentially life threatening?

Irresponsible as hell?

We'll talk, then you decide for yourself how complicated this subject is.

CHOLESTEROL

Let's start with what it looks like. Don't ask me why, I just think that's a great place to start.

White, waxy, fatty, globby (not a scientific term; my own). There it is. Imagine it . . . white, waxy, globby, sticky stuff traveling around in your bloodstream. It's some kind of ugly for sure, but just like fat, cholesterol is necessary. Cholesterol is important stuff. Essential to life itself.

The outer membranes of your cells would have a hard time living without it, and what would we do without the outer membranes of our cells?

You'll find cholesterol wrapping around nerve fibers as fatty insulation. The connection between hormones and Mr. C. (as we will be referring to cholesterol from now on, since it's a pain in the neck to type out the word cholesterol every ten seconds, and it's catchy) is very important. Hormones and Mr. C. Nerve Fibers and Mr. C. Cells and Mr. C.—connected, connected, connected.

Your body needs Mr. C. That's why it produces all it needs. Yep. Your body produces all the Mr. C. it needs. All animals do. The cow's body produces Mr. C. The chickie's body produces Mr. C. Your body produces Mr. C. All animals produce it. That's where Mr. C. comes from—the body of animals. There is no Mr. C. in the plant world. None at all. Ever.

Look at this. The old Mr. C. Content of Common Foods, right from John Robbins's book, right from "Food Values of Portions Commonly Used" (whatever they are).

Back to our perfect system. Your body. It needs Mr. C., and it produces all it needs. Oh, sure, there's a screwup every once in a while, but when it comes to our bodies and producing the right amount of Mr. C., it works just like it's supposed to work for the majority of us. (If you are one of the very small percentage of people whose body is manufacturing the hell out of it, ignore this chapter and call your doctor.) Our bodies, the animals that we are, produce all the Mr. C. we need. Well created, God. Bravo, bravo.

So what's the problem? How come the biggest issue in health these days is the number one killer, heart disease, which is directly connected with high blood cholesterol counts?

Doc McDougall says that there's nothing complicated about it and that having your cholesterol checked is

> "the greatest marker you have to indicate how much damage has been done to your body. It's easy, inexpensive, and a wonderful, accurate indication of the health you are in. It's a predictor of the future. A crystal ball—heart attack, stroke, atherosclerosis easily, easily foreseen with this one little test."

Well, that's handy, isn't it? A crystal ball to the future in the aisles of most supermarkets these days—one, two, three, quick prick, and you have the crystal ball of health telling you what's going on. Fascinating and something we'll be coming right back to, but I still have this question about our bodies producing all the cholesterol we need and how it ended up being such a huge health issue. Are our bodies going berserk and churning this stuff out?

♪ Why the extra cholesterol that's killing millions?

♪ Where's it coming from, Doc?

♪ That's all we hear about these days: high cholesterol, high cholesterol, high cholesterol. Watch out, it'll get you . . . as if it's coming out of nowhere.

♪ Does it just happen?

♪ Does it go hand in hand with age?

♪ Is it a given?

● ●

Cholesterol Content of Common Foods

ANIMAL FOOD Cholesterol Content (in milligrams per 100-gram portion)		PLANT FOOD Cholesterol Content (in milligrams per 100-gram portion)	
Egg, whole	550		
Kidney, beef	375		
Liver, beef	300	All grains	0
Butter	250	All vegetables	0
Oysters	200	All nuts	0
Cream cheese	120	All seeds	0
Lard	95	All fruits	0
Beefsteak	70	All legumes	0
Lamb	70	All vegetable oils	0
Pork	70		
Chicken	60		
Ice cream	45		

Source: Pennington, J., *Food Values of Portions Commonly Used*, Harper and Row, 14th ed., New York, 1985.

Left-hand side—cholesterol. How much? What foods? From high to low. Well done, "Portions Commonly Used" guys. Right-hand side—all grains. All vegetables. I think "all" is a very powerful word when it's in front of what foods we're talking about and behind the big zero. Zero, as in no Mr. C. anywhere in sight. This is not about "good" versus "bad" food. This is about Mr. C. Where the hell is it, and how can we learn more about it? This list of foods pretty much says it all, if one of the questions you've ever asked about this much-talked-about subject is how much Mr. C. and in what food?

Here's what I've been saying all along about memorizing. Who's gonna be able to keep track of the cholesterol level in egg versus ice cream? Again I say, if you have time for that, we need to talk about your getting a life. Come on, it's not that we are too stupid to remember or figure this stuff out, it's that we are busy, tired, have bills to pay, have kids to raise, and we want it understandable and simple.

As simple as it gets. Cholesterol comes from animals. Period. The end.

● ●

//y As you get older, does your cholesterol count go up?

//y This is a big confusing issue, Doc, and we need your expert advice. Make it simple. Help us understand.

"It's in our diet. The food we are eating. Animal products alone contain cholesterol."

So let's spend a second on this concept. If you eat animal products that have cholesterol in them, you'll get cholesterol in your diet. And saturated fat? Way, way back in the saturated fat discussion, the big connection was made between saturated fat and cholesterol. You eat saturated fat, and your body converts it into cholesterol. Two ways to get this stuff into your body. Excuse me, I'll let the good doctor finish.

"That's where it's coming from. You see, when you load in so much extra white, waxy, globby [my word, not the Doc's], your body can't get rid of it. You are putting in more than your body can carry out, so it builds up."

That's it!!
That's all!!
Other than the rare exception to the rule, the thing that's killing us is coming from our diet!! Just like fat!! We are killing ourselves??
Not sure what's so difficult to understand about that. In all the information that's out there, every article, news report, and expert opinion, why didn't you and I know that one simple fact? Cholesterol comes from animals, and we, the animals that we are, produce all that we need, and if we take in tons extra, we will have excess cholesterol, which causes all kinds of big, big problems.
You get that. If you take in more than your body can get rid of, then you've got a buildup. All I had to do was take off my clothes and look in the mirror at 260 to understand the buildup concept. Buildup city is what I was looking at every day. I guess that's what it would be like to look inside someone who has a high cholesterol count—lots of white, globby, gobby stuff floating around looking for a place to stick. Building up, clogging, closing in slowly, until bammo—no hole open for the blood to flow through. No blood, no life.
That's what I was thinking about on the plane with the meal that the Average Joe was eating. Nothing against plane food, although it's foul; nothing against beef, butter, or creamy dressing—just making the fat connection, that's all. Don't you see? You do have control. One very important thing you

can do if high cholesterol is your problem or if you don't want the problem of high cholesterol is stop eating tons and tons of extra cholesterol.

Who ever said we couldn't do anything about our health? When did we give up believing that we had something to do with how we look and feel?

If you're not sure whether you have high, low, or healthy cholesterol levels, just go grocery shopping, have a finger prick, and find out. Just look for the people in the white coats with the clean white tables, the slides of glass, and the little needles; they are all over the place these days.

Do you want to know where cholesterol comes from? It comes from animals. If you eat too much of it, it may build up. You know you shouldn't have too much of this stuff floating around. You live in the 90's; you're happening. Everyone knows it. But other than that, if you're anything like me, you probably don't know much more about this much-talked-about subject than that.

You'd think that after all the research and time spent on cholesterol in the last ten years the standard cholesterol counts would be pretty much hammered down. Healthy, unhealthy? Decided? Well, it's not. No chance when you get these scientists involved. There is big, big controversy here. If there is still any question about why the American public is so damn confused about all this stuff, let's just take a moment to explain to the AMA that when the "leaders" can't get it right, the troops are usually confused.

Here are both sides of the argument.

When you have your cholesterol checked, you are looking for the number of milligrams of cholesterol per deciliter of blood. It doesn't matter if you don't have a clue what a milligram or a deciliter is—I don't. Just know that what you are looking at is percentages. How much cholesterol is in a certain amount of blood. Period. Just like the fat percentages—how much fat is in

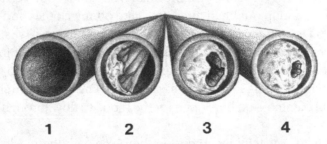

1   **2**   **3**   **4**

Your artery starts out like tube one, clean as a baby's bottom. When you eat saturated fat and cholesterol, and it starts to build up, it begins to look like the second tube. When you're looking at tubes three and four, you're looking at constricted, clogged . . . as in no blood getting through to your heart. Scary, scary, scary.

this much food. That's all you have to understand about how they decide what's normal or abnormal.

But in order to understand why there is so much confusion, you have to look at a whole different set of problems. It's beyond percentages when it comes to the experts fighting about what you and I should consider healthy or unhealthy.

Let's check out the difference in numbers, and you'll see what I'm talking about.

Normal range for the cholesterol count of the Average American was 210 just a few short years ago. But all that's changed, because those normal levels were maintaining the normal reality of heart attacks in our society. With these "healthy" range numbers we were averaging 1.5 million heart attacks a year, to be precise. Normal? Anything normal about that? So they changed it. The American Medical Association recently lowered the normal level. Now the numbers are:

Average American under thirty is 180 mg/dl.
Over thirty, 200 mg/dl.

Let's talk about what the numbers mean. The lower the number, the lower the risk of heart attack. Chart after chart, study after study shows that. They scream at us:

LOWER THE NUMBERS, LOWER THE RISK.

LOWER BLOOD CHOLESTEROL COUNT, LOWER HEART DISEASE RISK.

LOWER SATURATED FAT AND CHOLESTEROL, LOWER HEART DISEASE, STROKE, AND ON AND ON AND ON AND ON.

Remember the big losers in the heart-disease contest? Japan. And first and second place winners—Finland and the United States? That's what we're talking here—numbers in a killer game.

If it's true that the lower the number, the lower the risk—and it is—would it make sense to go low, low, low, thereby lowering, lowering, lowering the risk?

Why 210?
Is that the lowest you can go?
A safe number?
The best it can get?

How did the "people's health protectors" come up with that as a "safe" number?

What's totally safe?

What's out of the woods?

Is there a number that guarantees no risk of heart disease at all, unless your body totally whacks out and for some reasons starts producing tons of cholesterol?

Has anyone found such a number, and if so, what is it?

How far does Susan Powter, Food P.I., have to go to get this mysterious number?

Break into a lab in the middle of the night?

Hold a rally demanding the big safe number?

Hunger strike?

What will it take to get this number that could save lives?

I asked our friend Dr. John McDougall, knowing full well that we were discussing top-secret information that may take months to obtain.

"Sure there's a number that is a virtual immunity from heart disease. Every study done shows it. The AMA is very, very aware of it—it's a total cholesterol level of 150. Not difficult to get at any age, just don't eat cholesterol, cut way, way back on saturated fats, exercise, and except for a very rare case here and there, it'll happen."

VIRTUAL IMMUNITY FROM HEART DISEASE!!

IT'LL HAPPEN IF YOU DON'T EAT CHOLESTEROL AND CUT WAY, WAY BACK ON SATURATED FAT!! AND WE'VE NEVER HEARD THIS.

CALL THE GUYS WHO HAND OUT THE NOBEL PRIZES, THE INTERNATIONAL AWARDS, THE BASEBALL HALL OF FAME, ANYBODY WHO HANDS OUT A DAMN MEDAL AND TELL THEM WE'VE FOUND THE ANSWER. TELL EVERYONE YOU LOVE WHO'S DEALING WITH HIGH CHOLESTEROL, HEART DISEASE, STROKE, ANYTHING CONNECTED TO THESE HORRIBLE PROBLEMS THAT THERE IS AN ANSWER.

Run out and get everything that

Covert Bailey
Jane Brody
Annemarie Colbin
William Dufty
Francis Moore Lappe
Jim Mason and Peter Singer
John McDougall, M.D.
Earl Mindell
Gary Null
Dean Ornish, M.D.
Joseph C. Piscatella
Jeremy Rifkin
John Robbins
David Steinman
Andrew Weil

have ever written and give a copy to your doctor. Surely he/she will be glad to know there is something we can all do to help ourselves so that we do not die of heart disease. Right here in this food book, with the help of a few real experts in the field of heart disease and prevention, you and I have figured it out. Get ready for the awards ceremony? Ladies, pick your outfits and get your speeches written. What do you think? What should we do about accepting this thing? Not show up at the ceremony? Be cool like Al Pacino? Or just run up on the stage and give a forty-five-minute acceptance speech starting with our first-grade teacher and ending with all our relatives? The call's gotta be coming, because this is the answer, and it's so simple and easily understood! Wow, well done. Give credit where credit is due.

All I've ever heard—and I've been talking to a lot of people in the last few years about fat, health, heart disease, cholesterol—was the old 200–210 normal range. What's going on here? Is every heart patient in this country aware of this information? Are all those being treated for heart disease changing their diets dramatically? Solving the problem? Getting healthy?

My drama, my Private Dick excitement went right out the window—good news for sure—but it didn't take too much to find out about it. I was all ready to step out and investigate, and all I had to do was ask a question.

McDougall says it, but who else says what?

The AMA and the National Cholesterol Education Project say 200 mg/dl.

Dean Ornish says 150 mg/dl. (There it is again, that virtual immunity from heart disease number.)

After hearing this I called my father, because in 1987–88, at fifty-five years of age, my father had a cholesterol level of 210. He wasn't feeling great and was having prostate problems. Very common for men his age. To be expected, the doctor said. It's a given: After a certain age most people can expect these little life interferences, cancer, heart disease, not feeling too well.

So he went for a checkup. Right thing to do, but like his daughter, he didn't listen. (Where do you think I got this from?) The doctor's diagnosis was: Cholesterol count normal at 210. That was way back in the days when 210 was the standard; now with the "healthy" standard of 200, what's the difference?? Prostate should be looked at every couple of months. (My father was never going back for that one because he didn't like the examination, if you know what I mean.)

There was nothing he could do but hope the prostate didn't get any worse. No change in diet. No life-style changes. Nothing he could do except get examined once in a while—and what? Hope for the best? Live with not feeling very well? Pray that his prostate held up?

Thank God, instead of just accepting that rot, he started reading everything he could get his hands on about prostate, cholesterol, energy, etc. I'm proud to say that after watching what his grandson had gone through (which you still don't know about, but you will before the end of this book, I promise) he was open to hearing and trying some things that he may not have tried years before. (My son saved his life. Too dramatic? What do you think?)

So my dad changed the way he ate in a big way. He stopped eating cholesterol. Cut back on animal products. This is a man who grew up eating big, big beef. Australia and beef—what, are you kidding? Bacon, eggs, steak, whatever—he ate it. But with a cholesterol level of 210, he started not eating it. He started exercising and went back to the doctor's office for a checkup. His cholesterol count had dropped from 210 to 140. Remember the age we're talking here, fifty-five.

His doctor didn't believe the test and had him take it again. He thought there was something wrong with his machine. (You'll probably read in the *Globe* next week that my brother Mark says his father never had a cholesterol count of 210.)

START HERE START NOW

Some glazed doughnuts have almost thirteen grams of fat.

Substitute bagels with jam, honey, or some fat-free cream cheese,

if you like, for zero fat grams.

All we have to do is work toward making the transition to what we are eating, change a few things, get off the couch, and not worry ever again about heart disease or a high cholesterol count.

Now, you tell me what's so complicated. Did you have to have a degree to figure all this stuff out? I don't think so. And it boils down to connecting. Connecting that fat makes you fat. You get that? You see, I thought all my life that it was calories that made me fat. That's why I dieted forever. Didn't you think looking fabulous was about eating less? Sure, you and I both, and we were both wrong. All right, now you know that some changes need to be made.

- Saturated fat. Maybe you cut down a little and prevent heart disease because now you know the connection.

- Cholesterol. Simple, simple, simple. Animals, that's where it comes from. Your brilliant, wonderful body makes what it needs, and if you're really serious about cutting down on cholesterol, all you have to do is to connect it with saturated fat and for the rest of your life, cut way, way back on fat and don't eat cholesterol.

- Oh, the hydrogenation. Snack foods—full of it. You gotta read the labels. Choose the brands that don't include hydrogenated oil so you can live longer than the food.

Fat is done.

The food I was eating (past tense now) was loaded in FAT! . . . All my cravings can be satisfied in a low-fat way!

—*Jeanette, Wellington, Utah*

So what does it take to get lean, strong, and healthy? Looking at the facts and learning how to think differently. Let's not pretend for a second that there isn't comfort in what we all grew up with: the rewards, the punishments, the excuses. You want to know how far I took my excuses? How about using my ex-husband and the horrible things he did to me as an excuse for years? Been there.

The old gotta-have-a-degree to understand. Done that.

God forbid I made a decision and made a mistake. Lived in that fear.

And the kids! God forbid we make a nutritional decision about the kids.

And then there's the big line I hear over and over again: What if I fail again? As with all the other diets and food plans I tried before. What if I fail again??

Let me tell you something. This is about one thing. Going from dawning to doing. (Quote me on that, would you?) Has it dawned on you that fat makes you fat? Well, you gotta make some changes.

And how do you do that? How are you supposed to apply this to your life? Your husband, the kids, going out to eat, the parties, the restaurants, traveling, your life!!!

I'm telling you the truth when I say that once you understand this and then learn to apply it to your life, you will lose as much weight as you want to lose. You'll get the energy back that you've missed for years. You'll look and feel better than you ever have imagined you could. You'll get it, you'll use it, and you will love it.

● ●

Where's the Big Fat?   ¡"!

Oh, just before we move on, I want to give you this chart. I went to the grocery store and did the fat formula on a few things to give you an idea of fat contents. See you in transition. . . .

FULL OF FAT (80–100%)

Butter	100%	Coconut	85%	Bologna	81%
Salad Oils	100%	Cream, light	92%	Almonds	81%
Black Olives	97%	Avocado	88%	Frankfurters	80%
Cream Cheese	90%	Pork Sausage	83%	Spareribs	80%
Walnuts	87%	Sesame Seeds	84%	Egg Yolks	80%

VERY BIG FAT (60–79%)

Half and Half	77%	Brick Cheese	72%	Bacon	78%
Duck (w/skin)	76%	Sunflower Seeds	79%	Goose Meat	
Salami	76%	Pumpkin Seeds	77%	(w/skin)	65%
Peanuts	76%	Porterhouse Steak	63%	Ground Beef	67%
T-bone Steak	64%	Cashews	75%	Ice Cream (16%)	64%
Liverwurst	75%	Ham	61%	Tuna (oil packed)	63%
Cheddar Cheese	74%	Swiss Cheese	66%	Eggs	64%
Blue Cheese	73%	Ricotta Cheese	66%	Rib Roast	75%

BIG FAT (40–59%)

Dk Chicken		Goat's milk	54%	Caviar, sturgeon	52%
(roasted w/skin)	56%	Round Steak	41%	Sardines,	
Mozzarella		Rump Roast	52%	Atlantic	49%
(part skim)	55%	Soybeans	47%	Stewing Beef	47%

BIG FAT (40–59%) (continued)

Salmon, Sockeye		Whole Milk	49%	Lean Ground Beef	58%
(red)	49%	Ice Cream (Reg)	48%	Leg of Lamb	54%
Yogurt (reg)	49%	Tuna White (in oil)	47%		

MEDIUM FAT (20–39%)

Cottage Cheese	39%	Lt. Chicken		Ice Milk	29%
Cherry Pie	39%	(roasted w/skin)	35%	Bean Burrito	28%
2% Milk	35%	Low-Fat Yogurt	24%	Bass (freshwater)	30%

LOW FAT (0–19%)

Oatmeal	16%	Cabbage	18%	Green Peas	16%
Garbanzo Beans	14%	Cauliflower	7%	Apricots	7%
Kale	13%	Eggplant	7%	Bulgur	4%
White Tuna in		Asparagus	12%	Artichoke	3%
Water	13%	Celery	6%	Barley	7%
Lettuce	18%	Cucumber	11%	Cantaloupe	6%
Strawberries	4%	Turnips	6%	Pineapple	8%
Grapes	3%	Green Beans	6%	Rye, light	2%
Turnip Greens	11%	Spaghetti	5%	Wild rice	16%
Chestnuts	10%	Whole Wheat	5%	Grapefruit	2%
Mushrooms	8%	Brown Rice	5%	Peaches	2%
Apples	4%	Pears	5%	Papaya	3%
Blueberries	7%	Cherries	13%	Beets	2%
Lemon	11%	Oranges	4%	Prunes	1%
Cabbage	11%	Bananas	4%	Potatoes	1%
Rye, dark	7%	Carrots	4%	Chives	0%

SANDWICHES

Reuben	56%	Egg Salad	40%	Turkey Breast	
BLT (w/Mayo)	50%	Cream Cheese and		(w/mustard)	16%
Tuna Salad	45%	Jelly	39%		
Chicken (w/Mayo)	42%	PB and J	36%		

DESSERTS

Cheese Cake	53%	German Choc		Macaroon	26%
Choc. Chip	48%	(w/frosting)	41%	Sno Ball	24%
Brownie	46%	Pecan Pie	40%	Twinkie	23%
Ding Dong	46%	Choc Cream Pie	38%	Animal Cookie	22%
Chocolate Eclair	43%	Tapioca	33%	Fig Bar	14%
Gingersnap	42%	Oatmeal Raisin	32%	Gingerbread	10%
Pound Cake	42%	Vanilla Wafer	31%	Angel Food Cake	0%

FAVORITE FOODS

Deviled Egg	75%	Meat Loaf		Beef/Cheese	
Egg Roll	65%	(w/reg gr beef)	55%	Lasagna	45%
Onion Rings	65%	Cheese Pizza	49%	Macaroni and	
Eggplant Parmesan	58%	Chicken Pot Pie	48%	Cheese	43%
Beef Taco	56%	Hamburger Helper	45%		

• •

CHAPTER 2
MAKING THE TRANSITION

What you've got in your hands is no ordinary food book. Recipes, sure. What would a food book be without recipes? You will get recipes out the yin-yang at the end of each section of this book. What you've got is a Chinese menu of everything you ever wanted to know about food. Stage one, stage two, and stage three—three levels for three different reasons.

Would you like to learn everything I learned to lose 133 pounds and keep it off while eating more than you've ever eaten in your life? What do you think of that?

How about your understanding fully what the husband, the kids, the boyfriend, the whoever can eat, eat, eat without ever needing to know it's low fat and healthy?

You will be able to tell yourself and your neighbor what to eat, or I'll give you Simon & Schuster's number—and you can write a book, I'll buy it, I'll read it, and we'll talk!

How about never being fooled again by some get-thin-quick rip-off plan, because you're smarter than the twelve-year-old counselor who's advising you??

Yeah, yeah, yeah, that's how this book has been laid out. There is no beginning, middle, or end. It's three levels.

LEVEL ONE

FAT, you've been there. You've gotten to know it:

Saturated

Unsaturated

Hydrogenated

You know the difference. You know which one has to do with your heart and which one ends up on your thighs.

Living with too much of it and trying to live without it—yeah, yeah, yeah. But what about cooking, shopping, the kids, the husband, social situations, restaurants? Portion control, assessment, the why and how we eat, your body? Help is here.

Easy, convenient, understandable ways to make the change, cut back on your daily fat intake, and not have you or the family notice the change . . . except that special change, the one when people who haven't seen you for a while look at you and scream:

YOU'VE LOST SO MUCH WEIGHT—WHAT HAVE YOU BEEN DOING? YOU LOOK FABULOUS!

Now, any low-fat snob reading this and thinking, "Huh, level one is just for beginners only," listen up.

You see, you may take six things from level one—or only two if you're an advanced low-fat snob—three or four from level two, and a couple from level three, depending on where you are and what you want from the big food connection in your life.

LEVEL TWO

What is it?

Getting to know your preservatives. . . .

Colorings

Additives

Hormones

Do these things have anything to do with your health, your energy level, or the way you're looking?

Spices, sauces, herbs.

A little more whole, nutritious, earthy kind of stuff. In stage two we're just stepping deeper into food. You know with me that the kids, husbands, friends, family, and you are always considered at each stage (notice I'm trying out different titles as we go—I don't like this level thing; sounds kind of self-righteous to me).

LEVEL THREE

Then when you are as low fat as they come and pesticide aware as hell, here comes *level three:*

Sex and food, connected? Sure.

Addicted? Food have anything to do with it?

You'll need more, you'll want more, you'll get more, more, more options. The finer details, the fun facts about food.

Holistic treatments using foods—effective or a waste of time and money?

Seaweed—how the hell could anyone possibly eat it, and why would they?

The answers to the questions, clearing up the confusion, the opinions are all going to be presented in the three different fat-to-fit, unhealthy-to-healthy, clogged-to-clear sections of this food book.

I've been saying for years this is really simple. I'm a housewife who figured it out, and if I could, you guys are free and clear. Fitness, wellness, lean, and healthy are for everyone. Let's talk food and do it so that it works for you without walking around confused as hell, without going back to school and getting your degree in nutrition, and without feeling hopeless, out of control, and as if there is no answer in sight. It's more than in sight—it's here, it's now, and as for the other stuff, IT'S OVER.

Fine, well done, Susan. Makes a lot of sense—but what do I do? Do I just keep eating my traditional meals, get my protein from red meat, eat my butter-and-cream sauce, and stay deaf, blind, and dumb to heart disease, cancer, obesity, degenerative disease of all kinds? Look and feel horrible, learn to accept as normal a low quality of life, and forget about ever trying to sort it all out?? Understandable way to think, because that's how most of us have been living. But no, you can't do that anymore.

You don't look well, and you feel horrible. You haven't felt well in a long time. Your friends and family are dealing with or are dropping like flies from heart disease, cancer, diabetes, all kinds of things, and you haven't had any strength left past five in the afternoon in years.

You have to change something.

It's time for a transition, and this transition is going to be slow and easy.

REASON FOR CHANGE

Thinking about making a change because:

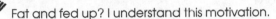

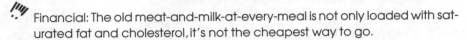

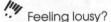

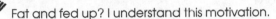 Financial: The old meat-and-milk-at-every-meal is not only loaded with saturated fat and cholesterol, it's not the cheapest way to go.

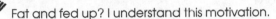 Health: After that second bypass, you may be fed up with the whole kit-and-caboodle (talk about saving some money—saving the whole country some money. Bring down those health care costs by not needing them—a thought and a political statement in one, pardon me).

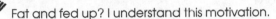 Feeling lousy?

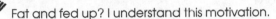 Taking twenty different medications just to get through the day?

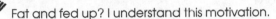 Never thought 50 would feel like 150?

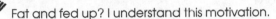 Sick of being sick and tired? (I have stolen someone's quote, used it twice already in this book, but it's a good one, so why not?)

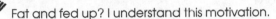 Fat and fed up? I understand this motivation.

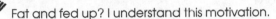 Just want to look good? (There it is, my reason for dropping the 133.)

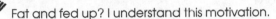 Want to be cool? Nothing wrong with that. It's very 90's to know what couscous is. (It's also very 90's to know every song that Donna Summer put out in the 70's, but hopefully that will pass soon—not Donna, love her, but disco.)

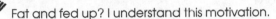 Want to understand what's going on around you? The changes you're reading about in every magazine you pick up? What's good for you, what's bad for you, what you can live without, and how? Fair enough is what I have to say about that—O.K., O.K., twist my arm, I'll write a food book, and we'll talk.

> I took the information I got from you and I began to make very small changes. . . . I dropped the mayo and the butter. . . .
>
> —*Jane, Athens, Alabama*

Changing the way you eat is a lot easier today than it was fifteen years ago. You've got the advantage of being socially acceptable now.

Let's go back in time ten, fifteen years, not so long ago, to Thanksgiving dinner sometime in the 70's (anywhere near the 70's is not too much to bear, even for a short travel back). You are in your Nehru collar, disco glitter, or whatever your preference was. (I was a mixture of both. The Nehru collar made me feel as if I were still a part of something important, and the disco worked well for the evenings of chasing boys, feeling cute and sexy, and dancing the night away. Consider me a 70's chameleon, but please don't ever refer to me publicly as that.)

It's you and the family in all your family's glory. Probably, especially in the 70's, totally dysfunctional—from the fashions to the families, the 70's were just one big dysfunction, don't you think?

Thanksgiving, U.S.A., Norman Rockwell city.

This year it's your turn to make the Thanksgiving dinner for the whole family. You've worked for hours in the kitchen preparing the feast. It's time to serve it to the hungry aunt, uncle, cousin, father, mother, brother, and sister who are sitting at the table, waiting to spend the next three hours eating and giving thanks. Now imagine fifteen years ago if you had come out of the kitchen with:

White meat turkey breast, broiled without the skin.

Potatoes, no butter, stuffed with vegetables, no cheese—dairy free.

Seven-grain bread.

Organic sweet potato pie with no oil, butter, or added fat.

A pasta dish or two thrown in.

Some spring water and fruit juice for beverages all around.

What do you think? Received well, this dinner of yours? Then go a couple of steps further and imagine that your guests:

Ate on recycled china.

Wiped their mouths with unbleached, recycled napkins.

Chewed each bite one hundred times.

Began their meal with a digestive meditation session and when finished . . .

Up, up, up for the after-dinner exercise session.

Remember, we've gone back only fifteen years. Not so long ago. This is not such a big stretch of the imagination we're talking about here. You and I both know that if you'd asked anybody over and suggested anything close to that fifteen years ago, you would have been:

A. Sent to the social leper colony.

B. Considered a 60's reject in a big way.

C. Chased out of town—depending on what part of the country you were in.

D. Found yourself without friends or relatives for the rest of your life, or at least until the 90's, some twenty years later—a long time to go without social contact.

If it was truly Norman Rockwell who laid out what it was supposed to be like, then I have to say that Norman lied. Probably not intentionally, but he lied just the same.

Not only did the perfect family not exist (why does every one of us understand the word dysfunctional?), but that perfect meal wasn't quite what it seemed to be, either. That holiday celebration meal, the meat-and-potatoes food we were all being fed, was killing us. We know that twenty years later. You've just checked out all the charts that have so clearly screamed the saturated-fat-and-cholesterol connection at us. You are not even halfway through section one but you're fully aware of the connection, which you weren't fifteen years ago, and neither was your mother.

See, we all grew up with the wrong info. Creating the bad habits. Making those strong emotional connections to all the wrong foods. Who knew that eating beef every night wasn't the luxury we thought it was? How were we supposed to know that the "diet" plate—burger (without the bun, of course), cottage cheese, and salad—wasn't such a diet plate? Do you think there wasn't a mom in this country who didn't think she was doing the best for her kids by giving them that super-high-protein diet? You think we had any clue what the price of that little pat of butter was?

You don't have to look back too far to see how much has changed when it comes to what we are eating, the way we are eating it, and the earth it's connected to. Paper, plastic—one of them connected to the forest somewhere in a rainy region, the other not!!

How wrong so many of the experts were about what we were putting into our mouths. Boy, did they confuse the hell out of all of us.

They all lied. They said it wouldn't die and it did. Disco died, thank God. The 60's—yep, the peace thing—died. I found out that the whole peace, love, and Woodstock concept wasn't all it was cracked up to be.

Sure, you go for years without caring about society, but how long can you live without makeup, a nice hotel, and a little cash in your pocket? Me? Not long!!

Create your own community? Eventually we've all gotta come back to the society that is and make it work. But the peace, love, and Woodstock 60's, the 70's, and our fifteen-year travel-back-in-time comparison all have something in common with the 90's, where you and I are right now in our food confusion.

Think about it.

Within fifteen short years we've been asked by those who set the standards to jump from a Norman Rockwell canvas, swing around, and take a walk through the 60's—this earth-consciousness stuff that's going on in the 90's is very 60's Woodstocky. Can't you see it? Throw in some low-fat eating aware- ness, disease prevention, herbal healing, environmental responsibility, and becoming fully aware of the rain forest and the natives living there. You've all but got to be a biochemist in the field of supplementation these days—an- tioxidant, schmoxident. And remember, the world is our family.

Thanksgiving, the all-American life-style, Barbie and Ken—it's all changed. Just in case anyone cares, if whoever created those abominations were to cre- ate a 90's version, think about what it would be. Babs would be a vegan. Ken would probably be a sushi chef. Ken behind a bunch of raw fish could be in- teresting, but we'll never know what he'd do with raw tuna, because nobody cares anymore. Babs and Ken, your standard was never attainable for any one of us. May they rest in peace.

This high-fat-to-low-fat, fewer-chemicals-and-preservatives, more socially aware, environmentally conscious change can be made. You can change your life-style without making the whole family walk out on you and your herbal remedies. Believe me, you can live in this world, in your community, in any part of this country, and function—without starting your own society, wearing funky clothing, or putting on the earth shoe version of Dr. Scholl's sandals (although I've just read that they are back in all their chunky glory).

So live in any level of denial that you want, but work toward making some changes so you can solve some of the problems that you don't want to live with anymore.

THOUGHT

When you hit the portion-control chart in this section, do it.

Try some stage two suggestions and feel free to run from whatever you want, whenever you want. It's called working within your life-style, your tastes, your physical considerations, and getting to your goal.

Experiment once a week with something different. Play with some dif- ferent decisions about what you're putting into your body and see how it feels (or tastes) to you.

You can even do it wearing tons of makeup while talking on your cel- lular phone, running your business, and searching for quality time. Take it from me, because that's exactly what I'm doing. You do it, your body gets leaner, you feel better, your life-style changes, and your choices change.

That's how you use this book.

> My husband said, "You know what? We've finally done it. We changed our eating habits for life."
>
> —*Jo, Colorado Springs, Colorado*

Thirty-six years later I've figured out that transition is a constant unless you're ten feet under. The process of change goes on every day in our lives, and as far as I'm concerned, as long as I'm moving forward, it doesn't matter what I have to go through to get there. Listen to me. You'd think by now I understood the old saying, Be careful what you ask for, because you just may get it.

Food and change, transition and Nic. Hand in hand. When I think about it, the ex-husband and food have been two of the biggest calls to action, movers and shakers, in my life.

Food. . . . the big connection started years ago, and never in my wildest dreams (and I've had some wild ones) did I think it would lead me to this: writing a book on food. Who's to know where your change/transition will lead you, so jump on board, hang on, and let's roll forward—my motto for life.

I figured when I was thinking about doing this book that you'd probably want to start with fat. I didn't start there when it came to the food connections in my life. It took me years and years to put this all together, and gaining 133 pounds was (this is hard to admit on the printed page) not the first thunderbolt I received to the head when it came to food and how it affected my life.

I went through hell and back, and through more food experiences than you can ever imagine. Of course you'll hear about every one of them before we're finished, but for now let me tell you that my food experiences go from my cervix (yeah, we're talking female reproductive system) to my son's health. But above and beyond my personal stories, I wanted to start where I thought you'd want to start. My cervix wouldn't be the place.

Getting fat was my finale. From figuring out that the sugary cereals weren't the best way to start the day to writing a book on food took sixteen years of reading, questioning, not believing what was out there, and getting struck by food lightning over and over again. (Amazing . . . it's not that I can't believe I'm thirty-six—I have no problem with the age thing; hell, I'll scream to the world that I'm thirty-six, because I'm having more fun now than I ever had in my life—it's just that it's a long time and it's hard to imagine that I've done anything for sixteen years. But I have, and it's the food thing!!)

What touched my soul and changed my life forever, branded the message into my brain like nothing else could? My health? Absolutely not!! My son's health? That certainly moved me forward, but in my life the 6.0 earthquake (not a funny description when you think about my reality—sitting at a table in Los Angeles typing this) was GETTING FAT.

Plain and simple. Gaining 133 pounds on better food than my Texas neighbors could ever think about eating. Hey, I knew about those preservatives, chemicals, and that nasty stuff in the meat they were eating. I was way ahead of the know-what-you-are-putting-into-your-mouth game. You see, my food connections from way, way back taught me a thing or two about all the info you're going to be reading about in section three. But do you think for a second that it made a difference in my life as I was hitting 150 pounds, 195, 210, 245, 260? Looky, looky what was happening to me. I was getting fatter by the second, and it never dawned on me that it had anything to do with what I was putting into my mouth. I swear. Other than the big diet connection, which happened every other Monday, taking food away and starving—the Monday morning diet commitment—I never thought about what I was putting into my mouth.

I knew it was too much.

I knew that food was the enemy.

I knew for sure that I had a control problem—I couldn't seem to stop eating and did all the wrong things—but I didn't think it was WHAT I was putting into my mouth, my body. And this is the same P.I. mind that's leading this investigation of ours. Are you feeling comfortable, secure, led by the best??

Haven't you convinced yourself that it's some deep emotional issue you're dealing with that's causing the old twenty, thirty, fifty, or whatever pounds to creep onto your body?

Don't you think it's genetic? Or how about the old "it's just that you've had a couple of kids" reason? But then you find yourself looking at your youngest, who's twenty-five, knowing that's not the reason anymore.

This is just a way for me to bare my soul, deal in honesty, and prove to all of you that if a simple shallow gal living in the suburbs of Texas who's already been hit over the head with the food-and-health connection can figure this out and make a smooth, easy transition, then this is going to be a breeze for you.

Losing weight, looking better, and getting into the dress size you want is a strong, strong motivation—and a very worthwhile one, I might add. I've admitted that on national TV, and it made me two things:

1. A raving lunatic that nobody would listen to, according to the aerobic industry. Hey, you guys, what do you think now?

2. Honest, according to the American women who have watched, listened, and agreed that that is a great motivation.

There isn't a woman reading this book who doesn't want to look and feel good, and that's all I wanted at 260 pounds. Heart, who cared? Energy to get through a day would have been nice, but cholesterol? All I cared about was whether that had anything to do with how fat I was. Do you think for a second that I worried about cholesterol sticking to anything other than my thighs? No, I didn't. Shallow! Frighteningly shallow, but who cares?

I started talking and found out that hundreds of thousands of women wanted the same thing and had no clue where to start. Yeah, transition is scary and it takes time, but that was not the problem. The truth is that the real problem for you, for me, for all of us was that we didn't know where to start.

Here I was, fat, feeling horrible, depressed, tired as hell all the time, ached and pained, and every day things were getting worse. And I wondered: What was causing this?

If it's transition you want, this is exactly where it started for me—in the questioning. Did you hear that? Let's repeat it together, because it's a real beginning: THE QUESTIONING.

Why do I look and feel this way?

After going over all the emotional reasons why I was looking and feeling 260 pounds worth of horrible . . .

> Life in the toilet
> He had a girlfriend
> I was lonely
> Sad
> Isolated
> Frightened

. . . I finally got to another question: What was I eating? You'd think at this point a lightning bolt would have gone off in my brain connecting everything that was happening to my body to what I'd been through during the last sixteen years (of course you still have no clue as to what the hell I'm talking about).

Not what happened at all.

I thought about my cervix. Thought about my son. Looked at myself in the mirror and went and ate more fat. Thought and thought and thought. How did I put on an extra 133 pounds?

Was it something that was causing an allergic reaction?

Maybe something that made my thyroid go ballistic?

An herb, a spice with the side effect of morbid obesity?

Had the FDA missed something? Should I investigate?

FAT? Naw, couldn't be.

Maybe a chemical in the air-conditioning ducts was causing my body to swell . . .

FAT?

A cleaner I was using? Yeah, that's it. Something strong. A chemical reaction of some kind. FAT?

Killer pollen in the air? You know, the kind that causes an extra one hundred pounds to attach to your body?

FAT?

How about if I wore one of those white surgical masks that the truly allergic wear when they go out? It might help.

Something, something . . . something was causing this obesity and exhaustion.

BIG BLANK SPACE

IN MY BRAIN

(AS SEEN ON THE PRINTED PAGE)

Something I'm eating?

Maybe, but what?

High calorie?

Take away food.

Another diet.

Then failure.

Eating everything in sight for weeks.

Then another diet.

Failure.

Bingeing.

Gorging on . . . FAT, FAT, FAT, FAT, FAT.

No lightning bolts. The answer came slowly and painfully.

FAT. That's what was making me fat.

Tired . . . somehow connected to the fat? I didn't understand anything about that then, but fat making me/you fat—I was getting it.

Fat.

> I grew up eating butter, even on cereal, red meat, all the other bad, scary midwestern foods. My inherited life-style . . . I rarely eat meat anymore. . . . I feel better, healthier than I've felt in a long time.
>
> —*Lee, Everett, Washington*

Once I understood that fat was the problem and that the fat was coming from the end of my fork, I started toward one of the biggest transitions of my life.

I read everything I could get my hands on, and this is where the whole thing started, because the more I read, the more contradictions I found:

Non-fat.
Not true.

98 percent fat free.
Really 68 percent fat.

Butter is better than margarine.
Don't touch margarine.

Olive oil is good for you.
All oil is 100 percent fat.

Whole milk.
Skimmed.
Or 2 percent.
Each one is the best for you.

Unless it's organic, don't touch it.
Pesticides don't hurt you at all.

Beef, the best and only complete protein, iron, and strength source available.
Beans, better than beef.

Fiber cures cancer.

Fiber makes your stomach extend, and you look fat—stay away
from it.

Live without vitamins—you can't.

The biggest ripoff around—all you do is wee them all out.

Save the earth, it's dying fast.

Earth-save hysteria is created by the environmentalists who have nothing better to do. There's plenty of land left.

Saturated fat kills.

Drink milk for strong bones.

Contradictions about food everywhere you and I look.

Whoever is handing out all the advice needs us, the women of America,
badly. Someone has to be at these meetings translating this information from
the word *go* so that we don't have to go through the process years later with
a billion confused and misinformed people.

All right, ladies, it's time for us to unconfuse what's being taught in the
schools, what's being blasted all over TV, what's coming out of our doctor's
mouth.

Assistant to the big guys? Interpreter for the people? We're in. We have to
do it. You guys have made it very clear what's confusing you. I know what
confused the heck out of me. We may have to wait to take on the schools and
the American Medical Association, but if it's food we need to sort out, and
we do, it ain't so difficult—it can be done. The marriage, the child-raising I'm
still working on, but the food—that's done.

It's easy to make the change, and there are a million reasons to do it. You're
clued in to some things that are necessary for good health and looking great.
A little less:

Saturated fat

Cholesterol

And of course the big one (pardon that one): fat. Less fat in your daily intake.
Less fat in your life. Less fat on your thighs. Less of the stuff that makes you
Fat. FAT.

If you're a beef jerky kind of guy (stated generically—you know that by now) or the organic veggie sandwich kind of guy, transition is transition, and although it will take time, patience, a desire to change, on and on and on, the biggest transition—one that will bring you more results than you can ever imagine and one that is connected with food like no other—is where we are going to begin. And it doesn't take time, patience, or anything else, only the right information. It is FAT, FAT, FAT, FAT. All the other stuff you're going to be reading about, and there's lots of it, you decide what you want to do with it, how far you want to go. Your transition will take you as far as you want to go. That's your deal. But from talking about, breaking down, cutting back on, and learning more about fat—the thing that, when you take less of it into your body, your body will get leaner—you'll feel better than you have in years. Even with the smallest changes you make, your body will change. That, my friends, is where we are going to begin.

Transition from high fat to low fat, how's it done? There is no right or wrong way. Believe it or not, this was my big dawning. Remember, nobody was talking about this stuff when I was 260 pounds, and if they were, I didn't know about it. My dawning was about taking what I could understand, when I could understand it, and doing what I wanted to do whenever I wanted to do it.

(One moment, please. I think you can safely say that was one of the worst written sentences in the history of writing. What do you think? But the strange thing is that I know you understand what I'm talking about, and that's all I really care about. So onward.)

Nothing I did was based on loving myself enough.

No affirmations involved.

Just common sense.

Facts that I understood and could apply to my life.

You are about to step into the ABC's of changing forever. Changing your behavior without anything involved but facts. Fun. Don't you love it!! Can't wait to read on? Well, let's go.

CHAPTER 3
THE "HOW-TO" CHAPTER

The how-to of transition.

I want to emphasize here that your looking great really begins with your thinking differently. I know you're thinking about your stomach, your calves, your underarms right now and saying, "Susan, I get it, but give me something that I can do now that's gonna make me feel better."

I get it. I'm there. And I'm telling you it's about changing the way you think, and I'm about to tell you how.

The guide to making a change, the application for all your newfound knowledge, is going to start with Bob's cousin—Bob, my editor at Simon & Schuster, and his cousin Sachiko St. Jeor.

You see, when you're writing a book, everybody has a friend or relative who is an expert in the field that you're writing about, someone they are sure you ought to talk to, to get the information that's going to make all the difference. This is the kind of thing I avoid like the plague, because nothing is worse than having to tell someone that his or her friend or relative is an idiot and that there is no way on earth you'd use anything he or she had to say in your book.

So you can imagine what went through my mind when Bob called and said he had a relative—distant, but a relative all the same, a cousin—who was a nutritionist, and he thought I might be interested in talking with her about my food book. I love Bob, and we've gotten along famously through the writing of two books, but I gotta tell you, I was worried. My trust in Bob's instincts waned for a moment.

So I had a plan. I'd call his relative, do the interview—you know, throw your editor a bone, tell him his cousin is a genius—and not use any of the information.

I am, after all, the author.

I could say it didn't fit into my text.

The motivation wasn't there.

Having writer's block?

I had a million excuses lined up and ready to go before I even picked up the phone to call Sachiko St. Jeor (check out the name; pretty, isn't it?).

I am writing this chapter right after finishing my interview with Sachiko, even though I'm as tired as hell and it's interfering with making dinner for my family, because I was so inspired, informed, and motivated by this woman that I had to write now. Good call, my initial feeling about this working or not working, don't you think? Kind of like looking at those four boys from England who were named after a bug and saying, Naw, they'll never make it.

I almost threw Sachiko out the window, but I didn't, and I'm writing this all down before the phone receiver is even cold. First, a little more about Sachiko. She's a nutritionist at the University of Nevada. She teaches a program to doctors that is very unusual and very impressive: nutrition and healthy life-style. Sachiko says:

"What we eat has so much to do with how we feel and the state of health we are in. It's important that physicians understand more about food and learn to apply proper nutrition and life-style to their own lives. Many times the consumers ask the doctors questions, and the doctors don't know the answers. That's a problem. Medical students face many of the same problems that the American housewife faces when it comes to eating. They have very busy schedules, with no time to plan proper nutritious meals. Eating on the run, they find themselves making bad choices of foods, and they are suffering the consequences."

Don't you love this woman? She's smart and fair, and her comments made so much sense and were so understandable and applicable that I loved her instantly.

Sorry, Bob, I may like her more than I like you. You've got a very cool cousin.

Sachiko, my new best friend, isn't just any nutritionist, she's a behavioral nutritionist. That's one of the reasons I thought we'd clash a bit, because so many times in the past I've spoken with these "behavioral" people, and they ramble on and on about not loving ourselves enough to get strong and healthy. And whenever I've tried to bring up the practical questions or suggestions about getting low-fat, higher-quality food, some oxygen, and a little strength into our bodies while we are hating ourselves, they just don't get it. They fight tooth and nail for the need to use affirmations and spend years in therapy figuring out why we overeat, what pain we are covering up, whether we are loving too much or too little, and all the rest of the stuff they want us to heal or figure out before they think we can solve the problem of being overfat. It's hard to get these guys to stop and consider the benefits or advantages of eating, breathing, and moving.

According to the books on the shelf in every bookstore in the country, food is:

> A feminist issue.
>
> The solution to a healthy life.
>
> Absolutely the answer to whether you are tired or toxic.
>
> Definitely the key to the hyperactive child.
>
> Possibly the answer to all disease.
>
> Either your best friend or your worst enemy.

When you eat you are:

> Starving for attention, or
>
> Eating your heart out.

Ever eaten in your life? If so you are:

> A survivor of food addiction,
>
> On a deadly diet, or
>
> Deep down inside, dying to be thin.

Helllllllllp me!
Enough.
After reading a bazzillion books on food, I've decided that all of us are bloody lucky to be alive. I mean, with all the horrible food connections we have in our lives, it's amazing we've made it this far. Sure, obesity and dis-

ease have been proven to be connected with the foods we are eating. Yes, around every corner is help for some kind of eating disorder—thank God for that, and there are a million food books on the market. So what am I doing? Writing another one. It's high time just one more food book hit the shelves—don't you think?

You see, I'm not sure we'll ever really get to the bottom of why we eat. Who really knows why we do anything? The therapists have ideas, some very good ones at that, but with each new "jump out of the socially acceptable be-havioral closet" that we face as a society comes a new disorder, so I'm not sure we'll ever catch up.

Aren't you still on the mother-daughter connection? I am. Don't you still want to know if it's self-love or self-hatred that "forces" you to eat the cake at 3 A.M.? Never figured that out! Aren't you still wondering what childhood trauma set you off last night?

I thought a better way to approach this whole food mess was to try and understand food—as in what it is, why we need it, what it is that we need, and why we even bother with it at all. So I asked my son. Who better to ask than my nine-year-old son? The question was what is food. Here's what he said:

"Food is for eating so we can stay alive, and sometimes it tastes good, but not always, like when you have to eat things you don't want to eat."

BRILLIANT!

There it is. Food is for eating so we can stay alive. Well done and very true, but one moment, please.

Someone is making you eat things you don't like? Who? Not me, the right-to-free-choice parent. It must be the guy downstairs, your father (if you haven't heard about the upstairs, downstairs arrangement, you haven't heard anything yet), because forcing children to eat what they don't like, according to some authorities on this food-connection story, is where all the trouble begins. So we'll talk to daddy. But for now, it's why we eat, and my nine-year-old has summed it up brilliantly. Talk to a thirty-six-year-old who's been through hell and back, and you'll get a much more complicated answer. You see, it gets screwed up as we get older. How's that for Psychology 101?

That's not what I got from Sachiko. I got just what I wanted for you and me: a clue on how to make our transitions as easy as possible, how to get started—from an expert, a behavioral nutritionist expert. Tips that can help you jump-start your life-style change. Stage one transitional suggestions that you guys can really use. That's what I wanted. In your hands you have a road map paved in gold from this woman. One, two, three easy steps to begin your change.

"With three easy steps, which take very little effort, you can cut your daily fat intake by as much as 40 percent."

YIPPPPPPPPPEEEEEEEEEE—that's a big step for a lot of people, and our buddy, the behavioral nutritionist of all time, is right. Nobody's gonna scoff at a 40 percent drop in daily fat intake!! That's why I had to sit down and write about it immediately. I'd steal everything she said and call it my own if I weren't a responsible human being or the author of this book, or if this interview hadn't been suggested by my editor (you know, otherwise I could get away with it). But since I can't, I'll just 'fess up to thinking about stealing it, give Sachiko all the credit, and get on with the business of getting the info to you so you can begin to make the changes in your life that will make you leaner and feel better.

Welcome to stage one transitional change, now that you are clear about the fact that fat has gotta go, or at least be cut down to normal, healthy, and all that, and are ready and willing to watch your body shrink.

ASSESSMENT

"The best way to get started, the first thing we do here at the hospital, is to assess the diet of the person who wants to make changes. I would ask you to write down what you've eaten for a week, giving details of what type of foods, how much, when, what was going on while you were eating, who was there, how you were feeling."

The hair on the back of my neck—what little there is—stood up when the doc suggested this. Anyone who's ever read anything I've written or heard anything I've said on TV, in print, in seminars, on audio or video knows how I feel about the old diet-mentality technique of writing down everything you eat and analyzing it to death.

> Waste of time
> Diet mentality
> Bondage
> If you have time to write down everything you eat,
>   you need to get a life

Just a few examples of my public declarations against writing things down in the name of getting skinny. But after my chat with Sachiko, I see the light, a brighter, clearer light than I ever saw after chatting with some of the other, bonehead behavioral nutritionists in the past. (Sachiko is starting to take on a saintly tone. This, in the convent I was raised in, is not a good thing, so I'm toning down my love for Sachiko. I can't afford to do anything else to guarantee my ticket to hell. Just in case that makes no sense to any of you, let me explain: Declaring sainthood is something reserved for the boys in the Vatican, and they don't like anyone else doing it.)

But I gotta tell you that when Sachiko suggested writing everything we eat down, I had to know why. Why would anyone want to write anything down? What good could it possibly do? It is diet mentality, and diets don't work, so why bother? You know my transition was slow, but it was effective—and I never wrote anything down, I just started cutting back on the big one (pardon that pun): fat. Write down for what? was the question of the hour.

Sachiko quickly cleared up my confusion, and it all boiled down to (pardon the low-fat cooking reference): assessment.

"Writing down what you've eaten for a week is good for one simple reason. It gives you something to assess. To be able to look at what someone/you have been eating for the purpose of understanding, education, and planning helps make life-style changes easier. Having a look at what's going on, when and how much, gives you a good indication of things that need to be changed. Many times people have never stopped to think, never considered what they are doing or how it may be contributing to how they look or how they are feeling. Why you are eating. When you eat. What frequency. What's influencing you."

All right. Makes perfect sense to me. As long as there isn't the weighing, scaling, oppression-with-every-morsel-you-put-into-your-mouth diet mentality going on, what harm could it do? Maybe having a look or assessing can help. I was assessing the air-conditioning ducts, looking for allergies instead of checking what and how often I was eating.

Assessing the wrong things—it's a wonder I got this far, isn't it?

"A good example of assessing is if, after a week of documenting your information, you notice that every time Aunt Mimi comes over, you end up eating a couple of bags of chocolate chip cookies. That will show you a couple of things. There is a problem not only with the bags of cookies but also with Aunt Mimi's visiting."

So you bag (pardon the pun) the cookies and Aunt Mimi's visits once you understand that the two may be connected, is that it?

"Yes, I wouldn't have said it that way, but you're right."

I'm loving it so far, Sachiko, but if you're going to have a look at what's happening and why, then you have got to make it very clear to everyone reading this that it has to be done in honesty, and totally and absolutely free of guilt. That's really important, because if you write down, assess, figure out the Aunt Mimi connection, and then beat the hell out of yourself because you feel like an idiot and are mad at yourself for letting Aunt Mimi get to you, then you're not doing yourself any good. You'll be sitting in front of the fridge shoving food in for sure, and that's not what assessment is all about—right, Sachiko?

"This isn't about judgment, it's about awareness, understanding what you are doing. This is about you and only you. With honesty and no guilt, you can have a look, and you just might put some things together that you've never thought about. Things that will help you change your life-style."

Susan's and Suzi's Assessments

Trigger Event	Response	Suggestion
Mother-in-law calls from the bus station—surprise!	Run to market for food and cleaning supplies and eat four candy bars while driving home.	Pick up lots of gum, hard candy, and fat-free pretzels to stuff your pockets and tell your son that you'll increase his allowance big time if he doubles his trumpet practice at home.
Receive notice from bank: You are $600 overdrawn.	Sit at corner cafe to balance checkbook; two pieces of chocolate pie later, you see you are $850 overdrawn.	Return those unneeded satin pillowcases to the French Shop and cancel your weekend trip to the the self-empowerment seminar.
Dentist calls to tell you your son needs upper and lower braces.	Shove handfuls of Cheetos in your mouth while walking through the Yellow Pages looking for a second opinion.	Make a glass or cup of your favorite tea and have a low-fat muffin while you pick up the phone book.

Boss hands you a pink slip; the company is downsizing.	Facing future famine, you fatten up on a seven-course meal at your local diner.	Walk to the park and go swinging.
Kids are fed, bathed, prayed for, and in bed.	Head for the TV with a bowl of comfort: four scoops of ice cream with sprinkles.	Make a cup of hot tea to have with graham crackers and honey; forget the news and take a hot mineral bath.
Therapist tells you your inner child is hungry and sad.	You pick up four Happy Meals on the way home.	Fire your therapist, eat a couple of lollipops, and tell your inner child to take a very long nap.
Your dad sounds stern on the phone.	You hang up and polish off a jar of Jif with your fingers.	Call your local nursing home and make reservations for your father.
Announcement comes for upcoming high school reunion.	Wash down a bag of Oreos with three Slim•Fast shakes.	Call your friend with the coolest wardrobe and tell her you're on your way over.
Doing family dishes, you think of all the starving children.	You eat all the loftovers.	Make a mental note to call your local soup kitchen and volunteer the family for next week.
Your preschooler bit three of his classmates today.	Contemplate course of action over two Snowballs and a Ding-Dong.	Scan your child's immunization records to see if he's up to date on his rabies shots; or go to your nearest pet store and buy a muzzle.

• •

That's what you get when you ask a mom of three children, an out-of-the-house working mom, and a very good friend of mine—Suzi Kressler—to jot down a few trigger reactions. Funny? And true, true, true.

/␣␣ Have you ever thought about what you are eating?

/␣␣ How about when?

/␣␣ Frequency?

/Ⱳ With whom?

/Ⱳ How many times a day, and what ticks it off?

If you do—or should I say, when you do—there you are, one step ahead of the game and ten steps ahead of where I was when I decided to change my life.

Assessment. It makes sense.

BALANCE

Dealing with the problem. Understanding and seeing the connections, frequency, etc., are important and will shed some light on a lot of things, but the bottom line once you have a look is that you are probably going to see what I saw and what Sachiko sees all the time.

"The most common thing we see is the high-fat, low-fiber, lots-of-excess-calories-a-day diet. That's the problem most of us are facing in our eating."

Gotta spend a moment on the "excess-calories-a-day" statement. I must make it really clear here so we don't confuse the "increase your daily caloric intake" subject that I've spent three years trying to clear up—all but establishing it in the national media—with what Sachiko just said. When our expert on behavior and nutrition talks about lots of calories, guess which calories she's referring to? The fattest calories: fat.

● ● ● ● ● ● ● ● ● ● ● ● ● ● ● ●

All Calories Aren't Equal

One gram of carbohydrates = 4 calories.
One gram of protein = 4 calories.
One gram of fat = 9 calories.

● ● ● ● ● ● ● ● ● ● ● ● ● ● ● ●

If it's excessive calories a day that are causing the problem, and it is, we are talking excess fat calories. The fattest, the biggest, the killingest, the thigh-wideningest—fat.

You know that because you have read the fat chapter. We're there when it comes to knowing that we are eating too much fat.

Please, please, please don't get locked into the calorie thinking, the dieting. Don't close the book and go sign up at your local diet center, 'cause that's not what we're talking about—right, Sachiko?

"Yes, that's true. Dieting doesn't work. It's the fat calories that we are talking about."

(I had to clear it up. I needed you guys to hear it from our expert so you'd know no dieting, ever again.)

About this food and fat thing, Sachiko believes:

"There is no good or bad food."

Good or bad food is not the issue. It's much more about the overloading of the high-fat, low-fiber, high-fat-calorie foods that's creating one of the problems that many of us are facing: obesity. Overfat. Unfit. We are not getting the most for our money with our daily eating, not getting enough of the "foods that give us more":

"Too much of one thing is the problem. The imbalance that is created by our daily food choices. Imbalance when it comes to fat in our diet."

That's the real problem and apparently one you'll see clearly once you've assessed what it is you are eating, how much, and how often.

Well, if it's about balance, let's talk balance. This is not so far-fetched. It's not as if we are running to holistic medicine to solve the problem. You don't have to go through disease and a sick baby like I did to get down to the nitty-gritty. This is good, it's making sense, and it's certainly something I can relate to.

Let's talk about what it took to put on an extra 133 pounds.

Loads of fat and not much else.

When I look back, assess if you will, what I see is an enormous imbalance. Check this out:

Breakfast

Muffiny things.
Cakey things.
Gooey, chewy things.
Egg sandwichy things (didn't know then that I could get the same thing without the yolk and not get fat; maybe you don't either, so I won't ruin the surprise).

continued

Lunch

The salads loaded with the dressings, mayo, butter!
Sandwiches loaded with the dressings, mayo, butter.
Tuna fish soaked in oil, then tossed with tons of mayo.
The cheeseburger with fries . . . and don't forget the milkshake.

Snacks

The late-afternoon vending machine candy bar.
The bag of potato chips.
The movie popcorn soaked in butter.

Dinner

Fried chicken with mashed potatoes whipped with milk and butter.
Good ole southern chicken fried steak.
Barbecued ribs with a baked potato . . . tons o' butter, sour cream with bacon, and
    cheese (oh, the things we do to an innocent baked potato!).

• •

Forget about exercise—that never happened. In my little assessment, you
can't even think of including high-quality foods. Weeks went by before I even
thought about eating anything that was not processed.

When was the last time you ate something that grew from a tree and that
was the way you were eating it—as in whole, as in not concentrated, as in
not mushed, smushed, and with a million preservatives added??? . . . It may
have been a while.

Grain instead of a piece of bread.

The apple instead of the juice.

The potato instead of the French fries.

For me we all know there was a food imbalance. Add to that the emotional
connection to what I was living in, feeling every day—forget about it. I was
a total disaster, a mess! It's easy to see, even having just a quick look years
later, that I was left with an imbalance, something I may not have thought
about until Sachiko brought it up, but an imbalance all the same.

Easy to see imbalance when it stares you in the face, isn't it? Assessing is a
breeze once you understand how to do it and why, and it's obviously an important step, but only one of the first—because if you think assessment
stands alone, you're wrong. Assessment leads you to something just as interesting, which our friendly expert calls "pattern of intake."

Official sounding? Sure it is. Why do you think she's an expert? How it applies to you and your change is all I wanted to know when I heard the phrase, and here it is.

PATTERN OF INTAKE

"During the process of assessing how much we are eating, we often get some insight into why, as in Aunt Mimi and the cookies. Our food intake pattern is established by many things: childhood, scheduling, hunger."

If it's childhood trauma and food issues you want to talk about, you and I both know that we all have a story to tell. I mean, how many Aunt Mimis do you have in your life?

A conversation with your parents, even well into your mature 30's or 40's, may still send you flying to the fridge. Some of us don't even have to go "back"—the emotional connections of the present can send us right into the eat-all-night saga.

The Prince's twice-a-month visits used to send me into a whirlwind of eating.

Having to borrow money from my father because my alimony check didn't come in time could cause an eating frenzy that would last for weeks at a time.

And as I've said over and over again everywhere I go, to this day a fight with my husband can have me eating a hot fudge sundae within minutes.

Now the Prince and I have matured—me so very much, him not quite as much (only joking, ex, just had to throw that in). So it's not the Prince that sends me anymore, quite literally, it's a million other things.

> Sadness sends me
> Worrying about the kids
> Reporters
> Deadlines

So what's changed? Childhood and adult issues are connected to our patterns of intake. We know that, but I'm a little confused—scheduling? What's the deal with scheduling and our pattern of intake? This is something new and different. May as well ask the doctor, because she's right here.

SCHEDULING

"Scheduling, or lack of it, can very much dictate our pattern of intake. Lack of proper scheduling causes, in many cases, hunger—and hunger can override what we need or what we have committed to do."

Hey, you guys—like the diet you began yesterday that you've already blown.

Like the big commitment you made to losing weight when you picked up this book.

Have you ever heard me say (if not, I'll say it again): IF YOU HAVE EVER GONE ON A DIET, LOST WEIGHT, AND GAINED IT BACK, YOU HAVE NOT FAILED. YOU'VE BEEN SET UP TO FAIL. AND GUESS WHAT ONE OF THE BIGGEST SETUPS IS IN THE DIET SYSTEM?

How about not eating enough food?

"You skip breakfast [hold on, guys; how many of us are guilty as hell of this even before this explanation gets off the ground? Hands up], grab something quickly for lunch as you race through your day, and by the end of the day, when you get home or you're on your way home, your hunger is so high it can at that point very much dictate what you grab and put into your mouth or spend all night long eating."

BULLETIN . . .

It doesn't always have to be some big psychological problem that forces us to eat enormous amounts at dinner and continue through the night. Check it out. It can be something much simpler to resolve than the emotional issues. The big hunger setup. Who'd have thought? This is great.

A scheduling screwup as opposed to an emotional screwup. A hunger drive beyond all hunger drives—because you've run all day long and haven't stopped to fuel. This just may be setting up millions of us for the behavioral eating disorder that we face every night. If this is the problem, then certainly there is a commonsense approach to a solution, right back into sainthood with Sachiko.

"There is a very simple solution to this problem: Eat during the day."

Gotta jump in here. Think about this: breakfast, lunch, and dinner. Fuel your body at regularly scheduled intervals, and you won't be setting yourself up for that ferocious hunger drive you find yourself dealing with at 7 p.m. every night.

When I was dieting at 260, which was constantly, I could go for a couple of weeks without eating or dieting (whatever you want to call it) but I would eventually end up eating all night. Controlling it was never a problem for a while, but that "healthy meal" at the end of the day always ended up looking like a Roman feast, complete with the gnawing of the turkey leg that could easily last through the night. Know what I'm talking about?

That's where I always ended up, of course, believing I had a night eating problem. Some trauma must have happened at night that caused my inner child to eat and eat and eat the night away. Never for a moment thinking it had anything to do with the fact that I'd been starving myself for a couple of days and that I was still running a household, cleaning up nonstop after two babies, up and down with one or the other all night long, washing a hundred loads of diapers a day, and burning a heck of a lot of fuel that I wasn't putting back in.

Talk about pattern of intake. Talk about Transition 101. Talk about years of experience with food and no connection. Looking back now I assess and think (is that the same thing?): fuel? There was none when I was dieting. Forget about breakfast on a diet. Never did I stop to eat breakfast or lunch unless lunch was one of those yummy shakes—or how about those diet bars we've all lived on for months? Maybe a salad? But food, fuel? Forget it, it didn't happen.

I didn't eat because I hated the way I looked and felt and I was determined to change it once and for all, and I was dieting, damn it!! WOW. Put it together. Think about it. And if I wasn't dieting, you want an imbalance? Excessive fat calories? Pattern of intake, including every childhood and present trauma under the sun? Fat, I could give you fat.

Without knowing what the heck I was doing and certainly without Sachiko, I did start eating and stopped setting myself up for the pattern-of-intake hunger dive every night. And guess what happened to my night cravings?

Out the window!

All of a sudden I wasn't having as much trouble "controlling" my cravings at 11 P.M. Just like the doctor said, my not eating all day was absolutely part of what was dictating and adding to the difficulty I was dealing with during my late-night bingeing. How about you? Are you having difficulty controlling the cravings?

Something as simple as not eating during the day "can set you up for overloading with high-fat, quick, easy-to-grab foods at night." Overloading, otherwise known as:

Overeating

Stuffing your face

Bingeing

Eating all night

Pretty exciting, huh? Easy. Understandable. Simple to apply.

Well, if you think this is great stuff, wait until you hear the rest.

Not eating all day, bad scheduling, also sets you up for something else that's really, really hard to fight. Listen to this:

SIGHT AND SMELL

"Lack of proper scheduling, not eating, sets you up to be much more susceptible to sight and smell."

See why my whole family is waiting on dinner for this interview? This stuff makes sense, and I'm loving it. Think about it: If you are ravenous because you haven't eaten anything other than that quick lunch to keep you going, and at five in the afternoon a pastry floats under your nose (you've had pastries attack you, haven't you?) what do you think is going to happen?

Then think about this. You've eaten a huge, high-volume, low-fat meal that has satisfied your senses and filled your belly. Do you think your reaction to the pastry floating under your nose is going to be different?

Just a thought.

> Candy
>
> Cookies
>
> Drive-throughs

More tempting when you're ravenous?

Think about dying of thirst in the desert, because that's what kept going through my mind as our friend was explaining this new addition to our understanding of self-sabotage, hunger setup number 101, behavior screwup in a big way. Picture this:

Crawling along the desert sand, you're dying of thirst: mouth parched, lips cracked and dry. Someone appears (mirage, not just a hotel in Vegas anymore) and places a huge pitcher of ice water in front of your parched mouth and dry lips. What are you gonna do:

(a) Say no, thank you, I'd like to wait until I'm almost dead before I give in to this temptation, or

(b) Drink the water so fast that you puke?

Don't you think if you're dying of thirst that a glass of water is going to look, smell, feel, and be a totally different experience than having an ice cold glass of water while sitting in your living room?

Now I just know that there are hundreds of snotty behaviorists, therapist whateverists, reading this right now and thinking: How basic. What common knowledge. Who does she think she is?

Well, to all the behaviorists in the world, since I have your attention, I'd like to say:

WE DON'T KNOW THIS STUFF.

THIS IS NOT COMMON KNOWLEDGE.

IF I'D KNOWN ABOUT THIS SIGHT-AND-SMELL-ENHANCING STUFF, SCHEDULING, PATTERN OF INTAKE, AND THE DIETING THAT WAS SETTING ME UP FOR THIS KIND OF FAILURE, MY LIFE WOULD HAVE BEEN A WHOLE LOT EASIER—BECAUSE EVERY TIME I FAILED, I THOUGHT THERE WAS SOMETHING WRONG WITH ME. I THOUGHT I WAS THE FAILURE.

Then I'd like to say to all of you:

PPPPPPPLLLLLLLLLLLLLLLLLLLLLLLLLLLL!

(That, my friends, is sticking your tongue out on paper!)

This is what Sachiko is trying to tell us. The "recognizing and education" are going to help you identify what needs to be changed, and it does make a whole lot of sense.

So I've changed my ways, again growing up in the public eye—me and the members of the Brady Bunch bunch, we've all grown up right in front of your eyes.

If you are unfit, overfat, and hate the way you look and feel, it "probably took years to get there":

"It didn't happen overnight and it's not going to change overnight, but there are many simple steps you can take that will make an enormous difference in your habits, patterns, and daily fat intake that will change your health."

And, I might add, the way you look. Sachiko, as a doctor, has to care about your health, but what we are talking about and won't ever stop talking about is what size you want to be. Losing weight properly and permanently. Having the body of your dreams. Will these changes make your dress size drop? Reveal a collarbone? How about a firm butt?

The answer is YES, YES, YES, YES. Becoming more aware of the fat you are taking in, when, why, how often, maybe even connected to what or who, will help you make the changes necessary to cut back on your fat. If you cut back on your fat, you know what's gonna happen: Less fat means less fat.

Doing this just may be the best, the most important, the biggest step you can take to guarantee the firmest butt, the drop in dress size, and looking and feeling better than you ever did.

> The other day . . . I ordered a big chocolate chip cookie. I took one bite but didn't really like it. That was a bad choice. I'm becoming more aware of the food I'm eating and the choices I'm making.
>
> —*Suzy, Victoria, Australia*

I concede. Change my ways and give full credit to Sachiko. When you take a moment to think about it, how we eat, how much, and when isn't just connected with the deep emotional inner-child traumas that we all suffer from. Our behaviors don't come out of nowhere. Sure, there are emotional connections, but please, let's give an ounce of credit to some of the physical connections to why we eat.

There's a bread factory a couple of miles from my home in Dallas, and every morning when taking the kids to school, going to work, or on my way to get coffee at my local "get your morning coffee" place, it takes everything in my power not to break into the factory with pounds of cinnamon and sugar, sprinkle it all over the production line, and eat every slice that's baking.

The smell could drive you wild.

Mexican food? All I have to do is catch a whiff of the stuff and I've got movies in my head of tacos beckoning me to eat, eat, eat until I get the chance to eat it.

And another thing that needs to be established right up front in our food discussion is that eating fat tastes good. Anyone who says that chocolate isn't the best-tasting thing you've ever tasted is a lying son of a gun.

Come on. When you were a kid, wasn't that bucket of Kentucky Fried with those great white bread rolls and that cole slaw the best-tasting stuff ever??

Grill that steak over the open fire and wad on the barbecue sauce with plenty of fried onions.

The cheese, steak, and grilled-onion hoagie—what could be better than that??

If you want to understand why the cheese, steak, and grilled-onion hoagies are so compelling, then we gotta talk biology for a minute so . . . from behavior to biology, come on . . .

BIOLOGY

Ever thought about that thing inside your mouth (not the steak-and-onion hoagie), your tongue? Do you think it was created only to help you get your words out? If it's eating and the biology of it all that we are talking about, then we have to start with that big pink thing inside your mouth (interesting sentence?).

Did you know that the tongue is considered the most versatile organ in the body? (WOW. I know a lot of men who would disagree with that!) Versatile is not the way I thought about my tongue half my life.

> A curse.
>
> The organ with a mind of its own.
>
> The organ that could never stop functioning.

From the day I can remember, it's been the thing that I just have never been able to "hold," if you know what I mean. During my divorce from the Prince I would have considered my tongue the sharpest instrument in my body, not the most versatile, and now it's how I make a living: talking, talking, talking. Until I started writing this book and took a second to think about what happens when you put food into your mouth, never, ever did I think the tongue was as versatile and as talented as it is.

The tongue is our protector. It registers revulsion when food is spoiled or poisonous. Many deadly toxins are bitter, and the tongue is the detector that tells the body to spit it out. Check it out. Just watch any eighteen-month-old in a high chair when you give him something bitter. Across-the-room hurl, that's what breakfast, lunch, and dinner was dubbed every day in my house, three times a day, when the boys were young.

You know your tongue helps you speak—don't ask me how we know that, but we do. But speaking is nothing compared to what else your tongue helps you do. Consider it your tactile connection to texture and tastes (sounds like a commando, doesn't it?).

Cravings. If you want to talk cravings—and everywhere you look, someone does—you can't talk about the emotional reasons we eat without including Mr. Versatile in your discussion.

Actually, it's a twin thing we're talking about here. It's your tongue and your nose, both very much connected to the cravings that we spend all day feeling.

Yes, yes, yes, it may be a smell that was in your grandma's kitchen that evokes a memory that creates a craving for love, but it also has a whole lot to do with the tongue registering the taste and the olfactory cells in each nostril reacting to the smell of it—and bingo, you're gone. It's over. Your versatile organ, the tongue, may be a powerful tactile connector, but those olfactory cells in your nose respond thousands of times stronger to the smell of food, thousands of times stronger than your taste buds do—so together they work to help create the taste and smell you desire so very much, and together they can be hell to combat. Throw in a grandma memory, and most of us are buried ten feet under and carried away by the craving.

The emotional connection is there for sure, but the tactical, the things we can control, are all a part of it also.

If it's the mouth and food that we're talking about, then you gotta go right to chewing, because it all starts to go wrong—in the physiological sense, not the emotional—in the chewing. Here's what's supposed to happen, and you see if it does or not.

The food you eat is mushed and smushed by your teeth and mixed with saliva unless you're toothless, then your process begins in the blender. Saliva importance on a scale of 1 to 10? Saliva is way up there because it's almost as crucial to the process of your food becoming your fuel as anything is. You may have thought in the past that digestive enzymes were the most important, or you may never have thought about any of this. But let me tell you that it all seems to start with that wet stuff in your mouth. Saliva. It's the stuff in the saliva that begins the process of turning food into what it's really all about: FUEL.

The stuff that keeps us going. Feeds everything. Keeps the fire burning. Helps that engine run. Maybe if we balanced the emotional screwups with a little fact and physiology, we'd get somewhere with this subject. So what better place to start than in your mouth, with your saliva?

CHEWING

Very excited to be here with you right now, because no matter how screwed up our connections with food are, we can get somewhere with the fuel discussion. Headway, headway, headway in figuring out how we can regain some control of our eating. Start in your mouth.

Chewing can be the beginning of the end for many of us who live with digestive problems. How you eat—not why, but *how*—is what we're talking about.

You sit down to a meal—if you're lucky. Most of us eat in the car, in between meetings, out of a snack pack. Who sits anymore?

You may sit down to a meal only once in a blue moon, but whether you're sitting at a table or driving through, have you ever thought about how you eat?

First thing we usually do is gulp down a huge glass of ice water or soda, right? It's an automatic in this country. You sit to eat, and there's a huge glass of ice water sitting in front of you within seconds. Do you know that you have to beg for ice water in England? That's a little history-and-food combo right from the horse's mouth. Just got back from London, and that was one of the first things I noticed—no ice water to be found anywhere. Nobody understands the meaning of cold water there. First, saying "May I have a glass of water?" before or with your meal gets you the strangest stares, then they figure you're either out of your mind or American.

Only in this country is ice water a given at every table, and if you live in the South, as I do, you sit down to the biggest glass of ice water you've ever seen—maybe 'cause it's hot. I don't know, but I've never seen anything like the size of some of the glasses of water I've been served in Texas. Wait a minute, I must have lost my mind for a moment.

Texas = big

Bigger than anywhere

Bigger than anything

Even with a glass of ice water there's Texas pride involved.

So our meals usually begin with a gulp of ice water. Then it's time to eat. How do you eat? Ever thought about it? I've been thinking and watching. Sure, watching people eat—why not? Doing a book on food makes you aware of things you never thought you'd be interested in or aware of. You're reading this chapter, aren't you? Did you ever think you'd be talking about your saliva? If you take the time to think about it, you just may find that, like most of us, you sit down and

Gulp

Inhale

Mainline

Chug

Wash down your meals

Chewing? Saliva? When would that moist important stuff have time to even mix with the food that's in our mouths? The first part of digestion, chewing—skipped. Don't we eat as if we are running a marathon? When's the last time you really chewed your food? Maybe if you're lucky or on vacation you'll get one or two chews in, but for the most part our food goes right down whole.

You wanna know what the food experts say is normal, even necessary, for good digestion in the chewing department? In order to ensure that proper digestion takes place, we should chew each bite of the food we are eating anywhere from fifty to one hundred times.

EACH BITE FIFTY TO ONE HUNDRED TIMES!!!!!

Excuse me. That's all I'd do all day, with the amount of food I eat.

> Where's Susan?
> Chewing.

> We have a segment to shoot.
> She can't, she's chewing.

> Book deadline?
> No can do, she's chewing.

> The boys need dinner.
> Sorry, Mommy's busy chewing.

Spend a moment, please. Chewing is one of the most important steps in the process of digestion. Most of the time we skip it or do just a bit of it before we send the wads of foods we are eating down to the stomach. You can't blame us, because who knew it was so important? But now that we do, let's get real with this "chew each bite fifty to one hundred times" stuff, shall we? Willing to help our bodies get the fuel it needs? Absolutely. But come on . . . fifty to one hundred times—is there a compromise on that one?

I found one. Dropping the old 100 plus had very little to do with chewing or caring about saliva, believe me. But once I found out about the importance of chewing and then started considering the process just a little bit it made sense to me. I was interested in doing what I could to get my body the fuel it needed to give me the energy that I so desperately wanted. So here's what I did: I started becoming more aware of how many times I chewed and put some thought into chewing a few more chews once in a while. What does that take? Nothing! So try it.

Here's a thought. The next time you sit down or drive through or run into your office late for work with your next meal, take a second and chew your food. No big meditation needed. You don't have to give up your job and stay home and chew all day. It isn't one hundred times or nothing. It's about becoming more aware of something that is very important. You can help your body do the job it's so well designed to do, starting with something that's easy to start with. Instead of wolfing down all your food at once, chew it a couple of times. Maybe stop for a second or two, take a breath, then chew. Stopping for a second is always a good idea—not long, just a second, and think saliva. Sounds a little nutty, but, hey, it works. Becoming more aware of your body, reconnecting, thinking about it can begin by taking a second while you're eating to chew. Why not? Could it hurt? Seems to me that it could only help.

It's like the exercise stuff I've been talking about for a couple of years now. Level of intensity? Working within your fitness level, ever heard of it? Well, change your eating pattern or pattern of intake by building the steps necessary to make that change realistically and working within them. Same thing, building your level of intensity physically, or building your chewing fitness. Increase your level of intensity as you go, one fitness level at a time. One food change, one understanding, one assessment, one connection at a time. Hey, a new twelve-step program in the works.

The walk that I took at 260 pounds was just as effective as the workout I did this morning. Both burned fat, both increased muscle strength, and both changed my body. They were just done at different levels of intensity, because I was physically not as fit then as I am now. So what? Which was more important? Which was more effective? Which level of intensity made the most difference? Neither.

They were equally important and effective. The workout that I did this morning was a strong, high-level-of-intensity workout because I'm strong enough to do it now. The walk I took years ago at 260 pounds was as strong and as high level as I could do then. Both increased my fitness level, and both increased my physical awareness. Both moved (pardon that one) me forward in the direction that I so desperately wanted: a strong, healthy life-style. A different body. Leaner. Feeling better. Looking better.

Everybody's dawning is different. Getting fat was mine, and feeling fat and lousy may be yours.

For Joan, it was her husband's heart attack.

For Erica, it was the pains in her legs from the weight she was carrying.

Jessy couldn't stand shopping in large ladies' stores.

Monique was tired of feeling like a failure.

Thelma was so damn depressed that she didn't want to live her life that way anymore.

Everybody's got a different face-down-in-the-gutter reason to make a change. Then it's a matter of taking the steps necessary to make it happen.

Having a look at what is.

Looking at your body and deciding what you want to change.

Looking at your life and figuring out where the fat's coming from and what changes you are willing to make.

Thinking about what you're eating, when, and why, without an ounce of guilt attached—just what is.

You wanna keep the creamer in your coffee, but you're willing to do without so much beef.

You'll cut the chicken back to three times a week and go from five to three to two ounces. Slowly, slowly, you'll get that fat out of your life and off your body.

Pizza—never, ever give it up? But the cheese can go as long as you can always be guaranteed the extra onions and all the low-fat toppings you want.

START HERE START NOW

One-fifth of a pizza can have up to nineteen grams of fat. Order it

with no cheese or light cheese, add extra veggies, and you have only

about four grams of fat.

Do you see it? Taking the steps of recognizing, educating, and incorporating small, realistic life-style changes, no matter what the level of intensity of change, will make a difference in how you look and feel, and can make a difference in your life. Learning as much as you can about your pattern of intake just may be as important as some of the bigger changes you may make.

So go ahead, do what the doc said: Write down just a week's worth of eating and have a look at it. Think patterns, think frequency, and think the type of food—pay close attention here. Do what the doctor ordered. HELLLLLLLP me. I never, ever thought in my wildest dreams that I'd ever say something like that, but thanks to the commonsense and loving presentation of Sachiko, the saint, I say it now with such conviction. It just may help you, and helping you is the most important thing.

Now there's one special habit, pattern of intake, sense and smell sensitivity that you really need to pay attention to. I know, I know you know, but just in case it isn't clear, I have to say it one more time: FAT.

"One of the most important changes most of us can make is cutting back on our total daily fat intake."

Because we eat way too much of it, and it's the fattest calories we are eating, right?

Correct-a-mundo. Make it simple. According to Sachiko, the first thing to think about when it comes to making this big change in your life is fat, and the best way, the easiest way to do that is by substitution.

PORTION CONTROL

This may be old news to some, but now that I'm open to writing it all down, I'm seeing this level one transformation in a totally different light, so I want to go through all the steps, no matter how basic they may seem.

"Substituting lower-fat meats for high-fat meats is a big step for most of us when it comes to changing our life-style and does make a difference in our total fat intake."

And it's called PORTION CONTROL.
SUBSTITUTION AND PORTION CONTROL—THE BEGINNING OF THE END OF YOUR HIGH-FAT LIFE-STYLE.

● ●

Portion Control

	Fat Grams	
Ground Beef (4-oz serving)		
Six servings	142	
Three servings	71	
		Saves 71 fat grams
Salmon (3½-oz serving)		
Six servings	48	
Three servings	24	
		Saves 24 fat grams
Beef Bologna (1-oz serving)		
Five servings	40	
Two servings	16	
		Saves 24 fat grams
Beef Hotdog		
Five servings	81	
Two servings	32	
		Saves 49 fat grams
Chicken Drumstick (batter-fried)		
Five servings	57	
Two servings	23	
		Saves 34 fat grams
T-bone Steak (8-oz serving)		
Five servings	240	
Two servings	96	
		Saves 144 fat grams
Frozen Fish Sticks (3 per serving)		
Five servings	52	
Two servings	21	
		Saves 31 fat grams

continued

Ham Lunchmeat (1-oz serving)
 Five servings   15
 Two servings   6
              Saves 9 fat grams

Roast Beef Sandwich (on bun)
 Five servings   69
 Two servings   28
              Saves 41 fat grams

Breaded Pork Chop (4-oz baked/broiled)
 Five servings   147
 Two servings   60
              Saves 87 fat grams

Beef Short Ribs (5 per serving)
 Five servings   231
 Two servings   93
             Saves 138 fat grams

Brisket (4-oz serving)
 Five servings   171
 Two servings   69
             Saves 102 fat grams

● ●

"Going from an eight-ounce steak to a three-ounce steak does make a difference in your body. Eating a five-ounce steak instead of a twelve-ounce steak can reduce your daily fat grams from sixty grams to twenty-five grams."

Who's going to argue with that? Certainly not me, Susan Powter, Food P.I. It only makes sense.

"Another advantage of portion control is that you place less emphasis on the high fat, many times the center of the meal, such as meat, the staples that we have been raised with. They become less and less important, less of your total meal. It's things like this that can change our focus, our understanding, our old habits with food."

Well, count me in on this argument for changing your eating habits. How much of what we eat is habit, what's placed in front of us, what our family ate? We've been taught for so many years that without certain staples, a meal isn't a meal. What are we supposed to do? Step out into foreign territory? Go off on a health food tangent? Deprive our families of the protein and nutrients they need to live, while we figure out a different emphasis for the meal? No. Too scary. Not worth the risk. No chance of that ever happening. So we don't. Understandable, but not necessarily right. Portion control seems to be the ticket to this big, important change of focus. Easy now, go easy. Just take your time and think about this.

Our focus, understanding, and old habits with our food are something we all need to change a bit. Our friend is right. In the past, based on the wrong information, the emphasis has been on meat as the center of the meal. The bulk. What's a meal without the beef? You have the baked potato, the corn on the cob, the salad, the bread—all that, but it's the beef in the center of the plate that has made most of us feel we are giving our families what they need to live, the protein, the iron, the strength that they need to keep going. Until very recently, it has been the right thing to do.

> The wifely thing.
>
> The good mother thing.
>
> The responsible thing.
>
> Can't get full without it.

Certainly can't feel satisfied without it and can't feed that meat-and-potato guy who's bringing in all the dough without it.

Staring down at a three-ounce slab of beef versus twelve ounces makes, if nothing else, a visual difference and does help cut back on the big one: Mr. Fat.

Because we now know without a doubt that beef is loaded with saturated fat, and saturated fat makes you fat and damages your body in more ways than one. You gotta cut down, and portion control seems to be one of the ways to do it. Hey, when the beef becomes the smaller, less important, high-fat focus, and the corn on the cob, the pasta, the veggies—the higher-volume, lower-fat (more of it than you could imagine), non-saturated-fat foods—will slowly creep into the center, or focus, of the meal. All you gotta do is make the big fat boy less important and smaller. Good start. Now how about going one step further in this thinking—you may as well, you've gone this far, and it makes a whole lot of sense. Go ahead, jump on board. If the main component of your meals goes from high fat to much, much lower fat, what do you think is likely to happen? You will be less fat? The family will be less fat? Absolutely!!!!

Old habits are hard to change—we've heard that for years—but it's looking easier and easier as we go. You have to admit that in the last ten years we've gone from calling somebody who doesn't eat meat a hippie or a rabbit-food health nut to recognizing it as perfectly normal; it is now socially acceptable to cut way, way back or not eat it at all. Norman would be amazed.

It's not the social stigma of all times anymore to not do what everyone else is doing. The skinless Thanksgiving meal now is a sign of awareness, caring about your body, love for others and the planet. This would be a good time to start. Easy, easy, easy to glide right into the political correctness called portion control of the high-fat foods.

START HERE START NOW

Substitutes

Whole milk: Use skim milk.

Whipped cream: Use Cool Whip Light or half whipped cream and half whipped egg white.

Eggs: Use egg whites or egg substitutes. In baking, substitute mashed banana for 1 egg.

Mayonnaise: Use light mayo or non-fat mayo, or low-fat cottage cheese and whip in the blender.

Ricotta cheese: Use low-fat ricotta or fat-free ricotta.

Cottage cheese: Use 1% low-fat cottage cheese or non-fat cottage cheese.

Crème fraîche: Use light sour cream or fat-free sour cream.

Cream cheese: Use light cream cheese or non-fat cream cheese.

Milk, 1 cup for cooking: 4 tablespoons powdered soy milk in 1 cup water or 1 cup Rice Dream milk.

Use water or vegetable broth to replace oil for sautéeing.

Bacon or sausage: Use turkey sausage (check label).

Ground beef: Use Healthy Choice 96% fat-free beef or 90% lean; use half and add oatmeal or shredded potatoes or carrots.

Beef bouillon, 1 cup: 1 tablespoon miso in one cup of water or vegetable broth.

The next station on this changing life-styles low-fat train? Visible fats.

"Cutting back on the visible fats—gravies, butter, oil, creamy anything . . . just the most obvious, and those you can substitute [tying in those two concepts beautifully]—easily helps create a lower fat intake."

VISIBLE FATS

Now here's something I can really understand because this is exactly what I did. Finally we get to something that I did. I may have missed the first eight steps, but when it comes to getting rid of the visible fats, I'm there. Anything white and creamy was out as far as I was concerned.

It didn't take much for me to know what I was eating; maybe that's why I didn't write anything down. I was eating loads of fat.

When? All the time.

Why? Because I was miserable, lonely, angry, scared, feeling horrible—remember?

Why? (Double why on this one, because I gotta bring the ex into it.) Because my ex-husband was a terrible man.

Logical, right?

Well, since I couldn't get rid of him—he'd already left—I started cutting back on those obvious visible fats, the one thing I did have control of, and you'd better believe that it made a difference in my life. I started shrinking with very little effort, while never feeling hungry.

You know how you feel after the third cake—not slice, cake? Horrible! Try eating less.

There we are, cutting back—PORTION CONTROL.

Consider going for a lower-fat version of the cake—SUBSTITUTION out the yazooo.

Eat a high-volume low-fat meal just before you sit down to the cake. Head on into SCHEDULING and proper PLANNING.

See if the cake still looks as good—bammo, how about that SIGHT and SMELL intervention?

VISIBLE FAT? DON'T PUT THE ICING ON IT.

Don't butter the pound cake.

Leave the ice cream in the freezer or put some low-fat yogurt on top instead. Less fat in means less fat on. (HEY, call the advertising company about that one. What a logo—sell it for a fortune!!!)

You don't have to go the total low-fat life-style right out of the gate.

"When you think about and work with these stages of change, you can beat the game rather than set yourself up for failure."

If you decide at any point that you want to really go for the gold in this changing-your-life-style thing, there's plenty more you can do to make your life as low fat as possible.

PREPARATION

You want to go just a bit further because this stuff is so easy to understand? Fine, then it's time to think preparation.

Next step.

• •

Cooking Comparisons

CHICKEN	
Fried, with skin	45%
Fried, flour coated	23%
Roasted, breast without skin	19%
TURKEY	
Barbecued	25%
Roasted, light meat	20%
Hickory-smoked	15%
PORK CHOP	
Pan fried	73%
Braised	48%
Broiled	43%
FLOUNDER/SOLE	
Baked with lemon juice and butter	45%
Baked with lemon juice and margarine	45%
Cooked without added fat	14%

I checked out four things: chicken, turkey, pork chops, and fish. Just have a quick look at a few cooking techniques, and you can see really clearly how easy it is to cut down on fat. Chicken, fry it with skin, and you're talking 45 percent per serving; roasted without skin, 19 percent. Tell me that 26 percent fat per serving is not a huge savings. Turkey, all you gotta do is go from barbecuing to hickory smoking it, and you're saving 10 percent. Hey, hey, hey, pan-fry your pork chops or broil them, it's 30 percent less fat on your body—it's up to you. Bake your flounder or sole, fine. Bake it with butter, 45 percent fat. You do the math.

• •

"Roasting, broiling, steaming, and baking your lower-total-fat, smaller-portioned, well-thought-about-when-and-why-you-are-eating food just adds to the whole picture—lower fat in a big way."

Think about these:

Whole milk is 49 percent.

Use skim.

Oil is 100 percent fat.

Sauté in water or veggie broth.

Bacon or sausage your favorite thing in life?

Check your labels and replace that hearty high-fat breakfast sausage
   with lower-fat turkey sausage.

Can't live without whipped cream?

Check out all the lower-fat versions in your grocery store, or forget
   about anything with that many chemicals in and top your pound cake
   with non-fat yogurt.

Dr. Marc Micozzi, someone you'll meet later (you're meeting everyone
later in this book) said that if the first time you think about food is when you
sit down at the table, then it's too late.

The more you know, the more you find out about food in your life, the
easier it is to understand that it's important enough to put some thought into.
What we buy. Why we buy it. How much of the whole thing is done uncon-
sciously. Patterns, daily intake, fat percentage—why, when, how, enough
with it. If it hasn't dawned on you to assess and place a higher importance
on the food you put into your body after all you've read, then I've failed miserably. But I think you have, and now it's time to get as practical as you can
get with your new information and take it with you down the aisles of the supermarket. Go shopping. Yes, that's right: Think about food before it ever
gets into the pot. Shopping. You and I are going to the market.

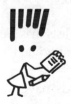

CHAPTER 4
SHOPPING

Can't talk food, can't even think food until you take the first step and go shopping. It's shopping I go once a week with the family, and it's that same once-weekly shopping trip that has me thinking Valium . . . only thinking, because it's the 90's, and that means deep breathing and meditation, not Valium. Hugs, not drugs, and all that. I may not take it, but I'd be lying if I told you that I didn't think about it every week when I take the WHOLE FAMILY grocery shopping.

Shopping isn't what it used to be . . . and it's time we talked about it. Try to make some sense out of what most of us face every week and understand it a bit, above and beyond the emotional traumas that follow you through the aisles. Shopping. The chapter and the reason, because it's bigger than you, me . . . We can't talk food without talking shopping, that's the way I see it.

Yes, things have changed for most of us. Time—gone. Convenience—in. And those things have absolutely affected the way we shop and what we are buying.

Our schedules and shopping lists may be different depending on whether you are a coupon-clipping stay-at-home mom or an out-of-the-house, working-three-jobs-to-keep-the-family-together-and-a-less-organized-because-of-it kind of mom. The cupboards have to be filled every however often (jumping right in and smashing the once-weekly myth) and the shopping trips made, and grocery shopping is grocery shopping, no matter how you look at it.

It's a big part of our lives, and if you think for one second that what you buy, how you buy, or what you pick up impulsively isn't planned, strategized, and laid out way before you or I ever get to the store, then you're fooling yourself, because it is. Check this out:

THE GROCERY STORE

The grocery store. The massive warehouse. The all-in-one shopping extravaganza that has taken the place of the mom-and-pop store.

The convenience and choices in today's modern warehouse markets are fabulous. Selection like you've never!!! If you want to know how much we have available to us, go abroad. Walk into any supermarket outside the United States, and you'll think you're in a hallway, not a grocery store. What's bigger and better than American supermarkets? Selection, price, and choices— we've got it all, and we're lucky as hell. But that doesn't mean we should leave our brains at the cart rack. Selection and savings, fine, but don't scrimp on your and your family's health by eating tons and tons of high-fat foods just because the food brokers place it, the advertisers make big pyramids out of it, and the checkout stand is designed to suck you in at the end of a tough shopping trip. It takes only a bit of awareness to change a whole lot of things. I'll tell you something: You need more than Valium to walk down the aisles of these new huge supermarkets today.

Where did they come from? Think about the first time you saw a "warehouse hypermart" in your part of the country, then think about how fast the twenty-seven others sprang up. For a while it seemed that the country was being taken over by superstores.

A lot has changed since World War II (wondering how World War II got into this discussion? Have a little faith and patience, and you'll see). We've come a long way from the old mom-and-pop store in all its romantic glory. Don't you remember:

The butcher cutting the finest cut of meat.

The young, eager-to-please stock boy working his way up the ranks, hoping one day to be the manager of the store.

Maybe you've even still got the small-town fantasy going on: the extended credit line when things got bad, during times of drought, locust plague, or just an all-out bad winter. Nothing screams American more than the mom-and-pop local grocery store, excluding apple pie, of course.

You think American when you think that, don't you?

Think we invented it, don't you?

Not so.

When you think market, shopping for food, you have to think Greek, Egyptian, and then cowboy. We've been trading gold for grain (pardon that little low-fat, high-volume reference) for a hell of a long time before Mom and Pop came along. We did, however, coin the phrase and should take all the credit.

> In 1869, the first A&P grocery store opened in New York City.

If you want to get a real feel for the open market, rent the movie *Aladdin* (as if you haven't already). Boys and monkeys swinging from poles, vendors yelling, princesses strolling the streets—those were the days when markets were markets. After the big one, World War II, Piggly Wiggly, Big Bear, and the A&P started sprouting (pardon the health food pun) up everywhere. The American supermarket was born, and the mom-and-pop store started to get a run for its money.

Knowing the manager? Forget about it.

Eager young man working his way up the ladder? How about hundreds of employees?

Stockers, pricers, checkout clerks, and big, big changes in the shopping habits of the American public.

If Mr. Piggly or Mr. Wiggly thought he had a big market, I do believe that the boys of that day would all roll over in their graves if they saw what's going on now. From A&P to something the size of the World's Fair. The supermarkets of today would swallow the grocery stores of the past and have old Mom and Pop for an appetizer. Here's where the Valium comes in. Who can walk into these things without being medicated? They are monstrous. The cart rack alone is overwhelming. Thousands and thousands of carts lined up ready for the shoppers.

The length and height of the aisles are astounding.

Have you ever looked up?

What happens if one of those skyscrapers of paper towel boxes begins to topple—industrial avalanche!

WOMAN BURIED UNDER POUNDS OF PAPER TOWELS AT FOOD WAREHOUSE . . . NEWS AT 11.

Whatever you want or need, it's in the American hyper/supermarket these days. Forget about the butcher, he's long gone, but any kind of meat you want is cut in any way you want it and covered in plastic in little styro dishes, waiting for you to buy.

Milk. No thick glass bottles with cream on top anywhere in sight. But how

about those ten-gallon cartons or one hundred different brands all screaming that they are better than the next—fortified, pasteurized, light, low, 1%,
2%, skimmed. You can get cases of everything, industrial-sized anything, pick
up some videos, get your pharmaceuticals, buy some jewelry, change the
tires on the car, and head home. That's shopping in the 90's, and you'd better believe that the boys who designed these monstrosities had a goal in
mind: to get you and me buying as much as they can get us to buy, without
us even knowing.

> I grew up with eating habits that got away from real food, so I didn't know what
> to do with some natural foods. . . . We (my family) eat better. . . . It's so easy. I've
> quickly become aware of how food manufacturers are producing food that is bad
> for us.
>
> —*Cindy, Mifflinburg, Pennsylvania*

Every section of your grocery store has its importance and power firmly
established before you or I ever get to shop it. What you grab and end up
putting into your body isn't just about what you like. Why do we like what
we like (talk about a sentence, but it makes sense when you think about it)?
How much are we being influenced without even knowing? Never thought?
Never cared! Understandably so—until, of course, we started talking food
and all that's involved. That's why we are here together right now, talking
distribution, food brokers, and eye levels, because they're important to your
fat detective training and career.

When I started writing this book, I starting thinking about things I'd never
thought or cared about in my life. The further I went with it, the more and
more amazed I became about how much is going on in the aisles of our supermarkets and how unaware we all are about something that we do once,
twice, or however many times a week. Understanding enough about what's
going on behind the scenes and being aware can increase our choices. If
looking left, right, up, or down can give us more options and release us from
the spell of the eye-level power that we didn't even know we were under,
then why not?

Finding out about some of this stuff just may give you some extra ammo
in the fight against the bombardment you face every time you walk down the
aisles of your neighborhood hyper/supermarket.

They know our buying habits have changed. They've studied our life-
styles. Convenience? They know all about it, and their system is something
to talk about.

Impulse buying out the yin-yang.

Advertising left, right, and center.

I just read that General Mills, the maker of Cheerios, spends more on advertising than any other food producer—$50 to $99 million annually. Isn't that a sin? I'm calling the Vatican to see if I can get that listed as one of the biggies. I grew up believing that wearing patent-leather shoes was a sin because it was the same as holding a mirror under your skirt so the boys could see your panties. Well, if patent-leather shoes are a sin, spending $99 million on those goofy commercials for Cheerios should be. I'm off, off to the Vatican.

In-store advertising can annoy you into buying. Those less-than-subliminal ads that run constantly in some supermarkets can make you run to the item hoping and praying that putting it into your cart will get the voice to shut up. It works: Studies show a 15 percent increase in sales when that voice speaks. The Cracker Jack man knew from the beginning what would make you buy: a free gift. What we did for the little printing set! I'd eat three boxes of the stuff just to try and get the rubber stamp and ink pad. Give 'em a gift, enter 'em in a contest. How many bowls of cereal have you eaten while reading the back of the box about the next contest?

I'll tell you what doesn't increase sales: those in-store demos you see all over the place, the lady who's trying to force you to taste the pigs-in-a-blanket that she's frying up in her electric pan. Yes, we try them, because we are hungry, but do you run to the pigs-in-the-blanket aisle and pick some up? Nope. These demos sell very little and cost a lot to put on; gotta pay for the space for the day, pay the person doing the demo, and then there's all those pigs-in-a-blanket that are given to hungry shoppers.

I have a little story about the Prince and me. You may have figured out by now that I'm totally dependent on including the Prince in everything I do. Healed? I don't think so!

So here goes . . .

Your food gets on the supermarket shelves a couple of different ways. Some manufacturers stock their own . . . oh, my, here's where the Prince comes in.

Guess what the Prince was doing when I first met him? As in first date, falling madly in love?

He was delivering beer for a major distributor.

A BEER DELIVERY MAN—WHAT COULD BE MORE ROMANTIC??

It wasn't food, unless you live in Germany, but he was delivering and stocking all the same. And I'm here to tell you firsthand how it's done. I know because I was there. Riding side by side with my Prince may have been against company rules, but it was our idea of heaven at the time. Silly me, if

I'd known how costly those little rides were going to be, would I have taken them? I'm saving that answer for my next book, *Learning from Past Mistakes: Do We or Don't We?*

I have seen the product taken from the truck—the Prince's huge arms glowing with sweat in the Texas sun. I saw him stack the boxes of beer, one on top of the other. I was with him when he made contact with the manager and brought his load in.

Wouldn't you consider this an eyewitness account of a manufacturer stocking its shelves?

Who says I'm not equipped to write this food book? Throw this story to the skeptics and laugh. HA HA.

I stood right there when he heaved his heavy load (a term I used later with the ex, if you know what I mean) from truck to shelf, and went home with him to soothe his weary body after a long day of stocking the bars in Dallas, Texas, with beer. (A public servant? Absolutely. In Texas, stocking beer is considered a public service. Just ask any cowboy. One of the most important jobs in the state . . . too scary a thought to even entertain.)

So I know distribution as not many people know it, and I had this feeling of familiarity when I started reading about your food and mine getting to the shelves of our local huge marts. Let's talk distribution for just a moment, shall we?

DISTRIBUTION

Some manufacturers still do deliver and stock their own products, but very few, because these days most of our food gets to us through supermarket warehouse distribution centers, big, big, big distribution centers. And—get ready for this—it's done by food brokers!

Can you believe this? Cool Whip dealers? I'm dying!

Talk about professions you never think about!!! Where do they teach this stuff? A Food Broker 101 college course?

Are there trade schools for food brokers?

Where's the Wall Street of food brokers?

I want to meet some food brokers and see what these guys are all about. Wherever they are and wherever they come from, they are the wheelers and dealers of the food you and I eat, and these boys have some power.

Food broker is the official title, and they buy and sell our food and vie for shelf space, and apparently it's a messy business. Think about it: Imagine how nasty the food broker business can get when things heat up between brands. Shelf space, where the product is sitting, has more to do with your and my buying it than you can ever imagine. . . . Can't you see it now, hit-men hired to knock over competitors' displays? Nasty tactics used to make sure that the mushy marshmallow mix doesn't get the same exposure as the cheese whip? Horrible things being done to grab the two most powerful spaces on that grocery store shelf—eye level, yours and your kids'?

You may be older, have the cash, and think you are making the decisions in your family when it comes to the food you buy, the food your family eats, but you're fooling yourself if you do. It's the kids who make most of the decisions about what goes into your cart, and the food brokers know it. They planned it this way. Sure, eye level—yours and mine—is a very, very powerful space on the shelf, but if you want to understand the power, the irresistible lure for kids, shop at their eye level the next time you go to the grocery store. Crawl around the supermarket floor, and you will be able to understand the spell they are under. You may also get arrested, but crawl around anyway—it's amazing.

The food brokers figured something out a long time ago: We buy what we see. If it's staring us right between the eyes, we are more likely to pick it up. If you don't believe me, look around the next time you're in the aisles. Cover some ground. Look left, look right, look up and down—you just may find some products you didn't know existed. You see, the guys sitting at that eye-level shelf space are very powerful. They've paid a lot of money to get there, and they are going to make sure their products scream at you to buy them. Fancy labels, low-fat, light, no-cholesterol claims everywhere. Whatever you want to hear, they'll tell you, because it's an expensive place to be. But watch out—once these boys figure out that you've figured it out, you just may find yourself at the bottom of a river with the marshmallow spread competitor tied to your ankles (dangerous business, this investigative stuff, but important to you and your family).

It's no accident that you have to wheel through the maze-of-goodies aisles before you get to the bread and basics aisle.

> Designed that way.
> Planned.
> Well thought out.

You think what's laid out just before you check out is by chance? Candy at kids' level. Think about it. After shopping at the Huge Mart, how do you feel? What's going on, no matter how well you've planned?

> The kids tired and hungry, screaming.
> You're so tired you could die.
> What are you gonna do? Fight it?
> NOPE.

You'll buy the children anything in sight, anything they want, to calm things down so you can get home, unpack the groceries, and get dinner started.

Have a look. What's right in their face at the worst time of the shopping trip?

> Bright, pretty colors.
> Products screaming yummy.
> Candy, candy, candy.

And buy, buy, buy is what we do. That's why the space just before the checkout counter is some of the most expensive and hardest to get.

I heard some great escape-that-checkout-stand suggestions from grocery-shopping Moms.

> While you're in the chip aisle, buy some low-fat potato chips, open the pretzels, grab a bag of whatever works, and start feeding them early.
> Buy 'em a toy in the toy aisle or get them a car in the used-car lot that's probably out back; keep their attention on a little craft project, not the gooey chewy stuff that's waiting for them at the end of the trip.

I bring my own food to the grocery store. Redundant, you may be thinking, but not at all. I used to bring what I knew my kids loved most and used the bribe through the whole shopping trip. Then just before we hit the most dangerous aisle in the store, I'd open the bag and hand it out. Of course while I was waiting in line I'd be picking up every magazine, a deck of cards, some Silly Putty, and a couple of those little sewing kits, spending five times the money I would have spent if I'd just bought the candy bar. But what the hell, the kids were eating high-volume, low-fat, great-tasting food while the family was going broke. Oh, sure, there's a design to the Huge Mart, and the smart shopper of today needs to be aware of more than label reading to get through a grocery trip unscathed.

But important as it is, it's not all you have to watch out for to walk away sane from your "local" grocery store these days. Before we talk label reading—and we will, because it's a big issue with me—I thought it would be nice if you and I walked through the grocery supermart together and talked options—and low fat, of course. And if we are going to do that, then we have to start with something that you probably never in your life thought about. Carts.

THE CART

Yes, that's right. The cart that you grab from those long, well-organized lines without even thinking, because there's a story there that amazed me when I read it, and I thought you might be interested.

The superstructure that can house everything that anyone could possibly want has been built, done deal, but I want to know why, why, why they can't design a cart with wheels that don't veer to the left. A cart with wheels that work.

Before I was writing a book, running a business, and doing a TV show, back in the organized grocery-shopping-list days of my life, a left veer on the cart didn't really bother me. Just a part of the process, and the boys and I dealt with it. On good days it could even turn into a little game or project—but NOW . . .

Running like mad, getting to the store with minutes to spare before closing, scribble pad in hand, starving kids unwillingly in tow, grabbing the steer-to-the-left cart can easily send me over the edge. It's during those times that I think Sylcan Goldman is trying to drive me crazy. You see, Sylcan invented the shopping cart in 1936. God knows what they did before that: baskets on the heads of the American housewife? Sylcan patented and sold it way back—with no baby seat; that was added in 1947. Before we continue, I want to know: What kind of name is Sylcan? Can you imagine looking at your new, sweet little baby boy and naming him Sylcan? Sorry, Sy, but it's not a name most of us would choose.

I wonder what Sy would think if he knew that his prized invention hasn't kept up with the times. How embarrassing. You walk into one of these massive shopping developments, and the cart that you invented veers to the left. Sorry, Sy, but as hard as I tried, I couldn't find the answer to why it happens, so for now it is just a part of our reality.

Face it, Sy: Most of your carts stink; they have to be reinvented. Until then we have to put up with the veer-left, no-room-for-more-than-two-kids, not-keeping-up-with-the-times carts that we have.

> I have altered all of our eating habits at home. My husband . . . laughs when I try new recipes, but he loves them. My girls do, too. My baby . . . loves caramel rice cakes.
>
> —*Lynn, Vernon Center, New York*

But when it comes to who's behind these outdated pieces of equipment, there's no question who wins. You see, I've read the studies and confirmed the fact that 70 percent of the grocery shopping done in America is done by women. Surprise, surprise, boys. And let me tell you that I'm fully aware of the 17 percent of the grocery-shopping men out there. (Who does the other 13 percent? Circus animals?) And I'm sure those 17 percent evolved males strolling the aisles of the supermarkets of America doing the grocery shopping are very, very nice guys, but you and I both know that the rest of the men in America:

(a) Do it all wrong;

(b) Buy all the wrong things;

(c) Are slow as turtles;

(d) Wouldn't know how to get all the ingredients together to make a meal if their lives depended on it;

(e) Can't think a week's worth of anything;

(f) Haven't had the experience necessary to perform the "art" of grocery shopping, keeping a house stocked with foods, feeding a family, organizing a pantry and fridge.

There isn't a man alive who can grocery shop properly. Oh, maybe one or two out there can do it well, but really, I am not being sexist or anything other than honest by suggesting that it's been a woman's job (political statement to follow) for centuries, and we've mastered the art. So you 17 percent, don't write angry letters to me saying I'm being unfair or stereotypical by not handing you a medal of evolvement, because I'm not gonna. We've been doing it for years; we are very, very good at it; we've been getting too little credit because it isn't easy; and that's just the way it is, bottom line. Ladies, you know what I'm saying, and before we continue I've got to stop and make my political statement about grocery shopping. Would you give me a minute, please? . . . It would be impossible for me to say "it's been a woman's job for centuries" without explaining, so please bear with me.

Women have been judged and valued for far too long on their ability to shop, whether it be for the children's school clothes or a ham—and it's over.

This is something that must change, because we do a bit more than shop, and changing it is . . . However, the bottom line is that when it comes to male or female behind the cart in the aisles of the American grocery store, we win, hands down.

In my family, I wear the pants behind the wheels of the grocery cart, and I usually take the whole family with me every week—the husband, the kids, and me. Don't ask me why, but I do.

The husband and I have been married for six years, and we've gone grocery shopping every week—most of the time twice a week, but for the sake of easy math, once a week for those six years. That means we've had over three hundred grocery shopping trips, three-hundred-plus times we've headed down the aisles of our local grocery store together. Same store, same aisles, for the most part, same groceries. You know what the kids will and won't eat, the snacks, the basics, and other than a creative whim, a holiday coming up, or a need to feed a relative, it's mostly the same stuff every week, right? So he has seen what kind of bread we buy and how many loaves we go through in a week three-hundred-plus times.

But on the rare occasion he's gone alone (usually because I was close to death and incapable of moving), he came back with the most amazing assortment of food you can imagine. Never once have I seen one of the old family staples; it's usually been stuff like:

Wild mushrooms.

The smallest bag of Trail Mix you've ever seen.

Imported beer from some far corner of the world—Icelandic Malt.

Frozen gourmet desserts—you know, the kind kids go wild over,
black cherry currant mint ice cream . . . useful foods!

The first couple of trips that the new husband made to the store were cute. But within months it took on a different tone. Livid? What do you think about furious? You see—and I'm talking to you right now as if you haven't a clue, but I know you do—when you're sick as can be and the cupboards are bare and the kids are wanting dinner, snacks, sodas, candy, cookies, and on and on and on and on, the husband comes home with gourmet coffee, some figs, and a few frozen dinners. . . .

It's during those moments, with the bare cupboards, desperately needing something more in the house to eat besides mint ice cream or wild mushrooms on rye, that his answers to the question, "Why can't you figure this out?" are never quite right. He just can't seem to explain to me why, after three hundred (and the number keeps increasing) trips to the store, he can't buy the right ingredients to make a sandwich or two. As hard as he tries, he can't figure it out.

So the husband, the kids, and I (amazing I don't drag the Prince along and complete our little family shopping group) are off to what for me is a psychologically traumatic journey.

YEAH . . . you get it. You've been there, and you know what I'm talking about. So that's where I found myself when the hub would go to the grocery store, and that's one of the big reasons we all go together. Always trying to teach Shopping 101, even after all these years, quality time with the kids (well, it's worth a shot), and the necessity of weekly grocery shopping all rolled into one. Now, do you understand why I think Valium every week??

In 1812, Brian Donkin, an Englishman, invented the tin can.

My shopping, the lists, the pattern, the kind of food I buy have changed dramatically in the last few years. But there's one thing that will never change.

I have a problem with stocking the fridge and cupboards, a really big problem. My fridge has to be overstuffed for me to feel there is enough food in the house. At this very moment my freezer is so overloaded with food that if you came over, you'd know this is childhood trauma at its best. Sometimes the vent at the top is so blocked with food that it can't get cold enough. Swear! True!

I overstock and fill the fridge to the point of ridiculousness because a full fridge that is opened and closed by people I love is a sign of love to me.

There it is—I said it—talked about something that's been bottled up for years. A fridge and access to it mean love to me. Done! Said publicly. Definite sigh of relief.

Let me take a moment and feel the empowerment that is sure to go along with that statement.

HAVING A MOMENT RIGHT HERE, RIGHT NOW . . .

Here we are acknowledging the fact that the fridge was, obviously, a big part of my emotional development, and it all started with, of course, my mother (wouldn't Freud be proud). My mother was a little intense when it came to the food/fridge thing. She wasn't very happy when we ate; it bothered her. She was very, very, very scheduled and rigid, and tromping through the house to the refrigerator, throwing the door open, and grabbing a drumstick didn't sit well with her at all. It's O.K. I can say that at thirty-six, but I have to tell you that she made an issue of it and responded in strange ways. Such as:

Wrapping food in white wax paper and labeling it.

Insisting that we "couldn't be hungry" even though we were.

Getting really, really angry when there was food eaten between meals. . . .

Which turned into:

My sneaking bowls of cereal late at night so Mom wouldn't know I was eating.

My brother and I (that was before he sold out to the *Globe*) grabbing food and running upstairs to eat.

All contributing, I'm sure, to my believing that a loving home is one with

an accessible full fridge. It also contributed to my grocery shopping extravaganza every week. You see, when I tell you that I come home every week
with bags and bags full of food, much more than is necessary, I'm not kidding.

But as I told you from the beginning of this book, I've worked like hell to
mature a bit in these last twenty-some-odd years, and as a result, my shopping habits have changed. My life has changed a lot, too; taking responsibility and growing up do it every time. A lot of energy has been spent on truly
trying to understand what my mom's issues were, and what I came up with
was that she was a human being, a woman of the 50's who did the best she
could with very little control over her own life while working within some
ridiculous rules about what a woman should or shouldn't be.

You and I may think that women have a long way to go, but when you
look back at what our mothers had to deal with, you have to feel sorry for
them. Mom may have handled the eating thing a little crazy, but she did the
best she could, and that's all you can ask from anyone.

That's just one level—it may be the deepest, but it's still only one—that has
influenced my shopping habits over the years. How about going from a stay-
at-home-and-work-my-butt-off mom to a career-out-of-the-house mom (not
for a second implying that being an at-home Mom isn't a career, because it's
the best career out there. Raising the next generation, what could be more
important?)?

An at-home coupon-clipping kind of gal, I was it. I'd clip every coupon in
sight, only to lose half of them, or I'd end up with a cartful of S.O.S. pads on
sale. I had hundreds of coupons every week, trying like crazy to be the wife
I thought I was supposed to be.

I scanned the papers every week, trying to figure out how these other
coupon heroes of mine did it. But standing at the checkout counter each
week, I never felt anything other than the big coupon loser up against these
women who cataloged, color-coded, and alphabetized their coupons and
ended up at the checkout line with the store owing them money. I swear I've
seen it, stood behind it, and gone home feeling the pain of it.

I failed in the coupon category miserably but excelled in the shopping list
category. Talk about pride. My shopping list was the most organized you've
ever seen. You want rigid, I'll give you rigid. Categorized—don't ask.
Amounts needed, brands preferred, menu suggestions beside each item—oh,
a list like no other in the neighborhood and that I took great pride in keeping updated.

Things have changed a lot because of some of the changes in my life. Now
if I can read the scribble on the eight little scraps of paper from the doodle
pad on the dashboard of my car (you know those damn things that never stay

stuck on) as I'm running through the store, while spending quality time with the kids as I shop—I'm proud.

Here's how it used to be.

The boys and I used to eat a big lunch and get ready for our shopping trip in the afternoon just after nap time. Never, ever did I go shopping with my stomach empty; you know what every article you read says about that:

> Don't go grocery shopping when you're what?
>
> Hungry.
>
> Or else what's going to happen?
>
> Buying everything in sight.
>
> Shopping with your stomach . . .
>
> You've been there a thousand times.

So, yeah, a lot has changed, but there are a couple of things that will never change, such as:

> Having to feed the family.
>
> Being responsible for putting the week's worth of food together for everyone.
>
> The pressure of it all when you insist, as I do, on taking the whole family.
>
> And the biggest lie of them all, the weekly shopping trip myth.

That once-a-week shopping concept is as big a lie as the fairy godmother. Nobody shops once a week. You and I both know that it's the run-back-to-the-store-four-times-a-week-to-get-what-you've-forgotten shopping trip that's real for most of us. Let's just tell the truth right here and now so that we can all stop feeling like unorganized slobs.

I'm always forgetting things, even in the days of the color-coded lists, with seven hundred organizers filled with the family's food needs. There were always those few ingredients for that special recipe I was trying that week, or the one emotionally connected warm fuzzy food that I didn't have enough of (usually needed right after one of the Prince's visits), or the extra diapers, bottles, mayo, whatever. Back in the old days I had the time to go back to the store—the energy, desire, strength, or hormonal balance was another issue, but time I had plenty of.

The boys are older now, so going grocery shopping with Mama, sitting in the grocery cart seat, isn't what it used to be. There were many weeks when grocery shopping was our main source of entertainment. When they were one and two, I could get away with it; they thought we were having big fun.

NOW, we've got to make one hundred stops before we get to the grocery store, and most of the time is spent with the kids staring at me in anticipation and asking questions like:

> Hey, Mom, when will we get home?
>
> Are we through yet?
>
> My friend is coming soon, and I could care less about food.

And how about this one that I heard the other day:

> Mom, Becky is calling me this afternoon. When are we gonna be home?

BECKY??? AS IN A GIRL, AS IN TALKING TO, DATING, EVENTUALLY MAR-RYING AND HAVING CHILDREN WITH. BECKY???

One of my sons talking to someone named Becky??? You could have shot me in the aisles and made me happier.

DON'T LEAVE ME, SON, AND RUN OFF INTO THE ARMS OF BECKY. And by the way . . .

> WHO IS BECKY?
>
> WHAT DOES SHE WANT WITH YOU?
>
> WHERE DID YOU MEET HER?
>
> WHAT'S GOING ON?
>
> WHAT CAN I DO??

Help me.
Guilt.
Confusion.
New trauma mixed in with the old. VALIUM??
So what'd I do?
Went into the longest spiel you've ever heard in my head about what had to be said at this very moment.
You really have to watch out for these eleven-year-old girls; I was one once . . .
Traumatic?

In 1894, Milton Hershey discovered how to make a bar of chocolate and began selling Hershey bars.

It's a miracle if we make it through the aisles without a major emotional setback or breakdown, but we do. Big market, Piggly Wiggly of yesteryear; good cart, bad cart. No matter where you go to get your food every week (or ten times a week), you, like me, have it ingrained in your brain that the best way to shop if you are going to stay out of trouble is by avoiding all the "scary" aisles.

Run from the cookie aisle.

Don't venture into the chips and snacks aisles.

Stay in the produce and fresh fish part of your store, and you'll be safe. Doody!!!!!

The women's magazines have been and are still sending that stupid message to anybody who wants to lose some weight, and they are wrong, wrong, wrong.

How long can anyone last in the produce part of the store?

BORRRRRRRRRRING . . .

And haven't they heard the thousand-year-old theory that the minute you tell someone they can't do something, whatever it is you said they can't do becomes the most important thing in their life?

If you want to become obsessed with snacking, all you have to do is tell yourself often enough that you can never go down the snack aisles in your grocery store, and watch what happens.

SNACK OBSESSED? YOU'LL NEVER WANT REAL FOOD AGAIN. IT'LL BE PROCESSED AND CORN CHIP–COATED FOR THE REST OF YOUR LIFE. GUARAN-DAMN-TEED.

To prove a theory I have, I made my own little market (not that I drew anything you see on the next few pages; I hired a graphic designer to do that because if I'd drawn our little shop, you'd have no clue what it is you're walking down).

If you know how many low-fat options you have in every aisle of your massive market and you can walk down them with confidence, without fear, and know that the choice is yours, your grocery-shopping life will never be the same. What do you think? Wanna go shopping and have a look at some great low-fat options?

I'm gonna start with the produce section so we can get it out of the way, right along with the diet mentality that the only things you can eat to lose weight are carrot and celery sticks. A public declaration right here and now: I hate salads. Celery sticks are disgusting. Carrot sticks have no appeal at all. And produce is not what I'm talking about when I, like a good Italian mama, say, EAT, EAT, EAT, EAT, EAT, EAT.

But produce is good. You can do a lot with veggies and fruits, and other than a few things such as avocados and coconuts, everything you look at is low fat . . . so it's not a bad section, if you know what I mean.

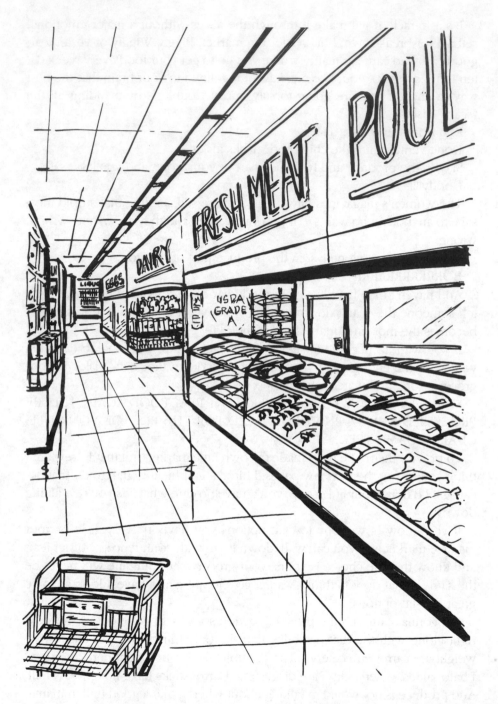

BRAND	ITEM NAME	CALORIES	PER SERVING FAT GRAMS	FAT%
DELI				
Peter Eckrich	Deli Lite Ham	30	1	30
Wilson's	Continental Deli Honey Cured Cooked Ham	70	2	26
Healthy Choice	Corned Beef	60	1.5	23
Healthy Choice	Pastrami	60	1.5	23
Healthy Choice	Oven Roasted Turkey Breast	45	0	0
Healthy Choice	Skinless Chicken Breast	45	0	0
Healthy Choice	Virginia Ham	60	1.5	23
Healthy Choice	Honey Ham	60	1.5	23
Alpine Lace	Cheddar Cheese	45	0	0
COOKIES/CRACKERS/POPCORN				
Keebler	Wheatables 50% reduced fat	130	3.5	24
Keebler	Townhouse Classic Crackers 50% reduced fat	70	2	26
Keebler	Golden Vanilla Wafers Reduced Fat	130	3.5	24
Keebler	Zesta Soup Crackers	60	2	30
Keebler	Elfin Delights Chocolate with Fudge Creme, 50% reduced fat	150	3.5	21
Keebler	Elfin Delights Cream Sandwich Cookie 50% Reduced Fat	150	3.5	21
Keebler	Elfin Delights Chocolate with Vanilla Creme, 50% reduced fat	150	3.5	21
Keebler	Elfin Delights Devil's Food Cookies, 50% reduced fat	70	0	0
Keebler	Honey Graham Selects Old-Fashioned Graham Crackers, Low Fat	120	1.5	11
Keebler	Cinnamon Crisp Graham Crackers, Low Fat	110	1.5	12
Keebler	Iced Animal Cookies	140	4.5	29
Keebler	Elfin Delights Caramel Apple Oatmeal Cookies, 50% reduced fat	70	1.5	19
Keebler	Zesta Fat Free Saltine Crackers	50	0	0
Keebler	Zesta 50% Reduced Sodium Saltines	60	2	30
Keebler	Zesta Original Saltines	60	2	30
Keebler	Club Partners Garlic Bread Crackers	60	2	30
President's Choice	English Style Ginger Snaps	130	4	28
President's Choice	A Family Arrowroot Cookie	140	4	26
President's Choice	Animal Crackers	150	5	30

continued

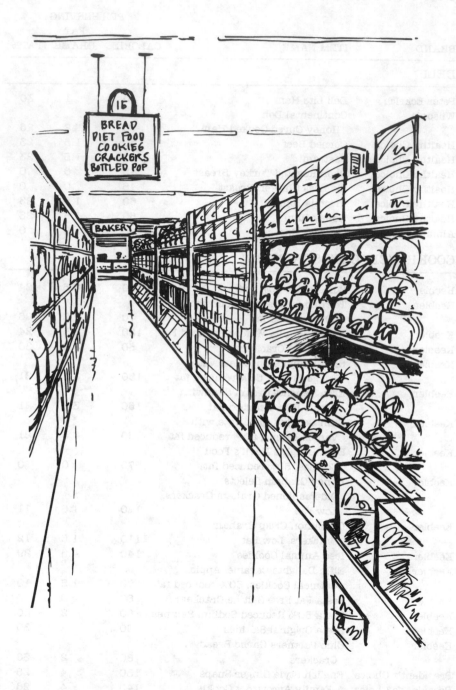

BREAD
DIET FOOD
COOKIES
CRACKERS
BOTTLED POP

15

BAKERY

BRAND	ITEM NAME	CALORIES	PER SERVING FAT GRAMS	FAT%
President's Choice	Cheese Top Hat Crackers	90	3	30
Mega	Animal Crackers	130	4	28
Nabisco	Famous Chocolate Wafers	140	4	26
Nabisco	Old Fashioned Gingersnaps	120	2.5	19
Nabisco	Premium Soup & Oyster Crackers	60	1.5	23
Nabisco	Honey Maid Cinnamon Grahams	140	3	19
Nabisco	Grahams	120	3	23
Nabisco	Nilla Wafers	140	5	32
Nabisco	Original Premium Saltine Crackers	60	1.5	23
Nabisco	Low Sodium Premium Saltine Crackers	60	1	15
Nabisco	Multigrain Premium Saltine Crackers	60	1.5	23
Nabisco	Unsalted Tops Premium Saltine Crackers	60	1.5	23
Nabisco	Fat Free Premium Saltine Crackers	50	1	18
Nabisco	Barnum's Animal Crackers	140	4	26
Food Club	Honey Grahams	120	3	23
Food Club	Fig Bars	120	3	23
Nabisco	Mr. Phipps Barbecue	130	4	28
Nabisco	Mr. Phipps Original	120	4.5	34
Nabisco	Mr. Phipps Sour Cream & Onion	130	4	28
Nabisco	Mr. Phipps Pretzel Chips Original	130	2.5	19
Nabisco	Mr. Phipps Pretzel Chips Fat Free	100	0	0
Nabisco	Mr. Salty Pretzel Twists	110	0.5	4
Nabisco	Mr. Salty Fat Free Twists	120	0	0
Nabisco	Triscuit Garden Herb	130	4.5	31
Nabisco	Fig Newtons	110	2.5	20
Nabisco	Fat Free Fig Newtons	100	0	0
Nabisco	Fat Free Fig Newtons—Cranberry	100	0	0
Nabisco	Fat Free Fig Newtons—Strawberry	100	0	0
Nabisco	Fat Free Fig Newtons—Apple	100	0	0
Nabisco	Fat Free Fig Newtons—Raspberry	100	0	0
Nabisco	Teddy Grahams—Cinnamon	140	4	26
Nabisco	Ritz Crackers, Reduced Fat	70	2.5	32
Nabisco	Garden Crisp Vegetable Crackers	130	3.5	24
Nabisco	Harvest Crisp Oat Crackers	140	5	32
Nabisco	Harvest Crisp 5 Grain Crackers	130	3.5	24
Nabisco	Reduced Fat Triscuits	130	3	21
Snackwells	Classic Golden Crackers	60	1	15
Snackwells	Cracked Pepper Crackers	60	0	0
Snackwells	Cinnamon Graham Snacks	110	0	0
Snackwells	Wheat Crackers	60	0	0
Snackwells	Chocolate Chip Cookies	130	3.5	24

continued

BRAND	ITEM NAME	CALORIES	PER SERVING FAT GRAMS	FAT%
Snackwells	Cheese Crackers	130	2	14
Snackwells	Double Fudge Cookie Cakes	50	0	0
Snackwells	Creme Sandwich Cookies	110	2.5	20
Snackwells	Chocolate Sandwich Cookies with Chocolate Creme	100	2.5	23
Frookie	Fat Free Banana Cookies	45	0	0
Frookie	Fat Free Cranberry/Orange	90	0	0
Frookie	Fat Free Oatmeal Raisin	90	0	0
Murray	Iced Chocolate Cookies—Low Fat	120	2	15
Murray	Iced Lemon Cookies—Low Fat	130	1.5	10
Murray	Gingersnaps—Low Fat	120	1.5	11
Pepperidge Farm	Fruitful Raspberry Tarts	120	3	23
Pepperidge Farm	Fruitful Peach Tarts	120	3	23
Pepperidge Farm	Fruitful Cherry Cobbler Tarts	70	2	26
General Mills	Crisp Baked Bugles	130	2.5	17
Popsecret	Pop Chips—Butter	130	3.5	24
Franklin	Crunch 'n Munch Butter Toffee Popcorn with Peanuts	140	4	26
Franklin	Crunch 'n Munch Caramel Popcorn with Peanuts	140	3	19
Rold Gold	Pretzels Tiny Twists	110	1	8
Eagle	Pretzels Sourdough Hard Bavarian	110	0	0
Planters	Pretzel Twists	100	5	45
Burns & Recker	Crispini-Sesame	110	3	25
Stella D'Oro	Fat Free Breadsticks—Original	60	0	0
Stella D'Oro	Fat Free Breadsticks—Garlic	60	0	0
Tostitos	Baked Cool Ranch Chips	120	3	23
Tostitos	Baked chips	110	1	8
Snyder's of Hanover	Sourdough Hard Pretzels	111	0	0
Guiltless Gourmet	White Corn Chips	110	1	8
Guiltless Gourmet	Nacho Chips	110	1	8
Smart Temptations	Original Chips	110	1	8
Louise's Fat Free	Potato Chips Barbecue	110	0	0
Louise's Fat Free	Potato Chips Vinegar & Salt	100	0	0
Louise's Fat Free	Potato Maui Onion	110	0	0
Louise's Fat Free	Potato Chips Original	110	0	0
Louise's Fat Free	Nacho Cheese Tortilla Chips	130	3	21
Louise's Fat Free	Popcorn, lightly salted	130	1.5	10
Weight Watchers	Smart Snackers Popcorn	100	1	9
Betty Crocker	Pop Secret By Request Popcorn	130	2.5	17
Orville Redenbacher	Butter Light Popcorn	140	5	32
Orville Redenbacher	Smart Pop	100	2	18

BRAND	ITEM NAME	PER SERVING CALORIES	FAT GRAMS	FAT%
Orville Redenbacher	Natural Light	80	0	0

FROZEN SNACKS

BRAND	ITEM NAME	CALORIES	FAT GRAMS	FAT%
Blue Bell	Light Ice Cream Vanilla	100	2	18
Blue Bell	Light Ice Cream Strawberry Sundae	110	2	16
Blue Bell	Light Ice Cream Vanilla Fudge	110	2.5	20
Blue Bell	Light Ice Cream Dutch Chocolate	100	2	18
Blue Bell	Light Ice Cream Cherry, Vanilla & Fudge	110	2	16
Blue Bell	Diet Strawberry	100	0	0
Blue Bell	Diet Neopolitan	100	0	0
Blue Bell	Diet Vanilla Bean	100	0	0
Blue Bell	Diet Chocolate	100	0	0
Blue Bell	Diet Orange Pineapple	100	0	0
Breyers	Frozen Yogurt Chocolate	150	4	24
Breyers	Frozen Yogurt Vanilla	140	4	26
Breyers	Light Ice Cream Natural Vanilla	130	4.5	31
Breyers	Reduced Fat Ice Cream Praline Almond Crunch	140	5	32
Healthy Choice	Premium Low-Fat Ice Cream Fudge Brownie	120	2	15
Healthy Choice	Premium Low-Fat Ice Cream Vanilla	100	2	18
Healthy Choice	Premium Low-Fat Ice Cream Rocky Road	140	2	13
Healthy Choice	Premium Low-Fat Ice Cream Bordeaux Cherry Chocolate Chip	110	2	16
Healthy Choice	Double Fudge Swirl	120	2	15
Ben & Jerry's	Frozen Yogurt Double Fudge Brownie	190	4	19
Ben & Jerry's	Frozen Yogurt Cherry Garcia	170	3	16
TCBY	Gourmet Collection French Silk Chocolate	150	4	24
TCBY	Gourmet Collection Chocolate Covered Cherry	150	3	18
Dole	Strawberry Sorbet	100	0	0
Häagen-Dazs	Frozen Yogurt Raspberry Rendezvous	130	1.5	10
Häagen-Dazs	Frozen Yogurt Orange Tango	130	1	7
Häagen-Dazs	Frozen Yogurt Chocolate	160	2.5	14
Häagen-Dazs	Frozen Yogurt Coffee	160	2.5	14
I Can't Believe It's Yogurt	Non fat with Nutrasweet Frozen Yogurt Razzleberry	100	0	0

continued

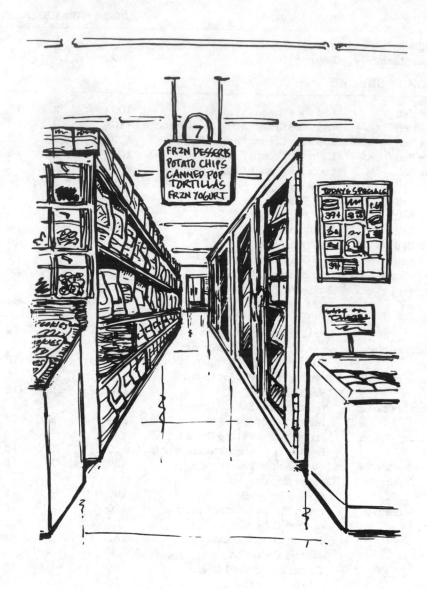

BRAND	ITEM NAME	PER SERVING CALORIES	FAT GRAMS	FAT%
I Can't Believe It's Yogurt	Non fat with Nutrasweet Frozen Yogurt Not Just Plain Yogurt	90	0	0
Blue Bunny	Citrus Snacks	50	0	0
Blue Bunny	Sweet Freedom Fudge Lites	70	0.5	6
Nestlé	The Flintstones Cool Cream Push Up	90	2	20
Nestlé	The Flintstones Original Push Up	100	2	18
Starburst	Low Fat Frozen Yogurt Snacks Strawberry	70	1	13
Starburst	Low Fat Frozen Yogurt Snacks Raspberry	70	1	13
Blue Bell	Mini Light Sandwiches	80	1.5	17
Klondike	Light Sandwiches	100	2.5	23
7Up	Spot Coolers	40	0	0
Popsicle	Ice Pops	45	0	0
Popsicle	Firecrackers	40	0	0
Creamsicle	Original Cream Bars	100	3	27
Fudgsicle	Original Fudge Pops	60	0.5	8
Dole	Fruit 'N Juice Raspberry	70	0	0
Dole	Fruit 'N Juice Strawberry	70	0	0
Dole	Fruit Juice Variety Pack	45	0	0
Welch's	Fruit Juice Bars	45	0	0
Luigi's	Real Italian Ice Cherry	120	0	0

CEREAL

BRAND	ITEM NAME	CALORIES	FAT GRAMS	FAT%
Nabisco	Team	220	0	0
Nabisco	Shredded Wheat 'n Bran	200	1	5
Nabisco	Frosted Wheat Bites	190	1	5
Nabisco	Shredded Wheat	160	0.5	3
Health Valley	Organic Raisin Bran Flakes	110	0	0
Health Valley	Organic Fiber 7 Flakes	100	0	0
Ralston	Corn Chex	110	0	0
Ralston	Rice Chex	120	0	0
Ralston	100% Whole Grain Chex	190	1	5
Ralston	Cookie Crisp	120	1.5	11
Post	Raisin Bran	190	1	5
Post	Banana Nut Crunch	120	3	23
Post	Alpha Bits	130	1	7
Post	Cocoa Pebbles	120	1	8
Post	Fruity Pebbles	110	1	8
Post	Great Grains Crunchy Pecan	220	6	25
Post	Great Grains Raisin, Date, Pecan	210	5	21
Quaker	Oat Squares	220	3	12
Quaker	Cap'n Crunch	110	1.5	12
Quaker	Cap'n Crunch Peanut Butter	110	2.5	20

continued

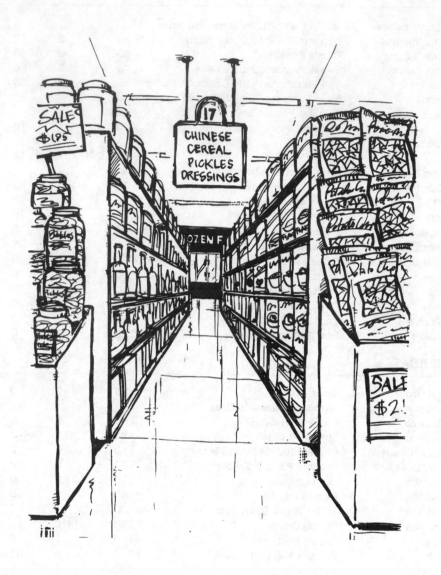

| | | PER SERVING | | |
| | | | FAT | |
BRAND	ITEM NAME	CALORIES	GRAMS	FAT%
General Mills	Kix	120	1	8
General Mills	Berry Berry Kix	120	1.5	11
General Mills	Cheerios	110	2	16
General Mills	Multigrain Cheerios	110	1	8
General Mills	Honey Nut Cheerios	120	1.5	11
General Mills	Apple Cinnamon Cheerios	120	2.5	19
General Mills	Wheaties	110	1	8
General Mills	Oatmeal Crisp with Apples	210	2.5	11
General Mills	Oatmeal Crisp with Almonds	230	6	23
General Mills	Oatmeal Crisp with Raisins	210	3	13
General Mills	Total Whole Grain	100	0.5	5
General Mills	Total Corn Flakes	110	0.5	4
General Mills	Crispy Wheats 'n Raisins	190	1	5
General Mills	Basic 4	210	3	13
Kellogg's	Cocoa Krispies	120	0.5	4
Kellogg's	Rice Krispies	110	0	0
Kellogg's	Special K	110	0	0
Kellogg's	Raisin Bran	170	1	5
Kellogg's	Corn Pops	110	0	0
Kellogg's	Smacks	110	0.5	4
Kellogg's	Corn Flakes	110	0	0
Kellogg's	Froot Loops	120	1	8
Kellogg's	Nutri Grain Golden Wheat	100	0.5	5
Kellogg's	Nutri Grain Golden Wheat & Raisins	180	1	5
Kellogg's	Nutri Grain Almond Raisin	200	3	14
Kellogg's	Low-Fat Granola without Raisins	210	3	13
Kellogg's	Low-Fat Granola with Raisins	210	3	13
Kellogg's	Frosted Mini-Wheats	190	1	5
Kellogg's	Nut & Honey Crunch	120	2	15
Kellogg's	Frosted Flakes	120	0	0
Kellogg's	Product 19	110	0	0
Kellogg's	Pop-Tarts Crunch Frosted Strawberry	120	1	8
Kellogg's	Pop-Tarts Crunch Frosted Brown Sugar Cinnamon	120	1	8
Kellogg's	Crispix	110	0	0

No choices? You have to stay only in the produce section? No way! I went shopping to give you an idea of some of the choices out there. I'm not endorsing these brands I'm just giving you an idea of where the fat is or isn't.

• •

So you have some options, but in order to qualify as the fat detective that you want so badly to be, you must have the ultimate weapon: the fat formula in your brain, ready to use along with your calculator. The piece of equipment necessary every time you go to the store.

LABEL READING

In case you don't or have no clue who I am (my first question is, Why'd you buy a book written by someone when you have no clue who she is?) or skipped chapters one and two, then let's cover the fat formula again so you have it down:

Number of fat grams x 9 = X

X divided by the total calories.

This will tell you what you want to know: how much fat per serving is in the food you are eating.

When you're talking shopping, should you believe what the labels say?

No, no, no, no, no, no. Don't do it. That will only get you more hidden fat than you can possibly imagine. Let's review or introduce, depending on where you're at with this label reading stuff . . .

Believing the labels will get you what? FAT.

Most things that say "98% fat free," "lean," "light," or "low fat" are what? A LIE.

Your weapon against the lie? The FAT FORMULA.

But no need to worry, you might be saying, because you've heard about the "new label laws" that have been passed by someone, somehow, during the last couple of years. There's no need for the fat formula. You don't have to do anything because it's been done for you.

WRONG

STOP

WATCH OUT

New label laws and David Kessler, the commissioner of the FDA, are joined at the hip.

Every major talk show, magazine, and newspaper that I've watched or read these days has featured this guy. Do you know who he is? Do you know what he looks like? Do you have a clue what he's talking about? Do the old labels that never made sense now make sense?

I've gotta tell you that I know this guy big time. Forget the fact that low-fat labeling means a lot to me. Don't even consider the fact that it's what I've been talking about nonstop for the last couple of years. Here's the real deal. For longer than you can imagine, I've been trying to communicate with David.

If you read *Stop the Insanity!* (pardon the personal plug), then you know that I've written to him. If you've ever seen me on national TV, then you know that I've asked him about this issue over and over again—with no response.

How about that $2.3 billion of taxpayers' money—that is, yours and mine—that was spent on the new labels?

Do they tell us what we want to know?

Davey, they don't.

Why not?

I've been asking, and you haven't been responding, Dave. Talk to me, Dave. What's the story?

If it's a story you want, then it's a story I've got for you about David Kessler. As I said, not many people have had the chance to see David until recently. It's as if only recently have they let him out of his cave to promote the wonder of the labels, and it took leaving the country for me to have a look at the man I've been speaking to for the last couple of years.

It was in London a few weeks ago that I first got to see him (don't I sound like the world traveler?). I'm lying in bed after a very long day watching one of the four channels they have over there. (Yes, four—as in three more than the one I was watching. Boy, if you ever want to miss something American, get used to having 150 channels to switch among and then have all but four taken away.) And there he was—David.

Not quite as handsome as I thought he'd be.

Had a nice air of trust, boy-next-door kind of thing going on, which is very commissiony.

I felt as though I was seeing my pen pal, long-lost lover, the man who was finally going to answer my questions. It was a moment, for sure.

Let's have a look at the work my long-lost lover has just done. The new labels on our food:

• •

American Cheese

NUTRITION FACTS

SERVING SIZE	1 SLICE	(21 grams)	CALORIES			70
SERVINGS		16	FAT CALORIES			45

AMOUNT/SERVING		%DV*	AMOUNT/SERVING			%DV*
TOTAL FAT	5 grams	8%	TOTAL CARBOHYDRATE	2 grams		1%
SAT FAT	3 grams	17%	FIBER	0 grams		0%
CHOLESTEROL	15 mgs	6%	SUGARS	1 grams		
SODIUM	290 mgs	12%	PROTEIN	4 grams		
VITAMIN A		6%	CALCIUM			10%
VITAMIN C		0%	IRON			0%

*PERCENT DAILY VALUES (DV) ARE BASED ON A 2,000 CALORIE DIET.

You turn Davey's new labels around and what you see is 5 grams of fat and right next to it, 8 percent, So you pick it up, go home, make your cheese sandwich, and all you've had is 8 percent fat. Oh, you know that there are 2 grams of total carbs, because Dave and his boys have made that clear, and 290 mg of sodium (yee hah, that's pretty damn high, isn't it?), otherwise known as 12 percent. Everything's listed, everything's fine.

Except for one thing. It's about as misleading as you can get. Let me explain.

Do the fat formula:

5 x 9 = 45

45 divided by 70 = 64 percent

So Dave, hear this, Dave. This food is 64 percent fat per serving. Your expensive new labeling is not telling us the information we want to know, unless we do the fat formula ourselves. Do you understand that, boys at the FDA?

Bologna

NUTRITION FACTS

SERVING SIZE	1 SLICE	(28 grams)	CALORIES			90
SERVINGS PER CONTAINER		8	FAT CALORIES			70

AMOUNT/SERVING		%DV*	AMOUNT/SERVING			%DV*
TOTAL FAT	8 grams	12%	TOTAL CARBOHYDRATE	0 grams		0%
SATURATED FAT	3 grams	15%	PROTEIN	3 grams		
CHOLESTEROL	20mg	7%	IRON			2%
SODIUM	270 mgs	11%				

*PERCENT DAILY VALUES (DV) ARE BASED ON A 2,000 CALORIE DIET.

Mr. Mayer, I'm looking at your label, and what I see is that total fat is 8 grams, then I see 12 percent. Above that—kind of boring, if you really look; not something you pay as much attention to—is something that says "Fat calories 70."

"Fat calories 70"—what the hell are you talking about? What does that mean to my health? "Fat calories 70" under "Calories 90"—what are you talking about?

I'm gonna do my fat formula.

8 x 9 = 72

72 divided by 90 = 80 percent fat per serving.

So now I've got 12 percent, something going on.

I've 70 and 90 going on.

And I've got what I want to know—that each serving of this food is 80 percent fat.

See, what you guys have done is confuse me more. Now I have three or four little games to play before I get what I want . . . and you're basing everything you're telling me not on total fat but on "daily value."

I've got your daily value.

You've taken something so simple and screwed it up.

Do the rest yourself; see what you think.

Check out these labels for yourself: You'll be amazed!

Green Onion Dip

NUTRITION FACTS

SERVING SIZE	2 TBSP	(31 grams)	CALORIES		60
SERVINGS		ABOUT 7	FAT CALORIES		40

AMOUNT/SERVING		%DV*	AMOUNT/SERVING		%DV*
TOTAL FAT	4 grams	6%	TOTAL CARBOHYDRATE	4 grams	1%
SATURATED FAT	3 grams	15%	FIBER	0 grams	0%
CHOLESTEROL	0 mgs	0%	SUGARS	less than 1 gram	
SODIUM	190 mgs	8%	PROTEIN	1 gram	
VITAMIN A		0%	CALCIUM		0%
VITAMIN C		0%	IRON		0%

*PERCENT DAILY VALUES (DV) ARE BASED ON A 2,000 CALORIE DIET.

Frozen Pie Crust

NUTRITION FACTS

SERVING SIZE	⅛ of one-crust (27 grams)	CALORIES		110
SERVINGS PER CONTAINER	16	CALORIES FROM FAT		60

AMOUNT/SERVING		%DV*	AMOUNT/SERVING		%DV*
TOTAL FAT	7 grams	11%	TOTAL CARBOHYDRATE	12 grams	4%
SATURATED FAT	3 grams	15%	DIETARY FIBER	0 grams	0%
CHOLESTEROL	5 mgs	2%	SUGARS	0 grams	
SODIUM	140 mgs	6%	PROTEIN	less than 1 gram	
VITAMIN A		0%	CALCIUM		0%
VITAMIN C		0%	IRON		0%

*PERCENT DAILY VALUES ARE BASED ON A 2,000 CALORIE DIET. YOUR DAILY VALUES MAY BE HIGHER OR LOWER DEPENDING ON YOUR CALORIE NEEDS:

	CALORIES:	2,000	2,500
TOTAL FAT	less than	65 grams	80 grams
SAT FAT	less than	20 grams	25 grams
CHOLESTEROL	less than	300 mgs	300 mgs
SODIUM	less than	2,400 mgs	2,400 mgs
TOTAL CARBOHYDRATE		300 grams	375 grams
DIETARY FIBER		25 grams	30 grams

CALORIES PER GRAM:	
FAT	9
CARBOHYDRATE	4
PROTEIN	4

26% Vegetable Oil Spread

NUTRITION FACTS

SERVING SIZE	1 TBSP	(14 grams)	CALORIES		35
SERVINGS PER CONTAINER		32	CALORIES FROM FAT		35

AMOUNT/SERVING		%DV*	AMOUNT/SERVING		%DV*
TOTAL FAT	4 grams	6%	CHOLESTEROL	0 mgs	0%
SATURATED FAT	0 grams	0%	SODIUM	50 mgs	2%
POLYUNSATURATED FAT	1 gram		TOTAL CARBOHYDRATE	0 grams	0%
MONOUNSATURATED FAT	1.5 grams		PROTEIN	0 grams	

VITAMIN A 10% (30% as beta carotene)

NOT A SIGNIFICANT SOURCE OF DIETARY FIBER, SUGARS, VITAMIN C, CALCIUM, AND IRON.

*PERCENT DAILY VALUES (DV) ARE BASED ON A 2,000 CALORIE DIET.

• •

From this you can see two things: that the new labels coming to a super store near you soon still require you to use the fat formula, and that old Davey doesn't do a very good job—typical of the men I pick, wouldn't you say?

Hey, FDA, how much fat is in this serving of food I'm about to eat? That's what you forgot to tell me.

I think you and I need to do something. Take the checkbook away from Dave, would ya? The guy just doesn't know how to spend our cash.

> I ran out and bought beans and spices. . . . My husband was working the pro-gram without really noticing until he had to pull his belt tighter.
>
> —*Bonnie, Lewiston, Maine*

Well, I don't know about you, but I'm tired. Shopping is tough, even on the written page, and we're almost done. There is just one little section of the grocery store that we have to talk about, because it's new—just added and very confusing to some people: the health food section. That aisle in the store that has stuff you can't pronounce. How about those rice cakes—would you ever buy them? When you see bags of beans and grains, do you have a clue as to what to do with them? I've gotta get something off my chest before we mosey down the health food aisle.

Just because it says health food doesn't mean it is low fat. The avocado sandwich? Nuts? Oil—virgin, pressed, and all very high in fat? But what's happening in the supermarkets all over this country, going hand in hand with the changes taking place at our Thanksgiving table, is the addition of the health food aisles in our grocery stores. No incense, no funky smells, and for-get about bulk bins. If you want grains, beans, rice cakes, low-fat, non-dairy, wheat-free cookies (something you may have been asking yourself about just last week—wonder where those wheat-free cookies could be?), soups by manufacturers you've never heard of but worth a try, crackers out the yin-yang, chips, energy bars, then this is the place to find it.

Try some of the stuff. Ramen, why not? Sauces different from anything you've ever seen in your life? Go ahead. Don't just walk down this aisle in fear, strut down, knowing one thing: All you have to do here is read the labels and decide what ingredients you want going into your body. Don't be fooled—but, hey, you've already got that down.

So here we go, summing up the old fat detective shopping tips and changing the way we shop forever.

- Be the ultimate fat detective.

- Read, read, read the labels.

- Look left, right, up, and down.

- Ask the manager for certain high-volume, low-fat brands.

- Request that they carry more low-fat anything.

- Make friends with the deli manager and suggest low-fat pasta, tuna, salad selections, oil-free anything, soups without fat, beans, rice dishes. You'd be amazed at how much you can change by sucking up to the manager of each department and making some high-volume, low-fat suggestions.

- Start a campaign. Tell the world that this is the only store in town trying to change.

- The bakery—same thing. Swear. You can get them to do low-fat versions of those muffins, banana bread, cakes. Why not? If we don't speak up, how are the owners, managers, food brokers of these places ever gonna know that we want things to change?

- Remember, there's power in numbers. Talk to your friends. Start a letter-writing campaign. Let the manager know that you're happy with the low-fat options.

See, there's nothing to it. All you have to do is become a radical, sign-waving, Congress-writing maniac. . . .

CHAPTER 5
EATING OUT

You've shopped, and you've learned more about fat than you ever thought you would or could. Forget about making a commitment, that's a given, because you're probably already dreaming about exactly what you're going to look like as you start getting leaner and leaner and leaner.

Over the years I've seen and heard about some amazing transformations in life-style that have led to the most unbelievable changes in weight, health, life. This is no longer my story, I've been upstaged in a big way. This is the story of thousands and thousands of women who are changing the way they look and feel. My weight loss and life-style change is nothing compared to so many other wonderful physical, emotional, and spiritual changes I've heard about over the years.

We are all different and have different goals and dreams. Each one of us has a different body that has different changes to be made in order for us to love the way we look and, most important, the way we feel. But there's something we all have in common, the same phobia. Over and over again I've seen and heard about it. The minute we start changing our eating habits—going from high-fat, clueless, what's-at-eye-level to low-fat, thought-about, aware-of-what-you-are-putting-into-your-mouth eating, we all get hit with a bad case of the FEAR OF EATING OUT. It never fails.

The what-can-I-eat-when-I-go-out question pops up every time because you're scared . . .

Scared that all this info means you'll end up in the kitchen all day.

Afraid that in order to get lean you'll have to quit your job and do nothing but cook.

Sure that getting lean, cutting back on your daily fat intake, means you'll never be able to go out to dinner with your friends again.

Desperately worried that you'll never drive through again in your life.

You're visualizing a future of long lists of food, lots of thought, and no convenience at all.

WRONG, WRONG, WRONG. Remember choices, ladies, choices. Living versus dying. Eating versus starvation. That's what this whole Stopping the Insanity—FOOD thing is all about. Food means:

> Food anywhere.
> Food always.
> Food forever.

And that includes eating out, because who eats in anymore?

When is the last time you baked your own bread? Do you even know bread needs to be baked, or did you just think it grew in slices on the bread tree and was picked, loafed, and put into plastic? Chives, basil, coriander— quick, what are they? When a recipe tells you to sprinkle a bit of fresh shiitake on your dish, do you have a clue what it is? Would you know fresh coriander if it hit you on the head? I wouldn't. I don't have an herb garden and never want one.

I tried like hell to bake bread. Hated it.

Veggie garden? Why, when the store has everything I want? Forget about this gourmet, garden-your-own, fresh anything—let's get real and talk about what America is really doing and how we can still do it and not all die of heart disease and suffer from obesity while we are on the way to clogging those arteries, shall we?

EATING OUT. That's what we are all doing in droves—but it's perfectly understandable why you think everyone in your child's play group understands holistic medicine but you.

Millet, known to all!

Kasha, everyone's favorite cereal!

Wheat grass on everyone's mind and in everyone's bloodstream, sucking bacteria and building their immune systems—everyone but you.

You think everybody gets this stuff because everybody is walking around pretending to understand. It's not politically correct to tell the truth anymore—MYTH SMASH NUMBER 1,000,000,000,000,001.

Nobody understands what homeopathy is. Holistic medicine is on the tip of everybody's tongue, but ask someone to define it.

Everyone is clueless about what vitamins to take, and nobody I've met bakes his or her own bread. It's just the thing to talk about right now, and once the media get their grubby little hands on something, they milk it dry. Who would know that better than me?

LEAN AND MEAN . . .

BROTHER SAYS . . .

EX-DANCER SAYS . . .

FITNESS GURU SCREAMS . . .

It never ends, but thank goodness you and I have the opportunity through books, seminars, tapes, etc., to chat, clear it all up, and get on with the truth. And let me tell you when it comes to America eating out, here are the facts on this one.

Let's take a little quiz about what's really happening at breakfast, lunch, and dinner in America. The best place to start is with fast-food facts and figures, because they are amazing, and they're the most politically incorrect thing to talk about when it comes to the food we are living on: the drive-through with the mostest.

(a) How many fast-food restaurants do you think there are in this country?

Seventy-five thousand. *Holy moly. Who'd have thought there were that many of anything anywhere! Who do you think is eating at all these fast-food joints? You gotta have a whole lot of people walking through each and every one of these places to keep them open.*

(b) How many people do you think McDonald's serves in a day?

Eighteen million people daily. *That's the size of China, isn't it? What's that times seven days a week? Is there a number big enough???*

(c) How much of the population eats daily at fast-food restaurants?

One-fifth. *THAT MUCH DAILY?*

HAAAAAAAAAAAAAAAAAA!!!! Nobody is eating out? And double the working moms of this country are suddenly going to stop driving through and go bake some bread? And let us not assume (sounded like a priest, didn't I?) that people who eat at fast-food restaurants don't care about how they look and feel, because they do. Is it that the working mother could care less about obesity or heart disease? Do you think that she's just fine with being overfat?

Being tired as hell is something she's fine with? NOOOOOOOOOOOOOOO
OOOOOOOOOOOOO.

Check out some of these fast food fat facts:

🎵 The typical fast-food-restaurant breakfast is bacon (81 percent fat), ham
(70 percent fat), or eggs (63 percent fat), all fried in butter (100 percent fat).
A big country breakfast with sausage at Hardee's contains 1,005 calories
and is 66% fat.

🎵 Fifty-five percent of the calories in a McDonald's Big Mac comes from fat.

We didn't ask but just assumed that whatever was in the food we were eating was O.K. So what if there were a few things in the ingredients that we
couldn't pronounce? I mean, we may have known that it wasn't the best food
in town, but did we know how high fat it was? We may not have known because we didn't want to up until now or because we had fallen under the
we-care-so-much-about-you-and-your-kids-and-wouldn't-do-anything-to-
harm-you-so-do-come-and-have-a-great-time-with-our-dancing-bears-and-
cartoon-characters-and-don't-ask-any-questions spell that most of these
places have us under.

It's similar to the label lies. For years we didn't ask, we just assumed that
whatever was in the food we were eating was O.K. Surely the food manufacturers wouldn't put anything in our food supply that would hurt us?

Surely?

Well, it's the same thinking when it comes to those cute little clowns, that
jumping-box guy, the friendly smiling faces at the counter. Without questioning, we've eaten and eaten and eaten, and the price we have paid is high:
obesity, heart disease, you or someone you love dearly having a heart attack.
Old Wendy (whoever the hell she is) isn't going to help you get through the
day when you don't have the energy to live your life. And Arby, what does
he know!

> Today I took my son to IHOP. . . . We split a bowl of oatmeal, two big bagels,
> and I had a pot of coffee. No cream cheese, and they were delicious! In my "past"
> life: cheese omelet, hash browns, bacon, and a big glass of whole milk. Now I felt
> full, healthy, and alive.
>
> —*Traci, Glendale, Arizona*

We have to find out the facts and make some simple changes—different
choices are necessary—if you want to get lean, strong, and healthy or if you
just don't want to consume a month's worth of fat in one meal. We'll talk. You
can't eat that everything-high-fat-on-the-plate meal every morning at your fa-

vorite diner without paying the price, but never eating again at a fast-food restaurant isn't necessary—it's not even a consideration. Why would it be?

Talk about a social outcast—no thanks. Anything with drive through is out for the rest of my life? It ain't gonna work. But guess what will? Thinking. Learning. Making different choices at the counter and cutting back on your fat intake. That's what works, and here it is. Examples of what is, what isn't, what could be, and what can't be. Then you decide. Fast living, fast times, fast foods . . . Sounds like another country-western song. (I've written the titles for at least two or three in just two books—amazing!)

Here's a list of the calorie and fat content of some of these fast foods. We'll go through it together, but before we do, we have to spend some time on the old calories-versus-fat subject in case you're not clear. We are not looking at calories; what we are looking at is fat per serving or fat per item. We went shopping together. Now let's go down fast food road together starting with Arby's.

ARBY'S

	Calories	Fat
Chicken Salad Croissant	460	70%
French Fries	246	48
Sausage and Egg Croissant	499	59
Regular Roast Beef Sandwich	383	42

It's not that I'm picking on this guy, it's that this list is in alphabetical order and it's the first one up. You can clearly see that the best choice here is the Roast Beef sandwich, coming in at 42 percent fat compared to the old Chicken Salad. (You'd think by the name that you're looking at a low-fat item; that's what most people think, that they're making a low-fat choice: 70 percent!! How's that for a heart patient?) A croissant rounds the corner at a whopping (hate to infringe on a competitor's logo) 70 percent. A perfect example of higher fat because of a few ingredients. When you are talking chicken salad on a croissant, where do you think the fat is coming from?

(a) The croissant;

(b) The mayo in the salad;

(c) Whatever else they put into the salad fixings to make salad.

The year 1683 brought us the invention of the croissant in Austria. Viennese bakers made the celebratory bun in a crescent shape, a croissant, to resemble the flag of Turkey, in commemoration of their holding off the attack by Ottoman Turks early that year. When a Viennese ate a croissant, he was eating the flag of Turkey.

ARTHUR TREACHER'S

	Calories	Fat
Cole Slaw	123	60%
Fish, fried (2 pcs.)	355	50
Shrimp, fried	381	57

I'm dying here because this example is going to blow your mind. You're at Arthur Treacher's (wherever the hell that is), and you order fried shrimp, knowing full well that you are going as far away from low fat as you can get. Fried shrimp: fat and cholesterol city! Just before you order, you decide to Stop the Insanity in your life. (A moment of truth and freedom from the bondage of high-fat life-style in Arthur Treacher's? Would you say I'm pushing it a bit on this one?) You have a change of heart (pardon the cardio reference in the middle of this high-fat conversation) and go with an order of coleslaw. You've just gone from 57 percent fat to 60 percent without even knowing it—and for what, coleslaw?

Obviously your best bet, if you can call it that, is the two-piece fish whatever. How could you lose, with 50 percent fat per serving??

BURGER KING

	Calories	Fat
Bacon Double Cheeseburger	515	54%
Double Beef Whopper with Cheese	935	58
Hash Browns	162	61
Onion Rings	302	51

What should be the lowest-fat item in the place is, again, the highest. Potatoes. There is so much you can do with them. You can eat them until you are so full you can't walk, unless of course you turn them into Burger King's hash browns. Look: The lowest calories, the highest fat . . . why? Because it's not the potatoes that are high in calories or fat, it's the preparation, as Sachiko says. As in drown them in grease, fry the hell out of them, and make them the highest fat item in the place!!

CARL'S JR.

	Calories	Fat
Bacon Cheese Omelette	290	87%
French Fries, regular	250	54
Scrambled Eggs	150	72
Zucchini, fried	311	55

HELLLLLLLLPPPP!!!!!

Scrambled eggs, 72 percent fat!! Haven't they heard of scrambled egg whites? The fried zucchini is the best bet on this menu of goodies because it has the highest calories going for it. Sounds strange, doesn't it? But that's the way it is. Highest calories, not much food—I mean, zucchini; after all, who could be satisfied with some zucchini for lunch—and the lowest fat percentage? Yuucckkkk . . . this is sad and gross.

Take a break with me. Running down this list tells you one thing. Think at the drive-through. Don't assume because you hear chicken that it's the lowest fat item. You read the labels in the grocery store to find out what's in the food you're eating in order to decide if it's high or low fat; do the same thing here. Nothing wrong with asking Bongo what's in the chicken salad.

Hey, chat up a storm with Ronald himself if that's what it takes to get the information you need to make the lowest-fat choice.

Forget even thinking about memorizing any of this. The saturated, the unsaturated, the Big Boy holding that big burger—you'll never remember any of it. But here's what you will remember: Think, ask, question, and make a lower-fat, higher-quality choice.

Let's keep going to the fast-food joints, because this is fun!!

DAIRY QUEEN

	Calories	Fat
Dilly Bar	240	56%
Fish Sandwich	400	38
Hot Dog with Chili	320	56
Onion Rings (3 oz.)	300	51

Didn't know they still existed. I'm not being a low-fat jerk by saying that; it's just that unless you live in a small town, you don't see a lot of Dairy Queens around anymore. When is the last time you saw one in Los Angeles? So any of you who do have a Dairy Queen in your town can write to me and explain what the hell a Dilly Bar is. Dilly? Short for what? Connected to what type of food—Dilly pickles? Dilly spears? Dilly weed? Dilly the herb? What are we talking about when we learn that the Dilly Bar is 56 percent fat? Since I have no clue as to what a Dilly Bar is, let's focus on the onion rings versus the chili dog. Not much difference in fat, not much difference in calories, but a whole lot of difference in volume, because how satisfying can a serving of onion rings be? Eat the dog, what the hell.

Next . . .

JUMPING WITH THE JACK

JACK IN THE BOX	Calories	Fat
Cheese Nachos	571	55%
Jumbo Jack Hamburger	551	47
Scrambled Eggs	719	55
Taco Salad	377	56

Did you know that the Taco Salad was higher in fat than the Cheese Nachos? See, this is what educating ourselves is all about—getting our heads out of the sand and becoming aware of what is, so that we can make different decisions or at the very least have some clue why we are so fat. It's pretty easy to see where all the fat that's hanging from our bodies is coming from. Most people don't go into their favorite fast-food restaurant and order only the Jumbo Jack Hamburger. It's that Jumbo guy, plus the fries, plus the soda, plus whatever, and maybe a taste of your friend's Taco Salad that the bazillion of people a day at fast food restaurants are eating.

MCDONALD'S	Calories	Fat
Chicken McNuggets	314	54%
Quarter Pounder	410	45
Sausage McMuffin	370	53
Cheeseburger	310	40
WENDY'S	Calories	Fat
Fish Filet Sandwich	460	49%
Double Hamburger	670	54
Taco Salad	660	50
Chicken Sandwich	430	40

Keep looking down the list; I have to get to the solution before I cry. It's very depressing sometimes looking at the truth, but knowing there is a solution is very empowering, and I need a little empowerment right now.

Consumer Reports has given us all the empowerment you or I need in the form of a wonderful list of everything out there that has a drive-through and what our options are . . . awareness city.

Check out the chart in the September 1993 issue. Percentage of calories from fat—easy to read and understand. Calories, something we are never going to be obsessed with again. Total fat grams, you can do the fat formula and check up on these boys if you want. Saturated fat grams, the stuff that sticks and clogs. Sodium milligrams, there if you need it. Price—WOW, these guys tell you everything. Weight, quality, and, the section I like the most, comments. They're the Siskel and Ebert of fast foods, the Rex Reed (whatever happened to that guy? We need to do a "where are they now?" on him) of burgers.

> It's about making choices. Over time I have found that I can eat anything I want (just high-volume, low-fat versions) and don't have to suffer. I have gone to restaurants and put together high-volume, low-fat, good-tasting meals while my co-diners are eating deep-fried fat and saturated fat. You know something, I really like the way low-fat food tastes! It's good, and I feel better eating it.
> —*David, Philadelphia, Pennsylvania*

Consumer Reports has prepared the list of all lists when it comes to fast-food eating. We don't even have to do any work when it comes to narrowing it down to the "best" of the worst. They have broken down and dissected fast food, and all the information you ever wanted to know is right there on pages 576–77 of their September issue. These are some of your low-fat options when you walk into your favorite burger joint. Run down the list and you'll see that the poultry and beef sandwiches run neck-and-neck (pardon the animal part reference) when it comes to calories from fat; you can go from 21 percent to 36 percent per serving. Then look at the total calories, which range from 320 for McDonald's McLean Deluxe to 142 for Burger King's Chunky Chicken Salad, down to 120 for Hardee's grilled chicken salad. Options, options, options, options—that's what we like.

The sodium is something you might also want to check out, because the ranges here are pretty steep. The Arby's Light Roast Turkey Deluxe (that's a longer name than most people in line for the throne have), a whopping (stealing a competitor's product name again) 1,262 to 230 for McDonald's Chunky Chicken Salad. But neither one of them does too well at the critics' corner.

"Little meat flavor."

Not very good when you're talking about a Roast Turkey Sandwich. And how about that chicken salad: "Unpleasant slippery coating" (GROSS, what do you suppose that is?).

I've never listened to critics. You taste it and decide for yourself if you like it; but this time when you eat it, you'll know exactly how much fat you're eating. We'll deal with the taste later.

Salads, pick and choose all the works—been done for you.

There's a surprise, listed under "Shakes": "So thick it must be eaten with a spoon" and it's 25 percent fat. It's a bargain, that Wendy's Frosty Dairy Dessert.

But wait, McDonald's low-fat milk shake—what's this? "Medicinal note due to slight taste of cherry and alcohol"—what's that all about? At 5 percent fat a pop, I'd like to know if there's alcohol in it before I give it to the family. Info like this from our friends at *Consumer Reports* is important if you want to make the highest-volume, lowest-fat choice for your family.

> I had no problem changing my eating habits. . . . I manage a seafood restaurant (a fish-and-chips place), and we deep-fry everything, even the dinner rolls, there! I used to live on that stuff, but not anymore! After eating healthy, high-volume, low-fat foods, I have no desire to eat that food anymore. It literally makes me sick!
> —*John, Fraser, Michigan*

Read on and get what you need, because this is good information. I'm going on to another day, another quiz from *Consumer Reports*. This one's called "Where's the Fat?" and it's the perfect way to illustrate how little we know just from looking and guessing. You can't just guess when it comes to the way you look and feel. You gotta be armed with the truth to fight this battle. Private eyes, food detectives, low-fat food guards: Take up your swords, grab your armor, and fight with me.

- The first item in our little quiz is a real surprise. Can you believe it? A McDonald's Hot Fudge Sundae being lower in fat than a Baked Apple Pie? Before you became a Food P.I., you would have been fooled easily by this one. Key words that would have gotten you:

  Baked. Everything baked is better, but not in this case.

  Apple. How bad can apples be? When they're sitting on top of a high-fat crust that we never think to question, they can be real bad. And all you gotta do is take the number of fat grams and the calories from *Consumer Reports* and then do the fat formula.

$$15 \text{ grams} \times 9 = 135$$
$$135 \text{ divided by } 280 = 48 \text{ percent fat per serving}$$

Would you believe that one lousy piece of baked pie can be that high in fat?

The Hot Fudge Sundae, as *Consumer Reports* says, has only three grams of fat—making up 11 percent of its 240 calories. Let me tell you guys, whether you eat fast or slow, if it's planned or unplanned, if your emotional connection is healed or still being worked on, the difference between 48 percent fat per serving and 11 percent fat per serving is what's going to make all the difference in the world on your body.

All the great suggestions that no doubt you are applying to your life are very important, but I want to say that the most important, the thing that's gonna make the most difference, is cutting back on fat. The rest we can deal with later.

- Some of the questions and answers in the quiz aren't as much fun. Who's to know which salad dressing at which fast-food place is lower in fat? I mean, that's something that you just have to memorize and know. No big clues or smashing surprises here—so just know it!

- Now here's something that Food P.I.'s really have to pay attention to. The Salad Bar at Wendy's can be a huge trap. Just like the *baked* in the apple pie, we assume when we hear salad that it's all fine, low-fat, and healthy. Not so, fellow low-fat consumers. If one of your choices for a topping is sunflower seeds, you figure natural; have to be good for your bowels or something. Fiber? Something. But look at what the *Consumer Reports* quiz says—would you have ever thought six grams of fat in every two tablespoons!!

  Amazing. Hey, all you guys who eat tons of toasted sunflower seeds at night while you're watching your movie with your spittoon cup by your side, do the fat formula. How about that 80 percent fat?

  O.K., you're mad now, aren't you? I've come along and told you a couple of things that you probably don't want to know. Enough with this educating yourself to get a better life-style and a stronger and leaner body. No more. Ripping sunflower seeds and apple pie? Why not just attack the game of baseball? It's downright un-American at this point.

  Take a breath. Digest this upsetting news. It's O.K., because finding out the truth isn't always easy. Get mad at me, I can take it. And whenever you're ready, let's get on with it.

- More bad news from our friends at *Consumer Reports*. You hear fish and think it has to be lower in fat than most things. What do you think now? The breaded and fried fillet sandwiches at the major chains are 40 percent fat. You want fat?

- Now check out the last item in our quiz. Chicken is chicken like fish is fish and apple pie is apple pie, right? NOT. It's the way you prepare it— what sauces you put on top of it and all the other things that go into the foods we eat. Skinfree Crispy—from Kentucky Fried Chicken—52 percent of its calories are from fat. My God, that's amazing, and not much better than the original recipe at 55 percent fat per serving.

You see, that's the key. Don't assume. That's what this little exercise teaches us. Start breaking things down.

ιω Bread, usually low fat (ask if you have questions—like the old Burger King Croissant sandwiches).

ιω Lettuce—you're safe there.

ιω Tomatoes. Fine for now.

ιω Pickles, onions, etc. You know there isn't a lot of fat there.

Then you get to the beef, chicken, roast beef, fish, whatever you have got in the center. You've got to break that down, no matter what the sandwich name says, like Skinfree.

> I went to a restaurant the other day. I asked if I could have a plate of steamed vegetables, and I told them I was allergic to all oils. I got the best low-fat meal of my life.
>
> —*Amber, Kimmswick, Maryland*

Since eating out isn't only about fast foods, once in a while we go to a restaurant and sit down to eat. I went out and got menus from every kind of restaurant you can imagine so that we could order together and you could get comfortable with asking the questions, making up your own concoctions, questioning the waiters and waitresses, and getting what you want for your hard-earned money and putting what you want inside your wonderful body. Because that's what ordering in a restaurant is all about. Question, question, concoct, concoct . . .

STEAKHOUSE

Yep, I'm heading right for the heart of the matter. Our first stop is the steakhouse, because I'm telling you that with a bit of common sense and the right info you can eat anywhere. I'm throwing all the cards on the table on the first trip out with you. Gambling, steakhouse, a bit of whiskey, they all go together, don't they?

APPETIZERS

This is a pretty fancy steakhouse, don't you think?

I'll have the shrimp cocktail.

Soup du jour—is it a veggie soup or something with no oil or butter?

This is the time to explain to your service person (how's that for the 90's) that you are going to die if you get any butter, oil, or vegetable spray, and it's really important for the future of their restaurant that you don't.

Salad city—these places usually have great salads or salad bars. Mix it up;

THE STEAKHOUSE

Appetizers

8.00	Sautéed Shrimp with Garlic Butter
7.50	Tarragon-cured Salmon with Cognac Mustard
7.50	Pan-seared Soft-shell Crab
7.50	Shrimp Cocktail
8.00	Escargot Vincenzo
8.50	Beef Carpaccio with Arugula and Parmesan

Soups

5.00	Lobster Bisque
4.50	Soup du Jour

Salads

5.00	Caesar Salad
5.50	Beefsteak Tomato with Cucumber, Purple Onion, and Roasted Pepper Vinaigrette

Entrees

17.00	Filet Mignon	7 oz.
21.00		10 oz.
19.00	New York Strip	12 oz.
24.00		16 oz.
18.00	Ribeye	14 oz.
28.00	Prime Porterhouse	24 oz.
26.00	Veal T-bone with Shiitake Mushrooms and Madeira	
18.00	Peppersteak with Green Peppercorn Brandy Sauce	

Special Entrees

20.00	Roast Rack of Lamb with Herb Crust, Roast Garlic, and Rosemary
42.00	Chateaubriand for Two with Béarnaise or Bordelaise
17.50	Roast Duck with Raspberry Merlot Sauce
17.00	Grilled Chicken Oscar with King Crab, Asparagus, and Béarnaise

Seafood

market price	Live Maine Lobster
market price	Catch of the Day
18.00	Grilled Salmon

A la Carte

5.50	Sautéed Mushrooms
5.00	Grilled Vegetables
3.50	Baked Potato
4.00	Creamed Spinach

Desserts

5.00	Crème Brûlée
5.00	Chocolate Torte
5.00	Fresh Berries Nestled in Puff Pastry with Whiskey Sauce
5.00	Ice Cream Crepe Caramel
14.00	Soufflé for Two

put tons and tons of your favorite stuff in it. Go for the vinegar dressing, and sprinkle some salt and pepper and some lemons on top. Great time to get a baked potato—a plain baked potato with salad stuffed in, some hot sauce, chives, onions. YUUUMMMMMMMM.

ENTREES

Holy moly, it's time to leave this place. Check out the prices!! Assuming someone else is paying, you'd go right for the lower-fat choices, and the lower prices—in this case, the seafood or chicken (think preparation here, and ask, ask, ask your waitperson)—or make up your own entree.

Easy to do: You already have the baked potato and the salad; you can easily add some corn on the cob (it's not on the menu, but you can ask; have the chef run to the store and pick you up some corn on the cob—he'll probably appreciate that), some grilled veggies, some rice, if you're lucky (they just might have it), and you'll have the highest-volume, lowest-fat entree around.

A LA CARTE

There's your baked potatoes, beat them to the punch. See if they can un-cream the spinach (steamed spinach with lemon and soy sauce and a little Tabasco thrown on top is heaven, and you can eat mountains of it) and shove that in your baked potato. And have the chef (at these prices you should be able to get anything you want; the chef should come out and do a dinner dance for you, if that's what you feel like having during dinner) sauté the mushrooms in water and spices. Bingo—take out the fat, keep the flavor, and eat!

DESSERTS

Sorbet—always ask for sorbet. Fruits. Get tons. If not, blow it off. After the meal you just ate, it's not as if you're going to be dying of hunger. Or go to your local low-fat yogurt shop.

Come on, the next stop on this eating train is:

The Kikkoman company began selling soy sauce in Japan in 1630—a long-lasting company!!

THE PUB

Much cheaper. Quick and lots of fun. Grab a few beers (no fat in alcohol, but if you have a drinking problem, and millions of us do, don't; have a non-alcoholic beer) and look at the menu with me.

APPETIZERS

These are my kind of appetizers—bulk. If they have black bean nachos, then they've got black beans. Ask about lard, chicken fat, and oil, and if they are free of all that, then make your own dippy thing. Some black beans with some lettuce, tomatoes, and onions; get the chips, but use them like a spoon, dipping them and eating from them but not eating them. You see, there's fat big-time in those damn chips that you can eat eight million of. If you really want to be a low-fat nut, do what I do: Smuggle your own low-fat corn chips into the restaurant. They'll never know, and if they find out and try to kick you out for bringing in your own food, you can start a revolution in the place, get everybody mad about being fed tons of fat and not even being able to have an option, blah, blah, blah. Just keep talking and demanding your rights and keep eating your low-fat chips with your hot sauce or black bean dip that you concocted and that won't make you fat. Don't worry about it, they'll get it eventually.

I've got you starting a revolution before we've even gotten to the main course. Have another beer and we'll eat.

ENTREES

You'll have to go for the basic grilled-without-oil-or-butter sandwich in our little pub. Grill that chicken, pile on the lettuce, tomato, and onions, ketchup, relish—add some mustard if you want—and bite into a great sandwich.

SALADS

It's probably best to ask for a plain salad unless the waitperson has the time to explain every ingredient in the chicken tarragon salad to you.

DRESSINGS

Be cool here, because you know these are loaded with fat. Make your own: Smuggle in some low-fat that you love. Can you believe all the rules we've broken in this place? It's been the criminal lunch-out. Why don't we

THE PUB

Appetizers

3.95	½ order 3.00	Black Bean Nachos with pico de gallo & sour cream
4.95	½ order 4.00	Blackened Chicken Nachos with pico de gallo & sour cream

SPECIALS

4.95 Marinated Pork Chops—A Spicy Taste Treat
4.95 Chalupa Combo (chicken, black bean, cheese)
     Handmade—The Flavor Of Texas

Tacos

3.95 Spicy & Crispy
3.00 Stuff-on-a-stick Pork or Chicken with chips & picante sauce

Sandwiches

4.50 Half pound Hamburger with grilled sweet red onion
     (with Cheddar Cheese .50 cents extra)
4.95 Grilled or Blackened Chicken Sandwich
4.95 Turkey, Bacon, Monterey Jack & Cheddar Cheese Club
4.95 Chopped Beef Sandwich—award-winning BBQ

All sandwiches served with Fries or Chips

Salads

3.95 Cacsar Salad
4.95 (with grilled chicken)
4.95 Grilled Chicken Salad
4.95 Chicken Tarragon Salad

Dressings: ranch, italian, blue cheese, honey mustard

Drinks

1.00 coffee, tea, pepsi/diet, dr. pepper, sprite

Draft Beer Pints

2.00 Budweiser/Bud Light   (at lunch .75) Shiner/Bass

Bottled Beer

2.00 domestic
3.00 imported
2.00 wine (Chablis, White Zinfandel, Cabernet Sauvignon)

Thank you for choosing The Pub.

just start busting up the joint (a very pub thing to do)? O.K., we're out of here and on to the next restaurant.

CHINESE

Everybody's favorite until the news reports recently blared out the fact that eating Chinese food is like eating tons of lard. Of course they didn't tell you anything else. No solutions. No way around it. Nothing you can do to avoid having heart disease after one night of moo-shoo anything. Don't you just love these guys? Do you wonder why we all walk around feeling like there's no point in trying? Everything gives us cancer. There isn't anything that's really low in fat other than veggies and fruit, and if that doesn't get us, then the chemicals will. So what the heck, why bother?

Understandable attitude, but not acceptable. Sure, the way most of this stuff is reported it's a wonder any of us care anymore. But they are wrong and irresponsible in the way they report the news about what's going on with food, exercise, the right and wrong of living a high-quality, low-fat life-style.

Yes, you can go to a Chinese restaurant and eat more fat in one sitting than you can imagine. You can go to Burger King and do the same thing. How about the local bakery? You can do yourself in there. Convenience stores can be coffins if you eat the highest fat things around. Or—and this is the "or" they always seem to leave out—you can go into any one of these places and get something lower in fat and live.

As in not be a social hermit. A self-righteous low-fat eater. Be someone your friends and family will still want to spend time with—that is, if you want to spend time with them. If not, go ahead and be a social hermit and use the "No, thank you, I can't eat anywhere or anything because I'm a low-fat-loving food P.I." for all it's worth. That's from *The 101 Ways to Dodge Your Family* book, coming soon!

I love Chinese food. Who doesn't? The other night my husband and I went out to eat Chinese at 1 A.M. I'd been at a meeting until 8 P.M., and the boys were hanging out with Nic. The husband and I spent some time talking and organizing schedules, and then before we knew it, it was midnight and we were both starving. So where do you go? To the open-till-4 A.M. Chinese restaurant, right along with all the bikers and other late-night folks.

I ordered vegetarian soup for four with one bowl. Mine, all mine. Spiced it up with some chili pepper and soy sauce, added some steamed rice, and ate it all as my warmup. Then right into the main dish—two of them, to be exact. Starting with the veggie fried rice—I know that fried means fried, but this restaurant knows and loves me and makes my fried rice with very, very, very little oil and lots of onions and scallions because I'm addicted to onions

Peking Palace

Fast Free Delivery

Soup

1.60	Chicken Noodle Soup	1.60	*Vegetable Fun Shee Soup
1.60	Chicken Rice Soup	1.35	*Vegetable Wonton Soup
1.35	Egg Drop Soup	1.60	Wonton Egg Drop Mix Soup
1.35	Wonton Soup	1.60	Hot and Sour Soup

Cold Appetizer

3.75	Cold Noodle with Sesame Sauce	4.95	Hacked Chicken with Multi Flavor

Hot Appetizer

1.35	Egg Roll	3.75	Chicken Dumplings, Steamed or Fried (6 pieces)
1.35	Spring Roll		
1.95	Scallion Pancakes	3.75	Spicy Noodles Szechuan Style
3.95	Shrimp Toast (4 pieces)		
3.75	Pork Meat Dumplings, Steamed or Fried (6 pieces)	6.75	Barbecued Spare Ribs
		5.50	Fantail Shrimp (4 pieces)
3.75	*Vegetable Dumplings, Steamed or Fried (6 pieces)	5.50	Roast Pork

Seafood

8.25	*Moo Shu Shrimp (with 2 pancakes)	9.25	Shrimp with Garlic Sauce
		9.25	Shrimp with Sa-Cha Sauce
9.25	Shrimp with Black Bean Sauce	9.25	Shrimp with Broccoli
		9.25	Shrimp with Snow Peas
9.25	Shrimp with Mixed Vegetables	9.25	Shrimp with Baby Eggplant in Garlic Sauce

Pork

7.25	*Moo Shu Pork (with 2 pancakes)	7.25	Shredded Pork with Peking Sauce
7.25	Sliced Pork with Black Bean Sauce	7.25	Sliced Pork with Scallion
		7.25	Sliced Pork with Zucchini
7.25	Shredded Pork with Garlic Sauce		

Chicken

7.75	Chicken with Sa-Cha Sauce	7.75	Chicken with Garlic Sauce
7.75	Chicken with Broccoli	7.75	Chicken with Mushroom and Snow Pea Pods
7.75	*Chicken with Snow Pea Pods		
		7.75	Chicken with Hoisin Sauce

continued

Chicken (continued)

7.75 Kung Pao Chicken	7.75 Chicken with Mixed Vegetables
7.75 Chicken with Eggplant in Garlic Sauce	7.75 *Moo Shu Chicken (with 2 pancakes)
7.75 Chicken with Black Bean Sauce	8.25 Lemon Chicken
7.75 Chicken with Hot & Spicy Sauce	8.25 Chicken with Walnuts

Beef and Lamb

8.25 *Moo Shu Beef (with 2 pancakes)	8.25 Kung Pao Beef
8.25 Beef with Broccoli	8.25 Shredded Beef with Garlic Sauce
8.25 Beef with Green Pepper and Onion	8.25 Beef with Scallion
8.25 Beef with Snow Pea Pod	8.25 Beef with Hoisin Sauce
8.25 Beef with Oyster Sauce	8.75 Lamb with Scallion
	8.75 Lamb with Sa-Cha Sauce

Health Food Section (All Steamed with Sauce on the Side)

9.75 Steamed Mixed Vegetables with Shrimp	7.25 Steamed Broccoli
8.25 Steamed Mixed Vegetables with Chicken	8.25 Steamed String Beans with Chicken
7.25 Steamed Zucchini	8.25 Steamed Broccoli with Chicken
7.25 Steamed Snowpeas and Waterchestnuts	9.75 Steamed Broccoli with Shrimp
7.25 Steamed String Beans	7.25 Steamed Mixed Vegetables

Vegetables

6.75 *Moo Shu Vegetables (with 2 pancakes)	6.75 Eggplant with Garlic Sauce
6.75 Sauteed Mixed Vegetables	6.75 Beancurd, Hunan Style (with mixed vegs.)
6.75 Sauteed Mixed Vegetables with Sa-Cha Sauce	6.75 Beancurd w. Black Mushrooms & Bamboo Shoots
6.75 Sauteed Mixed Vegetables with Garlic Sauce	6.75 Sauteed String Beans and Broccoli
6.75 Dried, Sauteed String Beans	

Noodles and Fried Rice

5.95 Special Fried Rice	6.75 Rice Noodle (w. choice of shrimp, beef, chicken, pork or vegetables)
5.50 *Fried Rice (w. choice of shrimp, beef, chicken, pork or vegetables)	7.50 Singapore Rice Noodle
5.50 Lo Mein (w. choice of shrimp, beef, chicken, pork or vegetables)	8.75 Subgum Pan Fried Noodles
	10.75 Seafood Pan Fried Noodles
6.75 Chow Fun (w. choice of shrimp, beef, chicken, pork or vegetables)	5.50 Jar-Jong Noodles (w. vegetable sauce)

and scallions. Then I ordered the veggie moo-shoo. No oil. Tons of flavor. Roll it all up in those Chinese flour tortillas, add some brown sauce with no oil, and who's gonna tell you that you aren't having fun? Deprived—what are you, nuts! I was so full by the time I finally stopped eating at 2:15 A.M. that I thought I was gonna die. It would have been a good time for a little romance, if you know what I mean. The kids with their dad, late-night time with the husband, but I was so full, I could barely move, let alone make love. The minute I took my makeup off, brushed my teeth, and my head hit the pillow, forget about it, I was gone.

It's pretty obvious how much fun going out for Chinese is with me, so when you go, think about me and order:

 Rice.

 Veggie dumplings, steamed.

 Moo-goo anything, grilled, boiled, without oil.

 Great fish plates in Chinese restaurants. Go to town: Order the chef's specialty and tell him how you want it prepared. There are lots of good soups to choose from, but watch out for those little bubbles of grease that float on top of every oily soup I've ever ordered in a Chinese restaurant. When you say to your waitperson, "Excuse me, this soup seems to have oil in it."
And the waitperson says, "NO, NO OIL."
And you say again, "Yes, there is oil in this soup."
And you get, "NO, NO OIL."
You can say, "Look, buddy, see these little bubbles floating all over this soup? Oil, oil, oil—that's what it is, nothing more, nothing less. Take it back and get me one without, PLEASE."

 Chicken with snow pea pods/mushrooms/bamboo shoots.

 Choices everywhere in your favorite Chinese restaurant. You just have to get used to ordering a bit differently, and they just have to get used to preparing it a bit differently.

> The restaurants see me coming and they cringe! If I don't see something on the menu that I choose to eat, I have them make it special or I substitute.
>
> —*Laura, Troutdale, Oregon*

I've never been anywhere that I couldn't eat out.

Cafeterias? Veggies, potatoes, fish, chicken, salads, bread, bread, Jell-O. I had to say that, because only in cafeterias do I still see that green Jell-O with the marshmallows in it. Why do they make that stuff??

Soup-and-salad restaurants are popping up all over the country. Great options. Soups, stews, potatoes with everything in the world piled high—inexpensive, quick, and everywhere you look these days.

Whoever said you couldn't eat out? Bake your own bread? Forget about it—not necessary. All you gotta do is think about what you're eating and make the best decision you can make at the time. Eat, enjoy and keep learning. Jill, Sally, and I just polished off a large pizza at 11 P.M. after a long, long day. The best thing I ever tasted because I was in the mood for pizza, didn't want the fat (so you know what I left off), and we made it so spicy that our mouths were on fire while we were eating it. What could be better??

CHAPTER 6

BEAR WITH ME

I'm going to ask you guys early in the game to bear with me, tolerate the upcoming tangent, and let me have my moment here. Consider this the be-kind-to-the-author section of this book. Put up with Susan. Let her have this one, because I'd like to spend a minute talking about something that's just a little off-center.

When information is being presented on a national level, as in the writing of a book, there is always an underlying feeling that caution is necessary.

> Be careful.
> Do some fence-sitting.
> Don't make too many big statements.

Being careful not to scare your reading, listening, or viewing audience. Sure, add some spice, but don't be too controversial. It's the feeling you get when you start out on projects like this.

Fair enough and absolutely understandable. Old Simon and old Schuster have invested some cash in the writing of this book, and I'm sure caution is always good (as though I'd have any clue about that!!).

What the publishers and radio and TV producers didn't understand until recently is that I'm talking to you, the women of America. I've been trying to tell them for a long time that because it's you, there's no need to go slow, fence-sit, or live in fear or caution, because you guys are brilliant. No need at all to be careful, because you want information and you don't want to waste your time with fence-sitting. We've had enough of that pretty, fluffy stuff to last a lifetime; now it's the gut we need to get to if we are going to make the changes in our lives that we want and need to make.

The way I figured it when I was thinking about this book is that we need to talk about everything, throw it all out on the table (pardon the pun), give it all to you. And if you read something you aren't interested in right now, you won't use it. You'll put it away and go back to it when you need it or are interested in it. Easy. Let you be the judge of what you want to include in your life and what you don't. Simple, simple, simple, and totally eliminates the fence-sitting.

As I'm doing the interviewing and research for this book, I'm being exposed (sounds like radiation, doesn't it?) to all kinds of concepts I never thought were connected to the food we put into our mouths and how it affects us. These are wonderfully challenging concepts that I want to share with you. I don't want to write this book without talking about them, so I created the "tolerate Susan's tangent" chapter to give me a place to do just that.

You know that guy I've been mentioning all along, Dr. Marc Micozzi? He's the one who got me thinking about this "bear-with-me" chapter. Dr. Marc Micozzi, M.D., Ph.D., is director of the National Museum of Health and Medicine, author of *Macronutrients: Investigating Their Role in Cancer* and *Nutrition and Cancer Prevention: Investigating the Role of Micronutrients* (I'm getting more and more impressed with each passing title), and a leading authority on antioxidants, oxidants, biflavonoids. (Impressed enough to give him a ring? As in call, not get engaged to him. Just what I need in my life, another husband. The expression "give him a ring" surfaced from my old Australian days. God knows what else is going to come out of my mouth by the end of this book.)

Our interview started off fence-sitty enough. Talking about fat, level-one transition, etc. Here's what the man with the most degrees I've ever heard of said about stage-one body-changing stuff:

> "If you want to change your body and get well, step one for most of us is losing weight. And losing weight doesn't mean dieting, it means watching what it is that you are eating."

There's a big statement!!! Hey, Doc Marc, with all due respect for all those titles, that's what you have to say? Yo, Doc, that's something I've been saying for years. You're making us yawn!!

> "I'm talking about total fat intake, because separating fats is not necessary unless you're talking about a health problem. Saturated, unsaturated, poly, or mono—don't worry about breaking it all down if what

you are dealing with is wanting to lose body fat—just cut back on your total daily fat intake."

Heard that a couple of times from some big, big names. Seems to be the consensus. Simple, understandable, will change the way you look and feel . . . got it. Now, right back to the conversation with the man I was liking more and more by the second.

"The best way to cut back on your total fat intake, change your body, lose fat, is to be realistic. If you are eating 50 to 60 percent of your daily intake as fat and you cut it down to the American Medical Association standard of 30 percent, it is going to make a difference. You can go lower in your daily fat intake, and that's very beneficial, but being realistic is important. So for many people who have been eating enormous amounts of fats, getting to 30 percent of their daily fat intake is good."

Another good beginning is:

"Cutting back on junk foods makes a big difference. Cutting back on snacky sugary foods is good because most of the time those foods are loaded with sugar and fat."

So kill two birds with one stone. That's a good beginning—a perfect stage-one suggestion.

But as we are talking basics, there's something in this man's voice that I really like. A sexual verve off to the left, you may be thinking. That would be controversial. That would be jumping right off the fence. Yep (not to the sexual verve, to the left)—yep to his voice, the kindness, the sensitivity, the sound of authority that resonated and made me, Food P.I., know there was something more than the standard "change what you are putting into your mouth" info. So I put on my jazz, lit my ciggy, and dug deeper. And boy, did I learn a thing or two.

"Working within your limits when you are making a change in your diet is important. Eating is a behavior, food is fuel. People don't eat nutrients, so why do we talk to people about what nutrients they need? They eat food, and there are so many social, cultural, and sentimental connections to the foods we eat that it's more complicated than just getting the fuel we need."

Think about it. From the backyard barbecue to the Christmas ham:

"The associations we make with food are very strong. In order to really make a change in the foods we eat and our life-style, we need to create new associations."

See, see, don't you see things picking up a bit with this statement? Make new associations with the foods we are eating? What's he talking about?

Not celebrating Christmas?
Never barbecuing again?

Naw, this guy would never do anything like that to us, but this connection thing has to be taken a bit further and discussed so we can break it down and figure it out for ourselves.

> Growing up, I lived in the typical German household—sausage, sausage, sausage, and everything was fried. I have changed my life. My kids wanted to go to McDonald's yesterday, I said O.K., knowing I could eat what I wanted. Guess what I wanted? To wait until I got home and eat the herbed rice and lentil casserole I made the night before.
>
> —*Susan, Snyder, Oklahoma*

Take a minute and think about the sentimental associations connected to what you've been eating all your life. All I've ever thought about were the negatives connected to the food in my life—bribed, manipulated, force-fed. Public Statement 106 from Susan Powter, Food P.I., said it over and over again. That's all the self-esteem experts seem to talk about—the pain associated with food. But what about the joy? The warmth? Love? The social sentimental connections?

Sure, it's hard to change behavior when you connect pain and suffering with it, but it's just as hard to change things when we've connected joy and social sentiment to it. If the best times of your life were Saturdays at the ballpark and if your closest moments with Mom and Dad took place just before you bit into that ballpark frank, what can you expect to feel when you find out that the ballpark frank is loaded with saturated fat, chemicals, colorings, and all kinds of stuff that you wouldn't feed your dog? You don't think it's going to be hard to say no to the ballpark frank? Yeah, you're gonna be fine sitting at the ballpark with your friends eating air-popped popcorn while they are chowing down on dogs? Commmmmmmmmmmme on!!!!!

So your strongest, most sentimental connection happens just before you take a bite of your dog. You're not ever going to stop eating franks even if your cardiologist tells you that you're gonna have the big one if you don't.

Oh, sure, if push comes to shove and you are going to drop if you take another bite, you may be able to force yourself to give up the food connected to the deepest emotions of joy and pleasure that you love, but you are always going to go to the ballpark feeling like the most deprived person on earth. Think about being the only person not eating turkey at the Thanksgiving table. So forget about changing the things we associate with big fun or the holidays. (What are you gonna do, start a national campaign to wipe out Thanksgiving? That'll go over well, don't you think?) But who's to say we can't change the food and the reasons it is connected to these warm, fuzzy, sentimental feelings?

It got me thinking about my sentimental, social connections with food. Where do I draw the line about what I'm willing or not willing to change in my life? What is socially acceptable when it comes to the food we are putting into our bodies? Why? What can we do to change some of the habits, the type of foods, or the socially acceptable connections to foods that are harming us—killing us, in some cases—and making a whole lot of us fat and unhealthy?

Notice how, when talking about my sentimental connections with foods, I went from first person to second person real quickly? It's because I don't have any—not sentimental food connections, we all have those, but a memory. None at all. If it's blocking out the first fifteen years of life that protects us from the inner-child turmoil, then consider me the most protected person on earth. I don't remember anything. Not an ice cream, ballpark, movie, or holiday experience—nothing! Brain like a sieve.

> Blocked to death.
> Inner child in hiding.

Whatever the reason, however you want to label it, I can't remember a damn thing when it comes to food-sentimental connections of my childhood except for what I've told you. Chocolate bar here and there. Lamb and mint sauce. Your basic wax-paper wrapping. That's about it when you're talking memories and food in my childhood.

But this concept of social and sentimental connections with food does make a whole lot of sense to me and is something that has to be very important when you're talking about food. I know that, and it probably needs to change a bit.

It's wonderful to bite into a ballpark frank with beer by your side, watching whoever hit home, but let's not live in denial about what it is you're biting into and how it affects your health. How about a higher-quality frank? Meat-free? Because as much fun as you may be having at that very moment, there's one association we haven't made because we didn't know it, and it's the most important, warm, fuzzy, sentimental connection ever: Respect for yourself. Caring for yourself. Giving yourself—through good food, high-quality fuel—the gift of health. Regaining control of your life by making your own choices, not having them made for you by a hot-dog manufacturer whose only goal is to sell a billion dogs a year.

Until recently we didn't know that everything we put into our mouths affects the way we live. How we feel is directly connected to whatever it is that we buy each week or eat every week behind home base. Remember the guy who said that if the first time you think about food is when you sit down at the table, then it's too late. This is not about stopping things that you love, or walking around feeling like the most deprived person on earth. This is about thinking before we eat, about improving the quality of our associations. Adding health and respect for our bodies to the picture.

> Our kids and husbands have no idea that they are eating better now.
> —Kelly, Kyle Ann, Rae, and Donna; Elgin, Illinois

Are you wondering at all why I'm talking ballpark franks with the women of this country? It's because I'm not talking ballpark franks as much as I'm talking changing associations. And who better to change associations with than the moms, wives, businesswomen, sisters, and daughters? The women, plain and simple. It's the moms who are going to influence the children and create new traditions, tastes, and social and sentimental associations. What's the matter with a Thanksgiving dinner that doesn't kill you? Why shouldn't that be normal and healthy? Why do we need to eat so much fat, cholesterol, and sugar that nobody can move for three days after the feast? Why? Was Norman's picture of how it all should be right? Or is it that we just never questioned it?

Is there a balance between saving the planet with every bite taken and just plain enjoying and eating well? Is it O.K. for the food manufacturers to flat-out lie to us and hurt our health deliberately? When did this become acceptable to us? Lying and cheating (the fifth country-western hit of the book, I might add)—acceptable and all-American? I don't think so.

Women can very much affect all of this stuff. Who do you think is buying the food? I'm not talking about how many times we do or don't sit down at a dinner table to eat anymore. Someone has to either cook it or order it in. Whether we all eat it together or not, we're eating.

Who's cooking?

Who's ordering out?

Who's stocking the fridge and the pantry every week?

The women. Please spare me the latest national survey about how much has changed. Don't give me the latest stats on how many men are now changing diapers, staying home, running the family, and doing the dishes more than once a week. You may have the most evolved man on earth, your guy may be willing to lend a hand often, but it's still the women of our country who come home from a twelve-hour day at the office and are expected to be responsible for getting the dinner ready, starting the laundry, organizing the kids.

Too often in too many households it's the husband who has the luxury of "unwinding" after a hard day at work. Let's just talk facts and leave out the reference to the very, very few households that are being run equally. When it comes to the double and triple duty that millions of working moms and wives in this country are pulling, it's still ten times the work and one-third the pay and credit that are the reality for most women.

But as overworked and pulling ten times the load as we are, guess what? We are in control and have the power to make some very important changes that will make an enormous difference in the health of our family, our community, our city, our country. True, true, true. What a thought.

Do you see it? Change the country by changing the food we buy for our families? I know, I know, it's a stretch, but just think about it.

> In 1893 the first completely electric kitchen went on display at the Chicago World's Fair, featuring a range, broiler, and teakettles.

As I'm writing this, I'm thinking about the changes in my home, in our family's traditions, since I dropped that 133 pounds and got well.

I may not be able to remember the first fifteen years of my life, but the last few are very clear. There have been so many changes. The traditions are the same—much better, as a matter of fact. Christmas still exists. Birthdays are big when you've got two kids. Who could not do Easter—the bunny and all? Good Friday has waned a bit, Ash Wednesday isn't what it used to be, but we have all the rest, and food is still the center and focus of many of them.

Easter just came and went with Easter candy, French toast for breakfast, candy, and baskets everywhere. My family goes to the ballpark all the time. Some weeks that's all we do in my family, with both boys big in baseball. We do eat hot dogs all the time. We do celebrate the victories with backyard barbecues. The boys' friends spend the night, and the food is nonstop. Food and sentiment reek from my house, but a couple of things have changed in connection with what kind of food and how we get it.

Why eat one little ounce of mixed nuts having seventeen grams of fat when you can have one ounce of unbuttered popcorn for a measly two grams of fat?

Taking food with us has become a standard in this house ever since I learned more and more about food. Once I confirmed the rumors about what was really in hot dogs, there was no way on earth I was going to eat them or give them to the two people I love most in the world. But don't ask me to give up one of my favorite meals: hot dogs with tons of sauerkraut, relish, mustard, onions, tomatoes, pickles, big fat bun (pardon that pun).

Why would anyone give that up? Just modify it a bit. You can easily go from high fat to low fat, chemical filled to not so chemmy, and still get the warm, fuzzy connection you had when you were a kid (or just last year, in my case, when all my memories seem to begin).

Take your food with you.

There is nothing wrong with that. Nobody really notices or cares. We just drink our own soda, bring our own dogs, eat our own candy—no fuss, no muss, lower fat and higher quality. When I found out about the lardy, yellow, fatty, chunky stuff that they load on the popcorn—this was way, way, way before the big popcorn scare came out in the press (ahead of my time, for sure?)—I started bringing my own to the movie theater. Against the rules? Sure it is, but who cares? We bring our own high-volume, low-fat, great-tasting popcorn, candy, cookies, and anything we want to eat when we go see a movie, go to the ballpark, go to a birthday party, friends' houses, family gatherings, whatever the occasion, because my children's and my health is important to me.

There's no deprivation; there is still the social and sentimental value of the experience, and a healthier, leaner body as a result. What more could anyone want? This way you get it all. Don't wait for the studies to come out, the news to be broken—all you gotta do is ask.

It's been real important for me to eat properly now, so my children will follow our example and grow up to be fit adults with good eating habits.
—*Cindy, Mifflinburg, Pennsylvania*

Ask Mr. or Ms. Concession Stand: What do you cook the popcorn in? Show me.

When they show you the pack of lard that they cook it in, you don't have to be a nutritionist to figure out that it's going to end up either choking your heart or on your waistline.

Come on, you know it's high fat, and you make the choice. Even if you choose to eat it, at least it's your choice. It's the robot acceptance—trusting people who are lying for profit and paying the high, high price of our children's and our health—that I have a hard time with. Don't even think about going to the movies and not eating popcorn or candy—what are you, crazy? You're gonna be grabbing someone's food within minutes. It's automatic. The lights go down, the music starts, the credits roll, and we all start dying of hunger for some crunchy, sweet, salty, and snacky things. Don't ever think you have to change that, but change the quality of the crunchy, sweet, snacky thing. Why the hell not, even if you gotta break a few rules to do it!! That's what I'm saying.

Here's where the universal (oh, I forgot to mention the universe; it's right after the country and then the world in the change-the-way-things-are statement a couple of pages back) principle comes in. If we, the women, the moms, the wives, the organizers of most of the events, social situations, and dinners at night, started to connect

> food with health
> food with the way we feel
> higher-quality fuel with a higher-quality life

and changed the associations, changed the whole kit and caboodle with these things that mean so very much to us all, can you imagine what the consequences might be?

Changes in the family's health?

Influencing the nation's connections to food and sentiment?

Consciousness connection with our planet (I'll explain that one later on)?

We could affect everything:

The money this country spends on health care.

Prevention. How about not eating the foods that contribute in a big, big way to those millions of heart attacks a year?

Hey, cut back on the fat and cut back on the adult and childhood obesity epidemic in our country, and the hundreds and hundreds of food connections that go hand in hand with the disease.

Sure, we can affect the country. When all the relatives come over for the Christmas ham or the Thanksgiving turkey, who's to say either one of them has to be on the table? What's the matter with trying something that is lower in fat, great tasting, and a little unusual this Thanksgiving or Christmas? Don't think you can affect the food manufacturers of this country?

Conscious shopping sure as hell will affect what these food boys are manufacturing, because when we stop buying the lies, they'll stop manufacturing them. It's all profit-driven, so stop putting the money in their pockets. Demand lower fat and don't buy high fat. Insist on higher quality by not putting up with crap.

Have we gotten far enough off the fence for you? This is the kind of stuff that nobody wants to talk about. When it is discussed, it's usually in the back of some health food store with a bunch of people eating sprouts and drinking moss. But there is nothing ethereal about this, nothing intangible. This is not theory, this is very practical, applicable information.

I'm using it. I live in the 90's. I have kids, a business, a husband, a life. . . . And changing the quality and the fat content of what my family and I live on has absolutely affected more people than I could ever have imagined in my wildest dreams. You have the power to make the changes. You can turn this craziness around and enjoy, trust, and create new associations with your food.

Thank you for bearing with me.

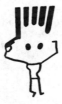

STAGE 1 RECIPES

BREAKFAST

Blueberry Pancakes

French Toast

Blueberry Muffins

Very Corny Corn Muffins

SOUPS

Minestrone Soup

Fish Stew

Potato and Vegetable Soup

MAIN COURSES

Fresh Tuna with Tomato and Pasta

Sesame-Chicken Nuggets with Oven-
  Roasted Potatoes/Fries

Chili

Beef Goulash

Spinach Lasagna

Steamed Fish

Beef Barley and Sautéed Vegetables

Turkey Chowder

Turkey Casserole with Vegetables

Turkey Loaf

Turkey Meatballs in Tomato Sauce

Chicken Fajitas

Chicken with Potato and Rosemary

Turkey Curry

Chicken and Sausage Jambalaya

SIDE DISHES

Roasted Vegetables

Spicy Red Beans and Rice

Barbecue Baked Beans

Corn, Tomatoes, and Lima Beans

SAUCES

Salsa—the Best Ever

Spicy Red Sauce

Orange Sauce for Broiled Fish

Mexican Green Olive Sauce

Mushroom Stew

Basic Tomato Sauce

DRESSINGS

Cucumber Yogurt Dressing

Balsamic Vinegar Dressing

Honey Mustard Dressing

CAKES

Carrot Cake with Applesauce

Chocolate Mousse Bars

Apple Blueberry Crisp

Chocolate Angel Food Cake

Upside-Down Plum Cake

Orange Sponge Cake

Blueberry Crumb Cake

Apple Bars

DESSERTS

Chocolate Meringue Kisses

Strawberry Ice

Rice Pudding

Strawberry Parfait

BREAKFAST

Blueberry Pancakes

1¼ c all-purpose flour	1½ tsp vegetable oil, preferably
¾ tsp salt	canola
3 Tbsp sugar	1¼ c 1% milk
2 tsp double-acting baking	1 c frozen blueberries
powder	
1 large whole egg, lightly	
beaten	

1. Measure and sift together the first 4 ingredients. If you do not have a sifter, gently shake the ingredients through a fine-mesh strainer.
2. Combine the next 3 ingredients in a separate bowl.
3. Place the frozen blueberries in a third bowl. Coat the blueberries with 1 table-spoon of dry ingredients. Do not let them thaw. This will prevent the blueberries from turning the entire batter blue.
4. Combine the wet and dry ingredients into one bowl. Mix together using a fork. *Do not overmix the batter* because it will make the pancakes tough. There should be small lumps (about the size of a pea) visible in the batter.
5. Add the blueberries to the mix and stir just enough to incorporate.
6. Preheat a large nonstick frying pan or griddle over medium heat. (A drop of water should quickly sizzle and evaporate when dropped on the pan.)
7. Drop ¼ cup of batter per pancake onto the skillet. When the top of the pancake is covered with little air bubbles, turn it over. When the second side is golden brown, approximately 2 minutes, remove from pan and serve.

Options
Replace blueberries with
   1 banana, thinly sliced
   1 apple, cored and chopped into small pieces, with 1 teaspoon cinnamon;
      the apple needs to be sautéed in a little water to soften.
   Strawberries or raspberries.

 Make a huge batch and freeze. Throw a couple in the toaster—instant breakfast!

Serving size	6 oz	Total fat	4 g
Servings per recipe	4	Saturated fat	1 g
Calories	265		

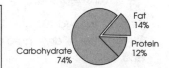

French Toast

2 large eggs	½ tsp ground cinnamon
2 large egg whites	8 slices challah bread, cut ¾
1 c 1% milk	inch thick; you may substitute
½ tsp vanilla extract	fresh white or Italian bread

1. Beat eggs and egg whites together.
2. Add milk, vanilla extract, and cinnamon to the eggs and mix well.
3. Soak the sliced bread in the egg mixture for approximately 5 minutes, until the mixture is absorbed.
4. Preheat oven to 350°. Arrange bread on a nonstick baking sheet. Bake for approximately 15 minutes, until the bread is lightly browned.
5. Or fry slices in a nonstick frying pan.

Options
Great with
> powdered sugar, sugar and cinnamon, jellies, maple syrup, lemon and powdered sugar, orange and powdered sugar, fruits, chocolate sauce, fruit pie fillings, and nonfat ice cream.

 Big favorite in our house—top with low-fat ice cream for a great dessert!

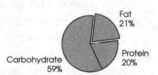

Serving size	6 oz	Total fat	6 g	
Servings per recipe	4	Saturated fat	2 g	
Calories	255			

Fat 21%
Carbohydrate 59%
Protein 20%

Blueberry Muffins

1¾ c unbleached flour	2¼ c frozen blueberries
2 tsp baking powder	1½ Tbsp canola oil
1 tsp baking soda	1 tsp vanilla extract
¾ c oat bran	1 medium egg
1 c applesauce	¾ c maple syrup
(unsweetened)	

1. Preheat oven to 400°.
2. Sift together all dry ingredients except oat bran. Add oat bran to dry ingredients and mix.
3. Toss blueberries with ¼ cup dry mix to coat.
4. In a separate bowl, mix applesauce, oil, vanilla extract, egg, and maple syrup.

5. Mix the dry and wet ingredients thoroughly but do not overmix. Add blueberries and fold gently into mixture.
6. Spoon into lightly greased muffin tin or use muffin papers.
7. Bake for 25 minutes, until muffins are golden. Cool and enjoy.

 Love, love, love these—very sweet with a yummy blueberry taste.

Serving size	2 oz	Total fat	2 g
Servings per recipe	18	Saturated fat	0 g
Calories	118		

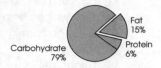

Fat 15%
Protein 6%
Carbohydrate 79%

Very Corny Corn Muffins

1 c unbleached flour	1 large whole egg
1 c yellow cornmeal	2 egg whites
4 tsp baking powder	1¼ c 1% milk
½ tsp salt	2 Tbsp canola oil
¼ c sugar	1 c canned cream corn

1. Preheat oven to 425°.
2. In a bowl, combine dry ingredients.
3. In another bowl, combine egg, egg whites, milk, oil, and corn.
4. Stir wet ingredients into dry ingredients until they are just moist. Do not overmix.
5. Lightly grease a muffin tin or use 12 paper muffin cups or use a nonstick muffin tin. Spoon mixture into cups.
6. Bake in oven for 20 to 25 minutes, until muffins are golden brown.

 Fabulous with soups and stews—really moist and sweet.

Serving size	3 oz	Total fat	3 g
Servings per recipe	12	Saturated fat	1 g
Calories	152		

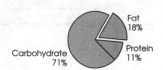

Fat 18%
Protein 11%
Carbohydrate 71%

Minestrone Soup

1 Tbsp olive oil	½ tsp black pepper, or to taste
1 c thinly sliced onion	6 c chicken or vegetable
6 cloves garlic, minced	broth
1 c diced carrots	1 28-oz can tomatoes with
1 c diced celery	juice
2 medium zucchini, diced	1½ c canned cannelini or
3 c shredded cabbage	Great Northern beans,
2 tsp oregano	rinsed and drained
1½ Tbsp basil	2 c water
2 tsp salt, or to taste	1 c elbow or ditalini pasta

1. Heat oil in large pot over medium heat. Add onion and garlic, and sauté until soft. Add carrots and celery, and cook for 5 minutes.
2. Add zucchini, stir well, and cook for 2 to 3 minutes.
3. Add cabbage and cook 5 more minutes.
4. Add oregano, basil, salt, and pepper. Cook 2 more minutes. Add broth and tomatoes, lower heat, and cook for 2 to 2½ hours, uncovered.
5. Add canned beans and water. Continue cooking for 15 to 20 minutes.
6. Cook elbows or ditalini in boiling salted water for 8 to 10 minutes, or until done. Add drained pasta to soup and stir well. Serve.

Wonderful on a cold winter night! Leave out the pasta and you can freeze it.

Serving size	18 oz	Total fat	2 g	
Servings per recipe	10	Saturated fat	0 g	
Calories	175			

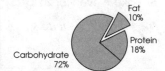

Fat 10%
Protein 18%
Carbohydrate 72%

Fish Stew

1¼ lbs. firm white fish filet (cod, red snapper), cut into 1½-inch cubes

5 medium potatoes (1⅔ lbs), peeled and sliced into ¼-inch slices

2 ripe tomatoes, peeled and chopped

1 large onion, sliced into thin rings

2 celery stalks, sliced

5 cloves garlic, minced

2 Tbsp chopped fresh parsley

1½ tsp. salt, or to taste

1 bay leaf

¼ tsp black pepper

¼ tsp red pepper flakes

⅛ tsp fennel seeds

2–3 inch piece orange peel (rind)

1 Tbsp olive oil

8 c water

1. Put fish on bottom of a large shallow pot. Cover with potatoes, tomatoes, onion, celery, garlic, and parsley.
2. Sprinkle with all the seasonings and oil.
3. Bring water to a boil.
4. Pour just enough boiling water into the pot to cover the ingredients.
5. Cook for 20 minutes, covered. Let sit for 1 hour, covered, for flavors to marry. Reheat if needed and serve.
6. Check the potatoes with a fork to be certain that they are done. Enjoy.

 Excellent! Even better the second day!

Serving size	16 oz	Total fat	5 g
Servings per recipe	6	Saturated fat	1 g
Calories	325		

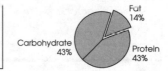

Fat 14%

Carbohydrate 43%

Protein 43%

Potato and Vegetable Soup

4 cloves garlic, minced	7 c chicken broth
1 large onion, chopped	2 c frozen peas
1 Tbsp canola oil	handful of egg noodles
3 medium russet potatoes, peeled and cubed	1 Tbsp fresh dill, or 1 tsp dried
	¼ c chopped fresh parsley
2 medium carrots, cut in half lengthwise and sliced	3 tsp salt, or to taste
	½ tsp pepper, or to taste
2 medium celery stalks, sliced	

1. In a large soup pot over medium-high heat, sauté onion and garlic in the oil for 7 minutes, or until soft.
2. Add potatoes, carrots, and celery, and mix well. Continue stirring for 2 minutes.
3. Add broth and bring to a boil. Lower heat and simmer for 30 minutes, or until the potatoes are ready to fall apart.
4. Add peas, noodles, dill, parsley, salt, and pepper. Cook 5 more minutes, until noodles are done. Correct seasoning and enjoy.

Option
Leave out the dill & parsley, and it's still the best.

 Tastes like "Mom's-great-old-fashioned-stew-on-the-farm."

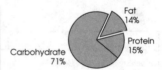

Serving size	17 oz	Total fat	3 g
Servings per recipe	6	Saturated fat	0 g
Calories	187		

Fat 14%
Protein 15%
Carbohydrate 71%

MAIN COURSES

Fresh Tuna with Tomato and Pasta

Sauce:
- 1 tsp olive oil, or spray some oil in pan
- 4 cloves garlic, chopped
- 1 onion, chopped
- 1 28-oz can crushed tomatoes in tomato puree
- 1 tsp salt, or to taste
- ½ tsp pepper, or to taste
- 1 tsp dry basil

Tuna:
- ¾ lb 1-inch-thick tuna steak
- 2 tsp olive oil
- 6 large cloves garlic
- ¼ tsp hot pepper flakes
- ½ tsp salt, or to taste
- 1 lb penne pasta

1. Heat oil over medium heat in a shallow pan. Add garlic and onion, and sauté until they turn light golden brown.
2. Add tomatoes, salt, pepper, and basil. Mix together and cook, covered, for 20 minutes. Stir occasionally so that the sauce won't stick to the pan. Set aside.
3. Heat oil in a heavy-bottomed pan that can hold tuna and sauce. Add garlic and cook for 2 minutes.
4. Add tuna and cook for 3 minutes, until side turns gray. Turn over and cook 2 more minutes. Break up tuna into 1-inch cubes with spatula.
5. Add sauce, hot pepper flakes, and salt. Cook for 6 minutes on medium heat. Adjust seasoning. Cook penne according to package directions. Serve sauce over the pasta.

 Try this, you'll love it.

Serving size	15 oz	Total fat	9 g
Servings per recipe	4	Saturated fat	2 g
Calories	403		

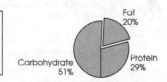

Fat 20%
Protein 29%
Carbohydrate 51%

Sesame-Chicken Nuggets with Oven-Roasted Potatoes/Fries

1 lb boneless, skinless chicken breast, cut into 1½-inch cubes	¾ c bread crumbs
	1 Tbsp sesame seeds

Marinade:	3 lg baking potatoes
1 egg white	2 tsp olive oil
¼ c soy sauce	½ tsp garlic powder
2 tsp garlic, chopped	1 tsp salt
2 tsp ginger, chopped	
1 Tbsp sugar	

1. Preheat oven to 400°.
2. Marinate chicken for 1 hour.
3. Mix bread crumbs and sesame seeds.
4. Remove chicken from marinade and let excess drip off.
5. Dip chicken in bread crumb mixture. Spray baking pan with oil and wipe off excess. Place chicken nuggets on baking sheet and bake for 20 minutes or until nuggets are golden brown.
6. Peel potatoes and cut into 1½-inch strips to look like a fat french fry. Toss with olive oil, garlic, and salt.
7. Spray baking sheet with oil and wipe off excess. Place potatoes in a single layer and bake at 400° for 40 minutes until crisp on the outside and tender on the inside.

Options
For Kids

     take out ginger.
     tastes and looks like chicken McNuggets.
     serve with fries or potatoes without garlic.

 Big hit with the kids—tastes just like fried chicken!

Serving size	11 oz	*Total fat*	6 g
Servings per recipe	4	*Saturated fat*	1 g
Calories	415		

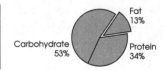

Chili

1½ c dried pinto beans, or 3 cups canned beans, rinsed and drained	1 large green pepper, cut into ½-inch cubes
1 medium onion, chopped	2 hot green chili peppers (jalapeños), chopped
1 bay leaf	2 tsp oregano
1 tsp salt	1 Tbsp cumin
4 c water	¼ tsp cayenne pepper
	2 tsp salt
1 Tbsp olive oil	2 bay leaves
1 lb lean ground beef	4–5 Tbsp chili powder
1¾ c chopped onion	1 20 oz can chopped tomatoes
2 Tbsp minced garlic	

1. Soak dried beans overnight in water to cover.
2. Drain beans and put in pot. Reserve liquid. Add onion, bay leaf, salt, and water. Cook over medium-high heat for 45 minutes, or until beans are tender but not mushy. Drain beans and save liquid.
3. In a large skillet over medium-high heat, sauté beef In 1 teaspoon oil until brown. Remove meat. Add 2 teaspoons oil and heat. Sauté onion, garlic, and peppers for 10 minutes.
4. Add the spices and sauté 5 minutes more.
5. Add meat, tomatoes, and beans, and cook for 45 minutes, until all the flavors are blended.
6. If the chili is too dry, add 1 or more cups of the liquid from beans and bring to a boil.

 Great over baked potatoes, rice, hot dogs, or low-fat chips for a chili pie.

Serving size	16 oz	Total fat	9 g	
Servings per recipe	6	Saturated fat	2 g	
Calories	441			

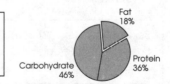

Beef Goulash

2 Tbsp olive oil
1 lb boneless chuck, cut into
1½ inch cubes
3 medium onions, sliced
6 cloves garlic, chopped
1½ Tbsp mild Hungarian
paprika
2 large tomatoes, chopped

2 medium green peppers,
cubed
1½ tsp caraway seeds
2 tsp salt, or to taste
4 c boiling water, or more if
necessary
4 boiled potatoes, cut into
1½-inch cubes

1. In a flameproof casserole or Dutch oven, heat the oil and sauté the meat until brown. Remove from pot and set aside.
2. Add onions and garlic, sauté until translucent, about 10 minutes.
3. Add paprika, heat through, then return meat to casserole. Add ½ the tomatoes, ½ the pepper, salt, caraway seeds, and 2 cups of boiling water. Bring to boil, cover, lower heat and cook for 1½ hours.
4. Add the rest of the tomatoes and pepper. Add another 2 cups of boiling water and cook for 45 minutes uncovered.
5. Check meat with fork for tenderness.
6. Serve with boiled potatoes (or noodles). Season potatoes before serving goulash over them.

Options
Add potatoes last 20 minutes of cooking for thicker sauce.
Add ½ can of low-fat cream of mushroom soup for richer, creamier sauce.
Thicken sauce with 2 Tbsp cornstarch dissolved in ½ cup water. Add to goulash while boiling last 5 minutes and stir until thick.

 Rich tomato sauce—just like your Hungarian grandmother used to make!

Serving size	21 oz	Total fat	8 g
Servings per recipe	4	Saturated fat	2 g
Calories	379		

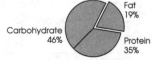

Fat 19%
Carbohydrate 46%
Protein 35%

Spinach Lasagna

1 lb lasagna noodles
2 10-oz packages frozen
  chopped spinach
2 lb fat-free ricotta cheese
1 whole egg
1 egg white
1 c grated Parmesan cheese
1½ tsp salt
½ tsp pepper
1 clove garlic, minced

1 tsp dried basil
¼ tsp ground nutmeg
½ lb part-skim mozzarella,
  shredded
½ lb fat-free mozzarella,
  shredded
4 c Basic Tomato Sauce (see
  recipe) or favorite nonfat
  zesty tomato sauce

1. Preheat oven to 375°.
2. Prepare lasagna noodles according to package directions. Drain and rinse pasta when finished.
3. Defrost spinach using a microwave or let it sit at room temperature. Do not cook spinach. Drain as much liquid from spinach as possible
4. Combine ricotta, spinach, whole egg, egg white, ¼ cup Parmesan, salt, pepper, garlic, basil, and nutmeg. In a separate bowl, combine the two mozzarellas.
5. Layer the lasagna in a lasagna pan (9 x 13 x 3) in the following order, going from the bottom to the top: 1 cup of tomato sauce, 1 layer of overlapping lasagna noodles, half of ricotta mix, one-third of mozzarella mix, one-fourth cup of Parmesan. Continue layering until all items are used up.
6. Bake uncovered for forty-five minutes. If top starts to overbrown during baking, cover. Let stand 5–10 minutes before serving.

 Rich and creamy. Can be mild, or zest it up with your favorite sauce.

Serving size	16 oz	Total fat	9 g
Servings per recipe	8	Saturated fat	5 g
Calories	429		

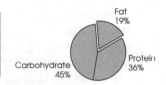

Steamed Fish

4½ lb whole sea bass (or any
  other low-fat fish), cleaned
½ tsp salt
½ tsp pepper
2 Tbsp chopped garlic
2 Tbsp chopped ginger

½ c soy sauce
⅓ c white wine
3 scallions, sliced with greens
  into 1-inch pieces
4 c cooked brown rice

1. Preheat oven to 400°.
2. Lay fish on the bottom of a large pan. Dry the inside and outside of the fish with paper towels.
3. Sprinkle inside and outside of the fish with salt, pepper, garlic, and ginger. Pour the soy, wine, and scallions over it.
4. Seal pan tightly with aluminum foil and place on the lowest shelf of the oven. Bake for 25 minutes, uncover, and test with a fork to make sure that the fish flakes. If not, bake 5 more minutes and test again.
5. Fish should come off the bone very easily, should be moist and flavorful, and should have quite a bit of sauce around it. Serve with cooked brown rice.

Options

Turn on broiler for 5 minutes to brown top when fish is fully cooked.

If pan is too large and there doesn't seem to be enough liquid, try doubling up on both the soy sauce and wine.

 A very rich, wonderful dish.

Serving size	18 oz	Total fat	8 g
Servings per recipe	6	Saturated fat	2 g
Calories	509		

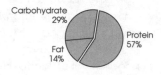

Carbohydrate 29%
Protein 57%
Fat 14%

Beef Barley and Sautéed Vegetables

1 c raw barley	2 tsp salt
4½ c water	½ tsp black pepper, or to taste
1 tsp olive oil	2 celery stalks, chopped
2 large onions, chopped	2 c carrots, chopped into
4 cloves garlic, chopped fine	small dice
¾ lb. beef chuck, cubed and	1 large green pepper, diced
trimmed of fat	2 c sliced mushrooms
1 tsp thyme	2 c beef broth
1 bay leaf	¼ c chopped parsley
½ tsp marjoram	

1. Wash barley with water until water runs clean. Combine barley with 3 cups water in pot and bring to a boil.
2. Cook for 30 minutes. Add 1½ cups more water and cook 10 more minutes. Barley should be tender but not mushy.

3. While barley is cooking, heat oil in a stewing pot, add onion and garlic, and sauté until soft. Add beef, spices, salt, and pepper, and cook for 10 minutes. Add carrots and celery. Cook 10 more minutes. Add green pepper and mushrooms. Cook 5 minutes, stirring.

4. Add beef broth, cover, and continue cooking for 1 hour, longer if necessary, until meat is tender. Add more water as needed to keep mixture juicy.

5. Add barley to beef-vegetable mixture. Stir for 2 minutes to blend and serve garnished with parsley.

 Rich sauce and full-bodied flavor—love those full-bodied low-fat dishes!

Serving size	17 oz	Total fat	9 g
Servings per recipe	4	Saturated fat	3 g
Calories	423		

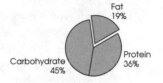

Fat 19%
Carbohydrate 45%
Protein 36%

Turkey Chowder

1 Tbsp olive oil	¼ tsp sage
1 large onion, thinly sliced	½ tsp garlic powder
¼ c chopped green pepper	6 c chicken stock or canned
3 medium carrots, diced	broth
3 medium potatoes, peeled and diced	3 c cubed cooked turkey (cook in water and use water for stock)
2 stalks celery, sliced	
1 tsp salt, or to taste	1 17-oz can creamed corn
½ tsp black pepper, or to taste	2 Tbsp chopped pimento from
½ tsp thyme	a jar
½ tsp basil	¼ c chopped fresh parsley

1. Heat oil in a large soup pot. Sauté onion and green pepper until onion slices are translucent.

2. Add carrots, potatoes, celery, salt, and spices. Mix well. Add stock and simmer for 15 minutes, until potatoes and carrots are soft.

3. Add turkey, corn, and pimento. Heat through but don't boil.

4. Just before serving, stir in parsley and adjust seasoning.

 Whoever said only clams could make chowder? . . .

Serving size	18 oz	Total fat	7 g
Servings per recipe	6	Saturated fat	2 g
Calories	304		

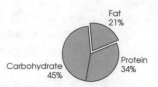

Turkey Casserole with Vegetables

1 Tbsp olive oil
1½ lbs turkey cutlets, cut into chunks
1½ c chopped onions
3 medium carrots, peeled and chopped
6 cloves garlic, minced
2½ c chicken stock or canned broth
1 c orange juice
¾ c canned crushed tomatoes

1 large red pepper, cut into strips
1 c rice
2 tsp chopped dried rosemary
1 small zucchini, cut in half and sliced
1 small yellow squash, cut in half and sliced
2 tsp salt, or to taste
½ tsp black pepper, or to taste
⅓ c chopped fresh parsley

1. Heat 1 tablespoon oil in a large deep skillet over medium-high heat. Sauté turkey chunks for 5 minutes, stirring frequently so they are lightly cooked. Remove turkey from pan and set aside (turkey should be partially raw).
2. Add onions, carrots, and garlic. Sauté, uncovered, for 5 minutes. Cover and continue cooking 15 more minutes.
3. Uncover and add stock, orange juice, tomatoes, red pepper, rice, and rosemary. Continue cooking for 15 minutes.
4. Add zucchini, squash, salt, and pepper. Continue cooking for 5 minutes.
5. Return turkey and vegetables to the skillet with the sauce. Cook 5 more minutes.
6. Serve garnished with parsley.

 It's worth the chopping . . . nothing like a good casserole.

Serving size	16 oz	Total fat	7 g
Servings per recipe	6	Saturated fat	2 g
Calories	390		

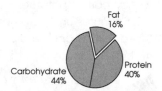

Turkey Loaf

1½ c chopped onions	1½ tsp salt, or to taste
2 tsp olive oil	¾ tsp black pepper, or to
1 to 1½ c chopped red pepper,	taste
or green pepper	2 egg whites
2 lb ground turkey	2 tsp dried basil
1 c chicken broth	¼ c chopped fresh
1 c bread crumbs	parsley

1. Sauté onions in 1 teaspoon oil for 5 minutes. Add red or green peppers and continue cooking 7 more minutes, until onions are soft.
2. Place onions, pepper, turkey, and the other ingredients in a bowl. Mix well.
3. Preheat oven to 350°.
4. Grease a 2-pound loaf pan with remaining 1 teaspoon oil. Fill with turkey mix and bake in oven until done, 1½ hours to 1¾ hours.

Options
Serve with bulgur and chick-pea salad.
You can slice as for sandwiches or use as an appetizer pâté.
Use the liquid for gravy; thicken with cornstarch.

 Perfect! Very easy.

Serving size	8 oz	Total fat	6 g	
Servings per recipe	8	Saturated fat	2 g	
Calories	263			

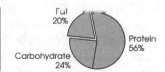

Turkey Meatballs in Tomato Sauce

Meatballs:
- ¼ c chopped onion
- 1 tsp chopped garlic
- 2 Tbsp bread crumbs
- 2 Tbsp chicken stock or water
- ½ lb ground turkey breast
- 1 tsp canola oil
- 1 Tbsp chopped parsley
- 1 egg white
- ¼ tsp oregano
- ⅛ tsp black pepper, or to taste
- ½ tsp salt, or to taste

Sauce:
- 1 large onion, chopped
- 4 cloves garlic, minced
- 1 Tbsp olive oil
- 1 large green pepper, chopped
- ½ c sliced mushrooms
- 1 tsp oregano
- 2 tsp basil
- 2 tsp salt, or to taste
- ½ tsp black pepper, or to taste
- 1 28-oz can tomatoes
- 2 Tbsp chopped flat-leaf parsley
- 1 lb spaghetti

1. To make meatballs: Sauté onion and garlic in oil until soft but not brown. Add 1 to 2 tablespoons bread crumbs if too sticky. If too dry, add 1 to 2 tablespoons chicken stock.
2. Mix with remaining ingredients in a large bowl. Form turkey into 1½-inch meatballs.
3. Preheat oven to 350°.
4. Wipe a large, flat tray with a little oil. Place meatballs on tray and bake in oven for 15 minutes. Set aside and make sauce.
5. To make sauce: Sauté onion and garlic in oil for 5 minutes. Add pepper and mushrooms, and cook for 5 more minutes. Add the spices, salt, and pepper, and cook for 2 minutes. Add tomatoes and cook for 20 minutes. Adjust seasonings.
6. Add meatballs and cook 10 more minutes. Add parsley, and sauce is ready.
7. Cook spaghetti and serve with meatballs and sauce.

 Give 'em to that meat-and-potatoes guy and you tell me if he can tell the difference in these meat—oops, turkey—balls.

Serving size	17 oz	Total fat	9 g
Servings per recipe	4	Saturated fat	2 g
Calories	644		

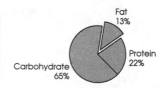

Chicken Fajitas

Marinade:

¼ c orange juice	1 Tbsp olive oil
¼ c pineapple juice	¾ lb onions, thinly sliced
1 tsp oregano	1½ large red peppers, thinly sliced
1 tsp cumin	1½ large green peppers, thinly sliced
1 tsp chili powder	
3 cloves garlic, chopped	3 cloves garlic, finely chopped
1 tsp salt, or to taste	
½ tsp black pepper, or to taste	¾ c salsa from a jar
	1 Tbsp cilantro (optional)
1½ lb chicken cutlets, cut into strips	8 corn tortillas

1. Combine juices, spices, and garlic into a marinade. Marinate chicken breasts for 30 minutes.
2. Broil or barbecue chicken for 2 minutes on each side, or until done. Set aside.
3. Heat oil in a large skillet. Add onions, peppers, and garlic. Cook for 15 minutes, stirring frequently. Do not overcook. Vegetables should be soft but not mushy.
4. Add salsa and cilantro. Mix well and heat through.
5. Warm the tortillas and serve with chicken and vegetables.

 Who doesn't love chicken fajitas? Try this version.

Serving size	18 oz	Total fat	12 g
Servings per recipe	4	Saturated fat	2 g
Calories	537		

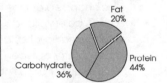

Fat 20%
Protein 44%
Carbohydrate 36%

Chicken with Potato and Rosemary

2½ lbs whole chicken, skin removed and cut into 8 pieces	2 bay leaves
	5 potatoes, cut into ¼-inch slices
8 cloves garlic, chopped	
1 tsp olive oil	2 tsp salt, or to taste
1½ c dry white wine	½ tsp black pepper, or to taste
1 tsp rosemary	3 c chicken stock

1. Preheat oven to 400°.
2. In an ovenproof casserole sauté chicken and garlic, uncovered, in oil. Lightly brown all sides.

3. Add 1 cup wine, rosemary, and bay leaves. Simmer for 5 minutes.
4. Remove chicken breasts and set aside.
5. Add potatoes, salt, pepper, and 2 cups of stock. Place in oven and cook, 1¼ hours, uncovered, until potatoes are soft and beginning to brown.
6. Add chicken breasts, remaining 1 cup of stock, and remaining ½ cup of wine. Heat through for 10 minutes. Potatoes should fall apart.

 Fabulous all-in-one meal!

Serving size	20 oz	Total fat	10 g
Servings per recipe	4	Saturated fat	3 g
Calories	446		

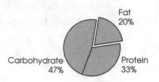

Fat 20%
Carbohydrate 47%
Protein 33%

Turkey Curry

1 lb turkey cutlets, cut into large cubes, or leftover roast turkey meat
1 Tbsp olive oil
½ c chopped onions
1 stalk celery, sliced
1 clove garlic, chopped
2 Tbsp curry powder
3½ Tbsp all-purpose flour

3 c chicken broth
1 tsp salt, or to taste
1 green apple, peeled and cubed
1 small green pepper, chopped
⅓ c raisins
6 dried apricots, cut into small pieces

1. In a large nonstick pan over medium-high heat, sauté turkey in oil until it changes color. *Do not overcook.* Total time should not exceed 6 minutes. Remove with a slotted spoon and set aside.
2. Add onion, celery, and garlic to the pan and cook until onions are translucent but not brown, about 6 minutes.
3. Add curry powder and flour. Cook with vegetables for 2 minutes.
4. Add chicken broth, salt, apple cubes, pepper, raisins, and apricots. Cook for 5 minutes.
5. Place turkey back in pan until warm.

Option
Serve with rice.

 For your International night, throw in a little taste of India.

Serving size	15 oz	Total fat	6 g
Servings per recipe	4	Saturated fat	1 g
Calories	319		

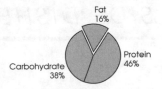

Fat 16%
Protein 46%
Carbohydrate 38%

Chicken and Sausage Jambalaya

4 oz smoked turkey sausages, cut into ½-inch cubes
1 lb skinless chicken breasts, cut into 1½-inch cubes
1 Tbsp olive oil
1½ c finely chopped onions
1½ c finely chopped green peppers
1½ c finely chopped celery

Seasoning:
2 bay leaves
1 tsp salt, or to taste
½ tsp thyme
1 tsp oregano
¼ tsp cayenne pepper
½ tsp Tabasco
1 tsp garlic powder

1 8-oz can tomato sauce
2 c converted white rice (instant)
3 c chicken stock
¼ c chopped scallions
2 Tbsp parsley

1. Sauté sausage in a large pot over medium-high heat for 5 minutes using 1 teaspoon of oil.
2. Add chicken and 1 teaspoon of oil, and sauté 5 more minutes.
3. Remove chicken and sausage, and set aside.
4. Add remaining 1 teaspoon of oil, onions, peppers, and celery. Sauté until lightly browned. Add seasoning and continue cooking for 5 minutes, stirring frequently.
5. Add tomato sauce and rice, and mix well. Cook for 5 minutes.
6. Add stock and bring to a boil. Reduce heat, cover pot, and simmer for 20 minutes.
7. Place chicken and sausage back into pot. Add scallions and parsley, and cook for 5 minutes.

 Great premenstrual dish—throw in extra Tabasco if you like it spicy.

Serving size	17 oz	Total fat	8 g
Servings per recipe	6	Saturated fat	2 g
Calories	455		

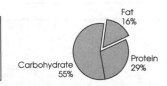

Fat 16%
Protein 29%
Carbohydrate 55%

SIDE DISHES

Roasted Vegetables

3 carrots, quartered lengthwise and then cut in half

4 medium zucchini, quartered lengthwise and then cut in half

2 small sweet potatoes, peeled and cut into ¼-inch circles

2 large onions, cut into 6- or 8-inch wedges

1 green pepper, cut into 1-inch strips

1 red pepper, cut into 1-inch strips

¼ c chopped garlic

2 Tbsp olive oil

2 tsp crushed rosemary

1 Tbsp kosher salt

1 tsp pepper, or to taste

Pam for spraying pan

4 c cooked brown rice

1. Preheat oven to 400°.
2. Cut vegetables and place in a large bowl. Add garlic, oil, spices, salt, and pepper. Use your hands to mix thoroughly.
3. Spray 2 sheet pans with Pam; wipe excess off with paper towel. Place vegetables in a single layer. Place one pan on bottom shelf of oven and the other on the top shelf. Rotate every 20 minutes to be sure they brown evenly on top and bottom. Cook for 45 minutes to 1 hour, checking every 20 minutes.
4. Serve with your favorite grain. This is good to eat as a snack at room temperature.

Options

Change seasonings to your favorites. You can also use string beans and mushrooms, left whole.

Eat plain or with pasta, in salads, on sandwiches, in fajitas, or add to any Italian dish. Or grill instead for a barbecue.

 Incredible! Great rosemary flavor.

Serving size	23 oz	Total Fat	3 g	
Servings per recipe	4	Saturated fat	1 g	
Calories	382			

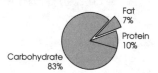

Fat 7%

Protein 10%

Carbohydrate 83%

Spicy Red Beans and Rice

1 Tbsp vegetable oil
2 large onions, diced
1 large clove garlic, minced
2 large green peppers, diced
3 celery stalks, sliced
2 bay leaves
½ tsp thyme
½ tsp cumin
1 tsp paprika
2 c canned crushed tomatoes

1 Tbsp cider vinegar
1 c vegetable broth, or more if necessary
1½ 15-oz cans red kidney beans, rinsed and drained
½ tsp hot pepper sauce, or to taste
1½ tsp salt, or to taste
4 c cooked rice

1. Heat oil in a large saucepan. Sauté onion, garlic, green peppers, and celery for 5 minutes. Add all the spices, tomatoes, vinegar, and vegetable broth. Simmer for 10 minutes.
2. Add beans, more vegetable broth if necessary, hot sauce, and salt. Heat through and cook for 5 minutes, until all flavors are blended. Cook rice according to package directions. Remove bay leaves before serving.
3. Serve over white rice.

 Staying with the cajun theme—thick and great.

Serving size	10 oz	Total fat	4 g
Servings per recipe	6	Saturated fat	0 g
Calories	348		

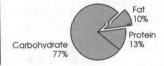

Fat 10%
Protein 13%
Carbohydrate 77%

Barbecue Baked Beans

3 tsp canola oil
2 cans pinto beans, rinsed and drained
3 medium onions, 2 chopped, 1 thinly sliced
2 large green peppers, diced
4 cloves garlic, minced
3 Tbsp prepared mustard

2 Tbsp chili powder
1½ tsp salt, or to taste
1 8-oz can tomato sauce
¼ c chili sauce
½ c cider vinegar
¼ c brown sugar
½ tsp hot sauce, or to taste
2 c vegetable broth

1. Preheat oven to 350°.
2. Heat 2 teaspoons of oil in a skillet. Sauté chopped onion, garlic, and green peppers until onions are lightly browned, about 10 minutes.

3. Add all the other ingredients except sliced onions.
4. Pour mixture into lightly oiled roasting pan using the remaining 1 teaspoon of oil. Arrange sliced onions on top. Bake for 1 hour, uncovered. The beans should look nice and brown.

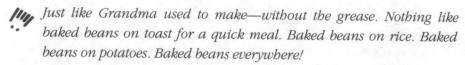 *Just like Grandma used to make—without the grease. Nothing like baked beans on toast for a quick meal. Baked beans on rice. Baked beans on potatoes. Baked beans everywhere!*

Serving size	14 oz	Total fat	4 g
Servings per recipe	6	Saturated fat	0 g
Calories	234		

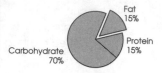

Fat 15%
Protein 15%
Carbohydrate 70%

Corn, Tomatoes, and Lima Beans

1 Tbsp olive oil
1 c chopped onion
1 large celery stalk, sliced
1 medium green pepper, diced
2 c 1-inch-cubed potatoes
2 c chicken broth
1 10-oz package frozen corn
1 10-oz package frozen baby lima beans

1½ tsp salt, or to taste
½ tsp black pepper, or to taste
¼ tsp Tabasco
2 tsp Worcestershire sauce
½ tsp oregano
1½ c canned tomatoes broken into pieces, with juice
2 Tbsp chopped parsley

1. Heat oil in a large stewing pot over medium heat. Add onions, celery, and green pepper until onions are tender.
2. Add potatoes and stir for 2 minutes. Add chicken broth, frozen corn, lima beans, and all the seasonings. Bring to a boil, cover, lower heat, and simmer for 30 minutes.
3. Uncover, add tomatoes and parsley, and continue cooking for 10 minutes.
4. Taste and adjust seasoning. Serve.

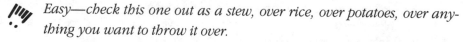 *Easy—check this one out as a stew, over rice, over potatoes, over anything you want to throw it over.*

Serving size	12 oz	Total fat	3 g
Servings per recipe	6	Saturated fat	0 g
Calories	186		

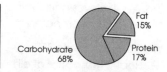

Fat 15%
Protein 17%
Carbohydrate 68%

SAUCES

Salsa—the Best Ever

- 5 plum tomatoes
- 5 tomatillos (available in Mexican shops; you can substitute plum tomatoes)
- 2 jalapeno peppers, seeded and cut into pieces
- ½ lime, juiced
- 2 Tbsp white vinegar
- ½ bunch cilantro, leaves removed from stem
- 1 medium onion, cut into pieces
- 4 cloves garlic, chopped
- 1 tsp. salt
- 1 tsp. salsa habañero or Tabasco
- ½ tsp pepper

1. Place all ingredients in a food processor. Chop but leave coarse. Use baked chips to dip.

 Easy—if you hate cilantro, leave it out. If you want it milder, cut out the peppers—here's what this one works with: baked chips, burritos, tacos, nachos, and over rice or an egg white omelet.

Serving size	2 oz	Total fat	0 g
Servings per recipe	6	Saturated fat	0 g
Calories	13		

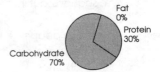

Fat 0%
Protein 30%
Carbohydrate 70%

Spicy Red Sauce

- 2 tsp olive oil
- 1 c chopped onion
- 2 large garlic cloves, chopped
- 3 c canned plum tomatoes
- 1 c water or juice from tomato
- 1 tsp salt
- 1 tsp cumin
- ¼ tsp ground coriander
- ¼ c dry red wine
- ¼ tsp cayenne pepper
- ¼ tsp black pepper
- ½ tsp chili powder
- 2 tsp tomato paste

- 1 lb cooked pasta

1. Heat oil in pan. Add onion and garlic, and cook until soft but not browned.
2. Add remaining ingredients except pasta and cook, covered, for 1 hour at a low simmer. It's ready to use on pasta or to zip up vegetables and beans.

Options

Add 3 minutes before complete (all, some or none):

1 c chopped artichoke hearts   ½ c steamed quartered
2 Tbsp capers   zucchini
½ c steamed quartered carrots

 Easy. The best spicy Italian sauce ever. You gotta try this.

Serving size	10 oz	Total fat	3 g	
Servings per recipe	5	Saturated fat	0 g	
Calories	144			

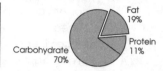

Fat 19%
Protein 11%
Carbohydrate 70%

Orange Sauce for Broiled Fish

2 c orange juice
½ c scallions, cut into ½-inch pieces
salt and pepper to taste
1 red pepper, sliced into 1½-inch strips

1 green pepper, sliced into 1½-inch strips
2 small tomatoes, peeled, seeded, and chopped
2 Tbsp fresh or 2 tsp. dry chopped coriander

1. In a small pan, combine orange juice, scallions, salt, coriander, and pepper. Cook, uncovered, for 10 minutes, until reduced to half.
2. Add peppers and cook for 2 minutes.
3. Add tomatoes. Check seasonings. Cook for 1 minute. Sprinkle on coriander. It's ready to serve over broiled fish.

 If you want to impress your friends, add some of this sauce over your broiled fish or chicken.

Serving size	8 oz	Total fat	trace	
Servings per recipe	4	Saturated fat	0 g	
Calories	82			

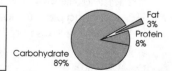

Fat 3%
Protein 8%
Carbohydrate 89%

Mexican Green Olive Sauce

½ Tbsp olive oil
2 medium onions, chopped
1 large green pepper, chopped
½ c chopped stuffed green olives
1 large lemon, juiced
1 Tbsp paprika

1 tsp ground coriander
1 c fresh orange juice
1 tsp salt
½ tsp black pepper
1 c brown rice; cook according to directions or use recipe in this book

1. Heat oil in a small pan over medium-high heat. Add onions and cook until soft but not browned.
2. Add peppers and olives, and cook 5 more minutes.
3. Add all other ingredients except rice and cook on low heat 6 more minutes.
4. Prepare rice.
5. Sauce is ready to serve on rice or fish.

 You thought you had to give up olives didn't you? This recipe cures the olive cravings. Here's a thought—use it as a sauce on vegetarian pizza.

Serving size	12 oz	Total fat	5 g
Servings per recipe	4	Saturated fat	1 g
Calories	264		

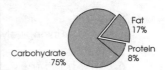

Fat 17%
Protein 8%
Carbohydrate 75%

Mushroom Stew

½ Tbsp olive oil
1 medium onion, minced
4–6 cloves garlic, minced
¾ lb wild mushrooms (such as portobello), thickly sliced into pieces ⅛ inch thick and 1 inch long
¾ lb fresh white mushrooms, thickly sliced

½ c red wine
½ c vegetable or chicken broth
1 tsp thyme
1 tsp crushed rosemary
salt and pepper to taste

1. Heat oil in a large pot (cast iron works great); you need plenty of room for all the sliced mushrooms.
2. Add onion and garlic, and cook over medium heat until they start to brown. This takes about 10 minutes. Keep stirring.

3. Add mushrooms, mix, and sauté for 5 to 10 minutes. The mushrooms should start to release their liquid. Add wine and broth, stir, and cook until it comes to a simmer.

4. Add thyme, rosemary, salt, and pepper. Cook on high until the liquid cooks down to half its original volume—about 15 minutes.

5. Serve over polenta, rice, or boiled mashed potatoes. Also good with Italian bread to soak up the juices.

 The other day I had this poured over mashed potatoes. It was fabulous!

Serving size	9 oz	Total fat	2 g
Servings per recipe	4	Saturated fat	0 g
Calories	125		

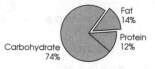

Fat 14%
Protein 12%
Carbohydrate 74%

Basic Tomato Sauce

2 tsp olive oil	2 tsp dried basil
1 medium onion, finely chopped	½ tsp dried oregano
6 cloves garlic, finely chopped	1 tsp salt
2 28-oz cans crushed tomatoes	½ tsp pepper
1 6-oz can tomato paste	1 Tbsp sugar or fructose
	2 Tbsp chopped fresh parsley

1. Heat oil in a saucepan over medium heat.

2. Add onion and garlic, and sauté until onion becomes very soft, approximately 10 minutes.

3. Turn heat to low. Add the next 7 ingredients. Cook, stirring occasionally, for 45 to 60 minutes.

4. Add parsley, stir, and cook 5 more minutes.

 Easy and better than anything in a jar. Impress yourself—make your own sauce!

Serving size	8 oz	Total fat	2 g
Servings per recipe	8	Saturated fat	0 g
Calories	83		

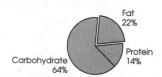

Fat 22%
Protein 14%
Carbohydrate 64%

DRESSINGS

Cucumber Yogurt Dressing

1 medium cucumber, peeled and cut into pieces

1 bunch scallions (5-6), cut into small pieces, including some of the green

16 oz plain no-fat yogurt (drain off liquid)

3 Tbsp lemon, juiced (about ¼ c)

1 tsp dried basil, or 1 Tbsp fresh dill weed

2 Tbsp chopped parsley

2 cloves garlic

1½ tsp salt, or to taste

½ tsp black pepper, or to taste

Place all ingredients in a food processor and blend until smooth. Serve over salad greens, pasta salad, or broiled fish. Dill is best for fish.

 If you hate dill or lemon (who hates lemons?), leave it out. Grab your low-fat chips and sit down and enjoy your movie!

Serving size	1¾ oz	Total fat	0 g	
Servings per recipe	10	Saturated fat	0 g	
Calories	22			

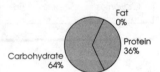

Balsamic Vinegar Dressing

8 Tbsp water

2 c balsamic vinegar

4 Tbsp dijon mustard (any fat-free version)

8 Tbsp lemon juice

4 cloves garlic, crushed

2 tsp salt

2 tsp oregano (dry)

black pepper to taste

2 tsp sugar

2 Tbsp parsley, chopped

Mix all ingredients together in a jar and shake vigorously.

 Try this for grilling, roasting, marinating, or over your salad.

Serving size	2 oz	Total fat	0 g
Servings per recipe	24	Saturated fat	0 g
Calories	8		

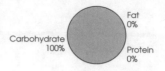

Fat 0%
Carbohydrate 100%
Protein 0%

Honey Mustard Dressing

6 Tbsp prepared mustard or to taste (non fat)
8 Tbsp honey

8 Tbsp lemon juice
12 Tbsp cider vinegar
2 tsp salt or to taste

Combine all ingredients.

 Anything you'd put a dressing on, put this one on.

Serving size	2 oz	Total fat	0 g
Servings per recipe	16	Saturated fat	0 g
Calories	54		

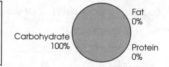

Fat 0%
Carbohydrate 100%
Protein 0%

CAKES

Carrot Cake with Applesauce

1½ c unbleached white flour
½ c whole grain pastry flour
1 c sugar
2 tsp baking soda
1½ tsp ground cinnamon
½ tsp ground nutmeg
½ tsp salt

1 c applesauce (unsweetened)
2 Tbsp canola oil
2 egg whites
2 large whole eggs
3 c grated carrots

1. Preheat oven to 350°.
2. In a mixing bowl, combine first 7 ingredients (all dry).

3. In another bowl, mix together applesauce, oil, egg whites, and eggs. Add the mixture slowly to the dry ingredients.
4. Beat together until well mixed. Add carrots and mix until they are integrated.
5. Pour into a loaf pan (9 x 5 x 3) and bake in oven for 1 hour 10 minutes, or until a toothpick inserted in the center comes out clean.
6. Turn cake out onto a rack to cool.

Option
Make a non-fat icing:

non-fat cream cheese, powdered sugar, non-fat milk, and vanilla extract made thick or powdered sugar, non-fat milk, vanilla extract, which is thin to drizzle on top.

 If you love carrot cake, you'll love this.

Serving size	3 oz	Total fat	3 g	
Servings per recipe	12	Saturated fat	0 g	
Calories	174			

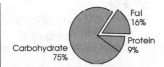

Fat 16%
Protein 9%
Carbohydrate 75%

Chocolate Mousse Bars

⅔ c unbleached flour
⅓ c unsweetened cocoa powder
1½ oz unsweetened baking chocolate
1 Tbsp canola oil

6 extra-large egg whites
1¼ c sugar
¾ c unsweetened applesauce
½ c plain nonfat yogurt
1 tsp vanilla extract

1. Preheat oven to 350°. Spray a 9-by-9-inch baking pan with oil and wipe off excess, or use a nonstick pan.
2. Sift together flour and cocoa powder. Set aside.
3. Melt chocolate in a double boiler. When melted, turn off heat and add oil. Mix until combined. Cool slightly.
4. Beat egg whites on high with sugar until very fluffy. Add applesauce, yogurt, vanilla extract, melted chocolate, and dry ingredients. Lower speed and continue beating until well incorporated.
5. Pour mixture into baking pan and bake for 20 to 25 minutes. The center of the mixture will feel firm and not liquidy when touched lightly. A toothpick inserted will come out covered with batter, not clean.
6. Cool and serve chilled. Cut into 16 bars.

THESE YOU WON'T BELIEVE! YOU GOTTA TRY THESE!

Serving size	2 oz	Total fat	3 g	
Servings per recipe	16	Saturated fat	1 g	
Calories	129			

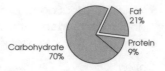

Fat 21%
Protein 9%
Carbohydrate 70%

Apple Blueberry Crisp

1 tsp canola oil

Filling:
4 medium Granny Smith apples, peeled, cored, and sliced
1 Tbsp lemon juice
1 tsp ground cinnamon
¼ c sugar
1 c frozen blueberries

Topping:
1 c rolled oats
⅓ c unbleached flour
¼ c brown sugar
4 tsp canola oil
½ tsp ground cinnamon
1 Tbsp orange juice

1. Preheat oven to 375°.
2. Lightly wipe a 9½-by-11-inch baking dish with 1 teaspoon oil.
3. Mix sliced apples with lemon juice, cinnamon, and sugar. Press into baking dish and sprinkle frozen berries on top.
4. Mix topping ingredients and sprinkle over blueberry mixture.
5. Bake for 30 minutes, until crumbs look lightly browned. Test apples with a fork for tenderness.
6. Enjoy warm or at room temperature.

 Try this one warm with low-fat ice cream melting on top—then you tell me if you're living in deprivation!

Serving size	4 oz	Total fat	3 g	
Servings per recipe	9	Saturated fat	0 g	
Calories	136			

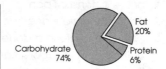

Fat 20%
Protein 6%
Carbohydrate 74%

Chocolate Angel Food Cake

1 c cake flour	½ tsp cream of tartar
¼ c cocoa	3 whole eggs
1⅓ c sugar	1 tsp vanilla extract
6 large egg whites	½ tsp almond extract

1. Preheat oven to 350°.
2. Sift flour, cocoa, and ⅓ cup sugar together. Set aside.
3. Whip egg whites until foamy. Add cream of tartar and continue beating until soft peaks form. Set aside in a large bowl.
4. Whip whole eggs with 1 cup sugar until creamy and golden. Add vanilla and almond extracts and mix until combined.
5. Fold whole egg mixture gently into whipped egg whites.
6. Fold dry mixture gently into egg mixture, until just combined.
7. Pour mixture into a 10-inch tube pan and bake for 40 to 50 minutes, or until a toothpick inserted in the middle comes out clean. Invert cake until cool.
8. Run knife around edge of pan to loosen cake. Remove bottom with tube. Run knife around the bottom of pan and around the tube. Turn cake onto plate.

Options
Serve with raspberry sauce: frozen raspberries and sugar to taste blended together.

 Note: Don't use a nonstick pan or flour on this one. The cake's gotta stick to the sides of the pan while it's cooking. Who doesn't love chocolate angel food cake?

Serving size	*2 oz*	*Total fat*	*2 g*	
Servings per recipe	*12*	*Saturated fat*	*1 g*	
Calories	*162*			

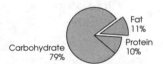

Upside-Down Plum Cake

15 prune plums, pitted and cut into pieces; can leave skins	2 large egg whites
½ tsp ground cinnamon	1 tsp vanilla extract
4 Tbsp brown sugar	½ c apple juice
1 c unbleached flour	6 Tbsp sugar
2 tsp baking powder	1½ Tbsp canola oil
	½ c applesauce

1. Preheat oven to 350°.
2. Mix prune plums with cinnamon and brown sugar. Place in a 9-by-9-inch baking pan, sprayed lightly with Pam.

3. Mix flour and baking powder.
4. Beat egg whites, vanilla extract, apple juice, sugar, oil, and applesauce together.
5. Combine flour mixture and liquid mixture, just enough so there are no lumps left. Pour over fruit and bake for 45 minutes to 1 hour or until browned on top and toothpick inserted in the middle comes out clean.
6. Cool on rack. Can be served warm or cold.

Options

Can be made with other fruits: pineapple, peaches, bananas, apples, pears, or nectarines.

 When we taste-tested this one, I ate the whole thing. I always say there's nothing like a good coffee cake.

Serving size	5 oz	Total fat	3 g
Servings per recipe	8	Saturated fat	0 g
Calories	151		

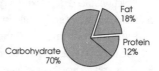

Orange Sponge Cake

2 c orange juice
2 tsp grated orange rind
2 Tbsp canola oil
1 c sugar
2 whole eggs

2 egg whites
1 c whole wheat flour
1 c unbleached flour
2 tsp baking soda

1. Preheat oven to 350°.
2. In a saucepan, bring orange juice and rind to a boil. Remove from heat and cool while proceeding with recipe.
3. In a mixer or by hand using a wire whisk in a large bowl, mix oil and sugar until creamy. Add eggs and egg whites one at a time. Continue beating until all the eggs are added.
4. In a separate bowl, combine flours and baking soda, and add to the oil, sugar, and egg mixture.
5. Add flour mixture to orange juice mixture, a third at a time, until just combined. Pour into a 10-inch tube pan lightly sprayed with Pam. Bake for 35 to 40 minutes, until a toothpick inserted in the center comes out clean.
6. Cool on rack.
7. Cut around sides of pan to loosen cake; remove bottom and center tube. Run a knife around the bottom and center tube to loosen cake. Invert onto cake plate and serve with lightly sweetened strawberries or raspberries.

Options
Drizzle powdered sugar and skim milk (vanilla icing) on top.
Serve with Amazaki Custard (recipe in stage 3).

 Easy, easy, easy. . .

Serving size	*4 oz*	*Total fat*	*4 g*	
Servings per recipe	*11*	*Saturated fat*	*1 g*	
Calories	*180*			

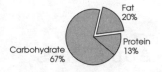

Blueberry Crumb Cake

2½ c unbleached flour
1 tsp baking powder
¾ tsp baking soda
½ c oat bran
½ c lightly packed brown sugar
½ tsp ground nutmeg
1 tsp ground cinnamon
3½ Tbsp canola oil
½ c applesauce
¼ c plus 1 Tbsp honey
1 c orange juice

1 tsp pure vanilla extract
5 large egg whites
pinch of salt
3 c frozen berries
3 Tbsp sugar

Topping:
¾ c unbleached flour
¾ c quick-rolled oats
½ c packed brown sugar
1½ Tbsp canola oil
2 Tbsp honey

1. Preheat oven to 350°.
2. Mix together flour, baking powder, baking soda, oat bran, sugar, and spices.
3. Beat oil, applesauce, honey, orange juice, and vanilla extract in a mixer. Combine with dry ingredients.
4. Beat egg whites with pinch of salt until soft peaks form. Fold into the batter. Spread into a 9-by-13-inch baking pan lightly sprayed with Pam.
5. Mix berries with sugar and spread over batter.
6. Combine topping ingredients until crumbly. Spread topping over blueberries.
7. Bake for 40 minutes, or until a toothpick inserted in the center comes out clean. Cool on a rack.

 Yummy and sweet. Love this warm for breakfast.

Serving size	7 oz	Total fat	7 g
Servings per recipe	12	Saturated fat	1 g
Calories	290		

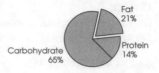

Apple Bars

1½ c unbleached all-purpose flour
1 tsp baking powder
¼ c honey
½ c lightly packed brown sugar
4 tsp canola oil
4 large egg whites
½ c applesauce
1 Tbsp apple juice

5 apples, peeled, cored, and thinly sliced

Topping:
1 Tbsp canola oil
¼ c lightly packed brown sugar
1 Tbsp apple juice
1 tsp ground cinnamon

1. Preheat oven to 425°.
2. Mix flour with baking powder in a bowl and set aside.
3. Beat honey, brown sugar, oil, egg whites, applesauce, and apple juice in a mixer. Pour into flour mixture and stir well.
4. Pour the batter into a 9-by-13-inch baking pan lightly sprayed with Pam and smooth batter. Arrange apple slices in lines across the dough, pressing them slightly into the dough.
5. Bake for 10 minutes, then remove. Lower heat to 375°.
6. Mix topping ingredients in a bowl. Drizzle over the apples in the pan. Return pan to oven and bake for 15 to 20 minutes, until a toothpick inserted in the center comes out clean.
7. Remove from oven and cool on a rack. Slice into bars.

 Reminds me of old-fashioned apple-strudel cake bars.

Serving size	4 oz	Total fat	3 g
Servings per recipe	14	Saturated fat	0 g
Calories	124		

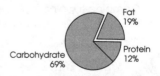

DESSERTS

Chocolate Meringue Kisses

1 Tbsp sifted cocoa powder	additional coca powder for
1 oz unsweetened chocolate, melted and cooled	dusting cooking sheets
4 extra-large egg whites	1 c granulated sugar
pinch of salt	1 tsp vanilla extract

1. Preheat oven to 300°.
2. Grease 3 cookie sheets lightly and dust with cocoa powder. Shake sheets lightly to completely cover with cocoa. You will need about 3 cookie sheets because this recipe makes 50 cookies, and you will want to bake them one after another.
3. Melt chocolate, then set aside to cool. (Melt chocolate in either a double boiler or on low power in the microwave.)
4. Beat egg whites with pinch of salt until soft peaks form. The eggs must form soft peaks or the cookies will not hold their shape.
5. Add sugar slowly and continue beating until very stiff and shiny.
6. Using a spatula, fold in vanilla extract, melted chocolate, and 1 tablespoon cocoa powder until incorporated.
7. Drop on cookie sheets 1 heaping teaspoon at a time. Space the mixture 2 inches apart. They will have the shape of chocolate kisses.
8. Bake for 30 to 40 minutes. Remove cookies immediately from cookie sheet. Cool completely and store in an airtight container.

 Easy and guaranteed to cure any chocolate cravings.

Serving size	1 oz	Total fat	2 g	
Servings per recipe	10	Saturated fat	1 g	
Calories	110			

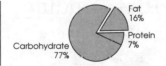

Strawberry Ice

1 c sugar, or to taste
2 c water
4 c frozen unsweetened
   strawberries or raspberries

½ lemon, juiced

1. This recipe should be made a day before it is needed.
2. Combine sugar and water in a saucepan. Bring to a boil, turn heat down, and simmer for 10 minutes. Remove from heat and cool.
3. Puree strawberries with lemon juice in a blender or food processor. Add two-thirds of sugar water, taste for sweetness, and add more if necessary. You may need to add sugar water before strawberries are completely pureed because of thickness.
4. Place mixture in a bowl, cover, and freeze for at least 2 hours, until mixture hardens. Beat in an electric mixer or food processor until creamy. Return to the freezer.
5. The next day, refrigerate for 30 minutes to soften before serving. Enjoy!

Option
Use organic strawberries and this becomes a stage 3 recipe!

 Sweet, creamy, and icy, great for the kids. Fabulous with non-fat chocolate sauce and fresh strawberries.

Serving size	12 oz	Total fat	0 g
Servings per recipe	4	Saturated fat	0 g
Calories	293		

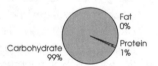

Rice Pudding

6 c low-fat milk
1 c white rice (*not* instant)
½ c sugar
   pinch of salt

1 c low-fat milk
3 eggs
1 tsp vanilla extract

1. Combine first 4 ingredients in a deep, heavy-bottomed pot over medium-low heat.
2. Let the mixture slowly come to a *soft* boil (it may foam up; that's O.K.). Continue the soft boil (too much of a boil will scorch the milk) for approximately 1 hour, or until almost all the liquid has been absorbed. The boiling will start making a "pop" or "slapping" sound. When it does, the rice is finished.
3. Remove from heat and add the last 3 ingredients. Combine well and let sit for 20 minutes. Serve warm or chilled.

Love this with cinnamon or nutmeg sprinkled on top! Add the warm fire on a cold winter's night and it's done!

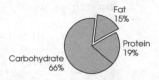

Serving size	9 oz	Total fat	4 g
Servings per recipe	8	Saturated fat	2 g
Calories	235		

Fat 15%
Protein 19%
Carbohydrate 66%

Strawberry Parfait

1½ c strawberries, very ripe fresh, puréed, or 2 10-oz pkgs frozen with juice
3 tsp plain gelatin

6 Tbsp sugar
4 Tbsp orange juice
½ c chilled evaporated skim milk

1. In a small saucepan, combine strawberries, 4 tablespoons sugar, and 1 teaspoon gelatin. Cook and stir over low heat until sugar and gelatin are dissolved. *Do not* let it come to a boil. Pour into large mixing bowl and place in freezer to chill.
2. Heat orange juice and 2 teaspoons gelatin in saucepan until gelatin dissolves. This can boil softly. Then keep on very low heat while preparing next step.
3. In small mixing bowl, beat skimmed milk on very high speed until it becomes frothy (about 3 minutes). While mixing, pour the warm orange juice mixture into the milk mixture. The milk will start to thicken and become creamier as the orange juice mixture cools. When this is accomplished, remove from mixer and set aside.
4. Take the strawberry mixture from freezer and mix on high speed until it becomes creamy (about 3 minutes).
5. Fold the two mixtures together until well incorporated.
6. Pour the parfait into champagne glasses. Chill for 30 minutes and serve plain or with fresh berries on top. If you need to chill it longer, take out of refrigerator 30 minutes before serving.

 Not quick or easy the first time, but definitely worth the effort for a special dinner.

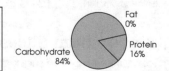

Serving size	5 oz	Total fat	0 g
Servings per recipe	4	Saturated fat	0 g
Calories	145		

Fat 0%
Protein 16%
Carbohydrate 84%

Remember when we were talking about holiday meals a few pages back? I just want to show how easy it is to change your traditional high-fat dinner into a low-fat feast. Here are some of my unofficial holiday recipes:

CHRISTMAS DINNER—BIG FAT

Relish Tray: Olives, slices of Cheese and Crackers, Stuffed
Celery with Cream Cheese, Deviled Eggs
Glazed Ham in All Its Juices
Candied Yams with Butter, Brown Sugar, and Marshmallows
Green Beans with Buttered Almonds
Buttered Dinner Rolls
Pecan Pie with Vanilla Ice Cream

CHRISTMAS DINNER—LOW FAT

Relish Tray
Glazed Ham Slices
Candied Yams
Creamed Mashed Potatoes
Whole Wheat Rolls
Fresh Green Beans and Onions
Angel Food Cake

Relish Tray
Fresh veggies (radishes, cucumber slices, cauliflower florettes, cherry tomatoes) with low-fat yogurt dip, pickles, baby corn, and artichoke hearts

Glazed Ham Slices
Top ham with brown sugar and pineapple slices. Bake (portion control here, eat a small portion of ham and load up on the potatoes and veggies).

Candied Yams
Slice yams lengthwise and lay in a casserole.

Make a mixture of fresh-squeezed orange juice, brown sugar, and cinnamon, and drizzle over yams.
Bake until heated through.

Creamed Mashed Potatoes
Creamed potatoes with skim milk and spice with chives

Warm Whole Wheat Rolls
Serve with honey instead of butter.

Fresh Green Beans and Onions
Steam to preserve vitamins and minerals.

Angel Food Cake
Serve with fresh berries and fat-free fudge sauce.
Options: Smother the cake with non-fat ice cream or strawberry sorbert.

THANKSGIVING DINNER—BIG FAT
• •

Whole Turkey Basted in Butter

Sausage Stuffing

Creamed Mashed Potatoes

Cranberry Relish

Waldorf Salad with Mayo and Sour Cream

Pumpkin Pie the Traditional Way (made with cream and whole

eggs and topped with whipped cream)

THANKSGIVING DINNER—LOW FAT
• •

Whole Turkey Breast and Gravy with Chestnut Stuffing

Mashed Potatoes

Beets in Citrus Dressing

Cranberry Relish

Waldorf Salad

Pumpkin Pie

Roast Turkey Breast

Roast your turkey breast according to directions.

Gravy

Defat the turkey juices, blend with some veggie stock, and thicken with cornstarch.

Chestnut Stuffing

Take your favorite low-fat dried breads (cornbread, sourdough, whole wheat), crumble and add chopped celery, onions, and spices. Moisten with low-fat chicken broth. Add a couple of egg whites. Fold in a big handful of chopped roasted chestnuts (chestnuts are very low in fat). Bake in a covered casserole until done.

Beets in Citrus Dressing

Cook whole beets in water until tender.
Rinse under cold water and slip off the skins.
Slice and put into a bowl.
In another bowl mix together: fresh orange and lemon juice (more of the orange and much less of the lemon), and a big pinch of ground cloves.
Pour over the beets and stir. Add a little salt and more pepper.

Cranberry Relish

Finely chop in blender or food processor fresh cranberries, a couple of fresh oranges with some grated orange peel, and a small handful of walnuts and sugar.

Waldorf Salad

Chop celery and fresh apples and add some raisins. Add a small amount of chopped walnuts.
Make a dressing by mixing together some non-fat or low-fat mayo with some non-fat or low-fat sour cream; add some salt and pepper and a squirt of fresh lemon juice.

Pumpkin Pie

Find a recipe for a low-fat pie shell or buy one.
For the filling, use your favorite recipe but substitute evaporated skim milk for the cream. Use egg substitute in place of eggs or use two egg whites for one whole egg.

HANUKKAH SUPPER—BIG FAT
• •

Brisket Smothered in Gravy Made from Juice Drippings

Potato Pancakes, Made with Whole Eggs and Fried in Oil,

Topped with Sour Cream

Kugel made with Whole Eggs

Cucumbers in Sour Cream and Chives

HANUKKAH SUPPER—LOW FAT
• •

Brisket of Beef

Potato Pancakes

Kugel

Peas with Tarragon

Cucumber Salad

Brisket of Beef

Make the brisket the night before.

Smear mustard over top and season with bay leaf, salt and pepper, and thyme.

Chop carrots, celery, and onions and lay on top of brisket. Cover and bake slowly according to directions.

Remove and cool. Refrigerate overnight.

Next day, scrape all of the fat globules off the juices, heat in the oven and serve.

Potato Pancakes

Finely grate potatoes and squeeze out all the juice.

Dice some green onions and mix with potatoes.

Wipe some oil in a nonstick pan.

Put a spoonful of potato mixture in the pan, one at a time, and cook until golden brown.

Serve with applesauce.

Kugel

Cook wide egg noodles according to directions.

Drain noodles and stir in grated onions and a couple of egg whites. Add salt and pepper.

Spoon mixture into a lightly greased casserole and bake uncovered until top is golden brown.

Variation:
Sweet Kugel Instead of onions and spices, add raisins, cinnamon, and sugar.

Peas with Tarragon

Steam some baby peas and sprinkle some fresh tarragon on top.

Cucumber Salad

Slice cucumbers very thin.

Add some sliced purple onion, vinegar, a little salt and pepper, and sugar.

Stage 2

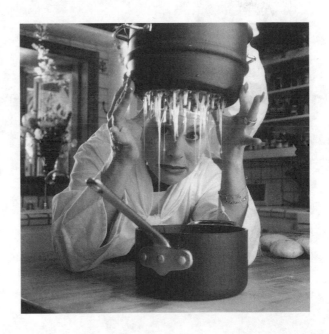

CHAPTER 7

HIGH QUALITY . . . WHAT ARE WE TALKING ABOUT?

Why stage two? What's in it, and why bother reading the rest of the book now that you've got the basics to a low-fat life-style down? Consider the book finished. With the information and recipes you have from stage one, what else could you need? Nothing!! You don't need more information than what you've got under your belt to change what's under your belt, if you know what I mean.

But maybe you want to know just a bit more about the stuff you used to hate that's now your best friend: food.

/// Interested in anything other than reducing your total fat and cholesterol intake?

/// Health? You wouldn't believe how much more involved the "health" part of what we put into our mouths is. We can, in stage two, go way, way beyond cholesterol and fat. Stage two, the reasons why.

Quality?

Ever heard of whole foods?

Know the difference between what's processed and what grows? Most of us don't.

You can't imagine once you crack this nut (pardon the very whole-food reference) what you'll find inside.

STAGE TWO IS

Loaded with info, lots and lots of emotionally charged discussions ahead. It tends to get a little heated when you find out about some of the stuff that's going into your body that you didn't know was going in, but that's what stage two of this book is all about:

> Discussion.
> Sharing information.
> Great-tasting food.

And it all gets back to my favorite issue: choice. Yours and mine. Adding information to our lives so that we can create more and more choices, choices that are different from what you may have now. Making some of those different choices helps give us back some of the control that we lose when we give all the power to someone else and just go along for the ride. (Do you think I've used the words "more" and "choices" enough in the last couple of paragraphs?)

Increasing the quality of what you're eating does increase the quality of your life. How could it not? You absolutely are what you eat.

You think the reason I wrote this book in three stages is that it just makes sense? I mean, three stages give you the opportunity to learn all this stuff slowly and open the door to take it one stage at a time, a concept that's worked well with all the twelve-step programs of the world. So what if instead of "stage" they say "day"? Who's thinking those kinds of details?

I'm here to tell ya, though, that's got nothing to do with why *Food* is being presented in three stages. It all boils down to one thing:

Denial.

Familiar with the word? I am. It's the way most of us choose to live until we are ready to hear what we haven't wanted to hear. With this wonderful three-part system, the Chinese menu of life-style changing, you can take whatever information you are ready to hear from whatever stage you are ready to hear it from, and keep the rest in the closet until you're ready to step in, digest (pardon that food reference pun) a bit more, and come out of the closet with a different understanding and maybe a few more life-style changes.

Hey, if it's meat you want to talk about in just a little more detail than you ever imagined, then walk down the stage two path with the rest of us.

Milk. Take your toe out of the water and throw your whole body into this discussion.

Dairy, the truth behind the udder. Come on . . . what harm can it do?

Stage Two.

One step further into the discussion. A mile or two down the road to
good health and better living.

That leap off the cliff of standard accepted info.

Oh, there'll be the charts and graphs, safe ground for most of us, and
there'll be the recipes—great, great-tasting food that you may never have
thought about. Foods that, until now, you may not have had a clue what to
do with . . . grains, beans, veggies!!

Here's the beauty of this whole thing: Anytime you want to run back and
live in stage one for a while, you can. No problem. Take just a little bit from
each section until you are comfortable, because you're gonna change the
way your body looks either way. The goal here is what's best for you!

If you want the whole truth and nothing but the truth, then read on. Swallow (pardon the eating reference) stage one whole, jump right into stage two,
while anxiously awaiting stage three. Just keep moving forward. Don't stop
getting the information that can help you look and feel the way you want to
look and feel.

AAAAHHHHHHH. Stage two—don't you love it?

> My idea of health food was that sponge stuff and some sprouts. Yech. I am now
> cooking legumes, lentils, brown rice, and lots of veggies and less meat. It is a good
> feeling to be eating healthy foods.
>
> —*Louise, Powell River, British Columbia, Canada*

Time to start, and start we will with a subject that's almost as confusing as
fat used to be to you: "health foods." "Healthy" foods. Don't you hate the
thought of them? Hear the phrase "health foods," and what do you think of?

Alfalfa sprouts?

Nuts and seeds?

Veggies left, right, and center?

Odd-looking people with odd beliefs, enlightened in another world's
thinking?

It's time for a 1990's "health food" update. Things have changed quite a bit
in the last couple of years. "Health foods" are getting a little bit more respect
now than ever before in their history. We—society, that is—have changed

some of our old stereotypes and prejudices about the sprout generation. We've changed our ways a lot since the life-style that so many of us dogmatically protected started to kill us and made us look and feel awful. It's getting harder and harder to protect it.

> Stand by your steak?
> Go ahead, cream on the butter.
> Smoke, smoke, smoke that ciggy.

We're all so aware of what's going on that we are thinking twice. We're still doing a lot of it, for sure, but at least we're thinking. Thinking and talking about "healthy" foods.

> "Healthier" life-style.
> "Healthier" everything.

And with all the talk, no more confusion? No, not so fast. If you polled a thousand people about "healthy foods" and what that means, you'd get a thousand different answers. Is it all good for you as long as it's under the "health food" umbrella?

Let me be the first to tell you that "health food" isn't always healthy. Just because it comes under that sprouted umbrella, is green, has a bazillion nutrients in it, and is "all natural," "from nature," and "connected to the rain forest" doesn't guarantee a couple of things that we know are "healthy."

Low fat? You know things high in fat are not the best things to put into your body if lean and healthy are what you're interested in. But lots and lots of "from nature" and "rain forest" foods are loaded with fat.

Food can come right from a tree and still be poisonous. How about those little red berries that everybody I've ever met has been told since birth not to eat? You can't just assume that because it comes from the ground it's the best thing you can put in your mouth. Or, more important, that it's gonna make your clothes fall off your body because you are "just getting so lean that you don't know what to do with yourself"—which is, need I say it again, the objective of this whole damn book.

The definition of "health" food can be as confusing as some of the labels on the side of your lunch meats, and if you don't think you can gain weight eating only "healthy" foods, take it from me: You can put on 133 pounds before you know it.

Wondering why I chose 133 pounds as the example of weight gain possible from eating "healthy" foods?

What do you think I did? 133 POUNDS ON THE NOSE EATING NOTHING BUT "HEALTHY" FOOD.

Pound cake? Sure. Cement trucks full of it.

Muffins? Yeah, a gravel pit full of them.

Cookies? I could have built a city on the amount I ate over a couple of years.

(Have you noticed an interesting connection with food, my weight gain, and construction going on here?)

But every single thing I put in my mouth during my ballooning up to 260 pounds was "healthy." Those pounds and pounds of pound cake that I ate? We're not talking commercial pound cake made with bleached white sugar, white flour, and additives. We're talking unbleached, whole wheat flour for me or nothing. Nothing had to be enriched because it was a "health food" pound cake.

Hey, not even an American Medical Association physician, with no clue about prevention, food, healthy, or anything associated with disease and food, could question unbleached whole wheat flour as healthy compared to bleached, enriched junk.

If it's the sugar that it all boils down to, and so often it did (nothing like sweet to soothe a broken heart), you could have taken your bleached white sugar and sat in your unenlightened home and eaten all you wanted, but me? No, no, no, I knew how important food was for my health. You could have come over any night of the week and found me munching on carob-coated peanuts by the bagful. You could have taken your Hershey chocolate and eaten all you wanted. I could have eaten most people under the table with my ten "health food" (high, high, high in fat) candy bars.

I'd gone through the fire knowing that how I was feeling was somehow connected to life-style, the food I was eating. I'd had two—not one, two— sons born with food allergies. Nobody could have told me back then that there wasn't a connection between what was going on in my life and the food I was eating.

Time to take a moment and talk about my sons' food allergies. I had one son in the hospital for months while I was pregnant with another baby and the marriage was breaking up. Yeah, you could say it was a slightly stressful time in my life, fair enough!!

IT WAS TURNING INTO MUSH BY THE SECOND.

I WAS LOSING MY MIND.

I WAS A WALKING HORMONAL EXPLOSION.

I COULDN'T DEAL WITH BLOWING MY NOSE, LET ALONE FUNC-
TION.

FORGET ABOUT IT—I WAS A GONER.

So my second baby was born. Perfect? Don't ask. This kid had, and still has, a face like the sun. He was Mr. Big Head, smiley, beautiful-baby-boy city. The best kid. The greatest disposition and Mr. Perfect. Everything going swimmingly—except, of course, for the marriage breaking up and my first son, just out of the hospital, still sick as they come. But even with all that going on, there was still the need to leave the house once every couple of months and do something with the husband.

So what do you do? Call Mom and ask her to baby-sit. The husband and I hadn't left the house or hospital for months. We were pulling one of those "if only we had a little time to ourselves, we'd be able to repair the crater in the middle of our marriage" kind of things. We went over to a friend's house just a few minutes from home (anyone reading this who has children close to-gether and hasn't left the house in forever understands that you don't go too far from home, sometimes for years; it just happens. Going anywhere past a ten-mile radius scares the hell out of you), and within minutes my mother called, hysterical.

> It's the baby.
>
> He's not breathing.
>
> Come!
>
> Someone help me!!
>
> HE'S NOT BREATHING!!!

It was one of those 911 calls that you never want to hear in your whole life. I knew immediately what was happening. Seizure. Same as son number one had. Allergies. Severe. Here we go again. . . .

Both boys are fine now, their "recovery" totally connected to food. Food, food, food, everywhere I look in my life it's staring right back at me. My sons are brilliant, beautiful, and the best kids in the world.

So picture this, I was sitting in Texas thinking about this, starting to figure out that what we are putting into our mouths has a very, very strong effect on our bodies, eating only "healthy" foods, and ballooning up to 260 pounds. Is there something wrong with this picture, or what?

You see, here is one of the big problems with "health foods." When you start talking "healthy" and "food" in the same sentence, you step into the murky waters that I have been dog-paddling through this whole book.

When you think "healthy" food, don't you think

 High quality?

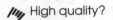 Low fat?

Whole?

Real?

Not processed to the point of not being able to recognize it?

No colors, dyes, preservatives?

Organic, if possible?

Free range, grain fed, and not stuffed into inhumane or inanimalane (WOW, there's a scary made-up word) conditions?

Responsible to the planet?

Isn't all that what goes through your head when you see the label "health food"? All of those things may be part of what makes up a "healthy" food, but here's the problem: "Healthy" doesn't necessarily mean low fat. It can be responsible to the planet and very, very high fat at the same time. Just think avocados—86 percent fat!

Definitely part of the "healthy" category are low-fat foods. But low-fat foods don't have to have anything to do with being good for you other than being low fat.

> Think soda.
> Think chewing gum.
> Think diet "meal" drinks.

These can be low fat foods, so in that sense they are "healthy." But they can also be total crap.

> Loaded with chemicals.
> Don't have to roam anywhere freely.
> Don't have to care less about our environment.

Forget about fiber or natural anything—other than being low-fat, "good" for your body doesn't even have to be considered when you're talking "low-fat," "lean," or the "new and improved, light" foods of today. Many of these low-fat, "healthy" foods are as far away as you get from anything your body needs to function properly.

> In 1925, Clarence Birdseye invented a method of quick-freezing food.

And if that's not enough to throw you into a tizzy, there's one more category of food that's got us scratching our heads. Think about the ones we know that are "good" for our bodies. "Healthy" for us.

Cholesterol free.

Loaded with fiber.

Sure you can have cholesterol-free foods that are good for your body—and loaded with rat poison. There are foods that work well with our bodies and foods that don't. Think about some obvious examples:

Coffee. Whether it's organically grown, hand-picked by Juan himself, or the standard American coffee that's processed with the most amazing chemicals you've never heard of, too much caffeine ain't so good for you. You've had mornings when you had one too many cups. Your whole body shakes. Your heart palpitates. You can't breathe. And you wonder why you drank so much. I drink coffee all the time, but it's not the first thing I grab in the morning anymore—food is. Then cutting back from four cups a day to one with some food—what a difference that can make in your clarity, in your energy, in how you feel.

Alcohol. Grains from organic barley or Thunderbird 20/20—too much is too much, no matter what. Who hasn't awakened with that head-exploding feeling one too many times and figured that out?

What we eat doesn't affect us? Here's a thought: include more of the foods that we know work well with our bodies and take in what we need not only to lose the weight but to gain the energy, fuel, gas (as in car engines—not what you get after eating cabbage) we need to live—isn't that possible?

But we are all just a tad confused because the labels—like the "98%-fat-free"-even-though-it-isn't-fat-free-at-all labels—have been abused. That's what's happening with the word "natural." Everything you look at is "natural." There isn't anything that has cholesterol in it anymore in any supermarket in this country. Everything is "natural." Everything is:

"Fiber filled"

"Low fat"

"Light"

"Natural"

"Healthy"

. . . you see? See what I've been dealing with? Come on—fiber-filled, enriched wood chips, or whatever you want to call some of the stuff that's added to foods because fiber is supposed to be "good" for your body? You, the reader, can truly sympathize with me, the writer, because you can probably see clearly now the very thin, thin line I've been walking—without a net. (I figured what the hell, if I was going to do this food thing, I may as well do it with the same courage I've seen over and over again on "Circus of the Stars.")

Bridging the gap. That's what we are going to do here. Talk low fat, good-for-your-body, and "healthy" together—and here's why. There are a couple of different ways to drop the old poundage, if you catch my drift.

COMBINING HIGH QUALITY WITH LOW FAT WITH GOOD-FOR-YOUR-BODY FOODS MAKES ALL THE DIFFERENCE IN THE WORLD.

Eating tons and tons of high-fat "healthy" foods got me to 260 pounds. So when I got on the scale and had my "moment of truth" seeing the number hit 260—forget about what that moment of truth felt like; you could have hit me with a sledgehammer anywhere, and it would have felt better—the only thing I thought about or was ever gonna think about again was low fat.

Forget about unbleached.

You can take your carob and stick it anywhere you want.

If you think I was ever gonna think about "health food" anything anymore, you are out of your mind, because it was low-fat-and-filled-with-anything-they-wanted-to-fill-it-with-as-long as-it-was-low-fat thinking that I was living, breathing, and eating from that day forth.

That's what I did—you've heard it before.

Cut back on anything white and creamy.

My total fat calories went from being 40 percent and up to 20 percent, then 15 percent daily.

Stopped eating tons and tons of fat and started walking.

Slowly, steadily I dropped a hell of a lot of weight. Eating crap, but low-fat crap.

> I do have to admit that I've been tuning into my body. . . . I can really notice a difference in the way I feel.
>
> —Lisa, North Bend, Washington

Losing weight and happy as a lark, that's what you could label me. But let me tell you what I noticed in my newfound, leaner-than-I-ever-could-have-imagined-and-eating-anything-as-long-as-it-was-low-fat life. This is hard to describe, but since I'm being paid to do so and it's very, very important for me to make this as clear as I can for you, I'll try.

Oh, I was lean and healthier than I'd been at 260, that's for sure, but when I ate the low-fat breakfast bar, I "felt" different from the way I felt when I ate the whole-grain cereal. Stay with me on this one, because we are getting into quality here, above and beyond dress sizes—how you feel, as in energy.

Which "fuel" lasts longer?

Which "fuel" gives you more for your chewing?

I found out the hard way (the biggest theme song in my life, "finding out the hard way"—country-western hit number 111,111,111) that eating just the low-fat foods without thinking about the quality wasn't the answer. Forget about "health foods"—we are talking quality, better described as:

Whole

Unprocessed

Real

We'll get further into this, but let's go on here. Losing the weight is good, and you can do it thinking only low fat, but you can do things you couldn't imagine by combining both: low fat and high quality. Our new title for foods that make you lean, strong, and healthy.

It's time to bring the nuns and the monks into our little discussion, because what I noticed when I ate the high-quality, low-fat food can best be described as clarity. When I was living on the low-fat-only kind of foods, I lost clarity. I had some energy—dumping 133 pounds will do it every time—but not that peak energy I knew was there. Sure, I felt better, but the "sluggish" feeling was still hanging around. Yes, yes, yes, things were so much better—but something was missing.

I figured since so many of the big events, the turning points in my life had been somehow connected with food, then maybe I should start there. (I was finally starting to put two and two together in my life without being clubbed upside the head with a baseball bat. Not bad after three or four major experiences with food and a whole lot of pain; doesn't take me too long.) Could that missing feeling be connected to what I was eating?

More clarity. That's what I wanted.

I checked out the foods I was eating. Had a look at what was going in and started to change a few things. Checked out the labels more closely than I ever had and wondered about the twenty ingredients I couldn't pronounce.

What were they doing to my body?

How were they connected with losing weight?

Could these twelve-letter words slow down the process of my body getting healthier, stronger, and leaner, or my mind getting clearer?

- **Sugar.** How about sugar? The amount I was eating in some of this low-fat stuff—was it helping, hurting, or not making a damn bit of difference?

- **Chemical sweeteners.** Did they help my body work efficiently? Did they make any difference?

- **High-performance fuel.** Is it or isn't it?

- **Processed foods.** Once in a while or all the time? Pastas, breads, bagels—could I substitute a bowl of some kind of grain or whole food for a bagel three mornings a week? Would it make a difference in the way my body looked and how I felt?

Before we continue let's make it real clear: I wouldn't even think about eating anything if I couldn't figure out how to make it fabulous—because after years of dieting and finally being able to eat, I was going to eat only what I enjoyed, something that tasted great and was exactly what I wanted—no more bland shakes, no more freeze-dried food, no more diet food. No matter what kind of clarity or crisper energy we're talking about, it's gotta be great food.

The more I thought about it, the more I read about it, the more I realized the high-quality performance connection to the high-quality foods, the further I went with the old high-octane (whatever that is) fuel-to-my-fire thinking. Can you imagine—me taking something as far as it could be taken??

How about eating more often something that grew from a tree or from the ground? (Of course, only after it got to the grocery produce shelf. If you think for a minute that I would ever get out in the field, pick a food, any food, and eat it, you don't know me very well. Check out my nails—do they scream farmer?)

Quality. I started thinking about the quality of the foods I was eating. Not because I was thinking about my body (my body looked better than it had in years) and not because I was interested anymore in joining the "health food" anything (I'd done that and gained a hell of a lot of weight).

But when I had something that grew from a tree once in a while, I felt better.

Clear.

Focused.

With energy that seemed to last longer.

You see, I started to have moments. I know, you're worried that I've lost my mind right now, and maybe I have, but hear this: It's going to sound like some dumb crazy universal thing, but I'm telling you the truth when I say that I heard birds sing for the first time in years.

The color of the sky looked bluer. (More blue? What's correct? It looked brighter.)

The sound of the children's voices changed. I heard the sweetness of my baby's voice when I walked into a room and he looked up and said Mama.

I was still experiencing the pain of the things I was going through. After all, it took me a while to get as mature as I am now. The marriage thing with the Prince, very painful. Going through the divorce, the monthly checks coming or not, the visits, the divvying up of our life together, sorting through the rubble of the explosion of my dream, all very painful for sure, but it was getting easier.

The Prince would come over to pick up the boys and it would hurt, but slowly there was another side to it. A balance. Somewhere else to go in the pain. When it hurt, when it got overwhelming, when I was scared, I could go to movement—exercise.

When I wanted to rush to the fridge and shove food into my mouth, it really, really did make a difference whether I picked up the low-fat piece of junk or the low-fat real, whole, long-lasting food.

Getting back to clarity, which I know is the wrong word but it's all I've got so I'm using it until I can figure out what the right word is. Awareness (new word), more energy, feeling better than I ever could have imagined.

Without changing a thing in the exercise I was doing, my body started to change when I included some of the quality foods. It became less doughy (as in breadlike, not like some cute animal in the woods). Even though I was more toned and stronger than I'd been in years because of the exercise, that extra inch of whatever fell away, and the definition of my body was totally different.

Call me nuts, call me whatever you want, but it's true. That's what made me commit to the highest-quality foods I was capable of eating. My body was looking more defined and better than in my whole life, and I'm gonna keep eating crap? Get out of here. It's a monk's breakfast full of whole everything or nothing for me if I'm gonna look this good without changing a thing!!!!

Whole foods left, right, and center in my life.

My new life motto: No, thanks, if it's not whole, I don't want to know from it. Sure, it was a bit of a change, but it didn't take long and it wasn't difficult (another one of my life's mottos). It took time, transitional time, but slowly the chemicals and the junk, the instant, canned, frozen stuff started disappearing, and the beans started to soak, the rice was a-cooking, and my imagination went wild with food possibilities, new combos of taste and texture and the pleasure of eating real food.

> Now I'm up to my ears in brown rice and couscous and find I'm loving it all!
> —*L.A., New Haven, Connecticut*

Strength. Endurance.

Stronger. Calmer. Clearer.

Easier to focus on things and make them work better for me.

I felt lighter even though I hadn't lost any more body fat. Same body, same fitness level, but something was changing inside. Didn't know what. Didn't care what. I just knew how I felt, and I liked it and kept right on doing it.

This is where you have to think monk, nun, guru-on-a-mountain for a moment. Do you get what I'm talking about here?

Things became crisper, cleaner, easier to see.

A balance.

A different dimension.

Eyes being opened wider.

That's what was happening. A healing. Who'd have thought about any kind of healing taking place when I started the low-fat thing? All I wanted was to drop some dress sizes and be able to move without feeling as if I was going to die. Healing!! Who cared? But it happened.

So . . . I joined a convent? (Didn't you expect me to say something like that? Didn't it sound like I was heading down some confessional spiritual path? Well, I wasn't. Forget about spirituality. That's not what I thought about at all.) Guess what I did?

I got selfish with the peace I was feeling. Loved the different dimension that had crept into my life without my ever knowing. Wanted more, more, more of this balance (there I go again abusing the word *more*). Loved the extra inch falling off. Was thrilled about the spurts of "extra" energy I was getting by adding a whole food only once in a while. Couldn't believe the clothes that were getting looser and looser. Who wouldn't desperately want to increase that kind of pleasure?

That's all I was thinking about at the time. Basically take this newfound balance and add more pleasure than pain to my life—how's that for a change? Sounded good to me. Don't you think it would be nice? How about increasing your choices when it comes to ways out of the pain, whatever the pain may be? Hey, adding options left, right, and center—why the hell not??

Go for it. How's that for taking the spirituality out of the experience of coming back to life, then screwing it up by bringing it right back to the practical? Well, pardon my surfacey side one more time, but that's exactly what I did. No big transformation experience for me. We're talking survival here—nothing more, nothing less.

START HERE START NOW

I love to sauté with non-fat vegetable broth. Here's a great cooking tip: Pour the can of broth into an ice tray and freeze. Then, when you want to sauté some vegetables, just pop out a cube or two and throw into the pan.

WHAT DO YOU DO?

Increasing the amount of what we all know to be healthy foods, grains, veggies, beans, and fruits, and decreasing some of the instant, processed (low-fat but still processed), chemical-filled junk—muffins, cakes, cookies, frozen, canned, packaged stuff—became my focus. Forget about all the theories that come from both sides of the story that do nothing but confuse the hell out of all of us. We'll soon know if it's true that wheat grass can cure the world or whether chemical sweeteners give us cancer. Why spend our time arguing over whether or not we can eat ice cream made with the same chemical that's in industrial cleaners and suffer no side effects?

The minute you start finding out about foods—real, low-fat, less-artificial-anything foods—you know there's no reason for all the discussion, the studies, the theories. Think about it.

◖ High fat is high fat, and ice cream made with whole milk is very high fat no matter how you look at it. Here's a good example. Have a look with me.

Peanut Butter Cup Ice Cream—All Natural!
NUTRITION FACTS

SERVING SIZE	½ CUP	(106 grams)	SODIUM	130 mg	5%
SERVINGS PER CONTAINER	4		TOTAL CARBOHYDRATE	27 grams	9%
AMOUNT PER SERVING			DIETARY FIBER	2 grams	8%
CALORIES	340		SUGARS	24 grams	
CALORIES FROM FAT	220		PROTEIN	7 grams	
% DAILY VALUE			VITAMIN A		10%
TOTAL FAT	24 grams	37%	VITAMIN C		0%
SATURATED FAT	11 grams	55%	CALCIUM		10%
CHOLESTEROL	70 mg	23%	IRON		4%

INGREDIENTS: CREAM, SUGAR, SKIM MILK, PEANUTS, WATER, EGG YOLKS, NONFAT MILK, COCOA BUTTER, CHOCOLATE LIQUOR, HYDROGENATED PALM KERNEL OIL, DEXTROSE, PEANUT OIL, SALT, GUAR GUM, CARRAGEENAN, SOYA LECITHIN, VANILLA POWDER

Ben and Jerry's. I hear they're really nice guys who care a lot about the environment. I'd love to go to their factory someday and visit. Good-tasting stuff, and fat? Have a look for yourself.

FAT FORMULA

$24 \times 9 = 216$

216 divided by 340 (total calories) equals 64 percent fat per serving.

Tastes good for sure, but you and I both know that you never, ever have just one serving of this stuff. I'll be the first one to admit that if I can't eat the whole pint of ice cream, why bother? We are talking nice guys that are selling very, very, very high-fat stuff.

◖ There are lower-fat choices. Choose them. Higher fat to lower fat, one problem out of the way. Let's look at a low-fat choice.

Rocky Road Premium Low-Fat Ice Cream
NUTRITION FACTS

SERVING SIZE	½ CUP	(71 grams)	CHOLESTEROL	LESS THAN 5 mg	1%
SERVINGS PER CONTAINER	4		SODIUM	60 mg	2%
AMOUNT PER SERVING			TOTAL CARBOHYDRATE	28 grams	9%
CALORIES	140		DIETARY FIBER	2 grams	6%
CALORIES FROM FAT	20		SUGARS	19 grams	
% DAILY VALUE			PROTEIN	3 grams	
TOTAL FAT	2 grams	3%	VITAMIN A		4%
SATURATED FAT	1 gram	4%	VITAMIN C		0%
POLYUNSATURATED FAT	0 grams		CALCIUM		10%
MONOUNSATURATED FAT	1 gram		IRON		0%

INGREDIENTS: WHOLE MILK, MARSHMALLOW (CORN SYRUP, SUGAR, WATER, MARSHMALLOW STABILIZER [VEGETABLE PROTEIN, GELATIN, DEXTROSE], NATURAL AND ARTIFICIAL VANILLA FLAVORING [FLAVORING, ALCOHOL, WATER, PROPYLENE GLYCOL, AND CARAMEL COLOR]), SUGAR, CONDENSED SKIM MILK, CORN SYRUP, CHOCOLATE COVERED ALMONDS (ALMOND PIECES, SUGAR, CHOCOLATE, COCOA BUTTER, COCOA [PROCESSED WITH ALKALI], NATURAL FLAVORS, LECITHIN, AND SALT), COCOA POWDER, MALTODEXTRIN STABILIZER (MONO AND DIGLYCERIDES, LOCUST BEAN GUM, GUAR GUM, XANTHAN GUM CARRAGEENAN STANDARDIZED WITH DEXTROSE), CHOCOLATE EXTRACT (CHOCOLATE EXTRACTIVES, ALCOHOL, WATER, AND ARTIFICIAL FLAVOR), CREAM, NATURAL AND ARTIFICIAL

VANILLA FLAVORING (FLAVORING, ALCOHOL, WATER, PROPYLENE GLYCOL AND CARAMEL COLOR), VITAMIN A PALMI-
TATE (CORN OIL, GLYCEROL MONOOLEATE, POLYSORBATE 80, AND VITAMIN A PALMITATE).

Healthy as they come and low fat?

Don't ever, ever, ever believe that label.

> FAT FORMULA
> 2 grams of fat
> $2 \times 9 = 18$
> 18 divided by 140 (total calories) equals 13 percent.

Yeah, that's low fat. So find the flavor you love and eat it. Remember, we're only talking low fat, not high quality. Just for fun, even though you don't care about anything but fat with this example, let's check out the label. Thirty-five-plus ingredients with no clue what at least half of them are. This brand says Healthy Choice. Healthy? Is everything in this low-fat non-food healthy? Alcohol? Carrageenan? What in the hell is that, and is it healthy? Maltodextrin—sugar? What is that? Propylene glycol . . . come on, healthy? Who knows? But we're talking low fat, and now that you've confirmed it, low fat it is.

If you go beyond just low fat and if saturated fat and cholesterol mean anything to you, it's simple: Choose a nondairy (there goes the saturated fat and cholesterol) brand of ice cream. And there you go, another problem out of the way. One final label for us to check out:

All Natural Fruit Sweetened Non-Dairy Frozen Dessert Raspberry Swirl

NUTRITION FACTS

SERVING SIZE	½ CUP	(78 grams)	SODIUM	10 mg	0 %
SERVINGS PER CONTAINER	4		TOTAL CARBOHYDRATE	26 grams	9%
AMOUNT PER SERVING			DIETARY FIBER	0 grams	0%
CALORIES	110		SUGARS	14 grams	
CALORIES FROM FAT	0		PROTEIN	0 grams	
% DAILY VALUE			VITAMIN A		2%
TOTAL FAT	0 grams	0%	VITAMIN C		8%
SATURATED FAT	0 grams	0%	CALCIUM		0%
CHOLESTEROL	0 mg	0%	IRON		0%

INGREDIENTS: WATER, BROWN RICE SYRUP (PARTIALLY MILLED), MIXED FRUIT CONCENTRATE, (PINEAPPLE SYRUP, PEAR AND PEACH CONCENTRATES), BLUEBERRIES, PEA STARCH, NATURAL FLAVORS, LEMON JUICE CONCENTRATE, FRUIT PECTIN, CAROB BEAN GUM, GUAR GUM.

Nondairy Example

Zero fat grams. That's a good low-fat sign.

Water, brown rice syrup, mixed fruit concentrate—high-quality ingredients, and how about that dairy? Anywhere in sight? Nope. Great tasting. Nondairy. Zero fat grams. If you want the best example you can get of high-quality, low-fat foods and enjoy food again (the way I like to live), try a pint or two of this stuff, with the bananas laid out just right, three different flavors of the low-fat, nondairy stuff, with the low-fat chocolate syrup heated and poured on top.

Or how about some low-fat, high-quality graham crackers? Take the little crunchy biscuit, put some of this stuff in the middle, add the graham cracker top, a little chocolate syrup or . . . How about that low-fat cone and a quadruple cone of this? Or a couple of scoops in your favorite low-fat root beer soda, and—you guessed—time travel city. Or throw in a blender, add your favorite fruit juice concentrate, some ice, a banana or two, whip it up, and sit down to a cold creamy smoothy. Or just grab the pint, get under the blankies, put on your favorite movie, and go to town, knowing that you've improved the quality, gotten rid of the saturated fat and cholesterol, don't have to even think about adding 64 percent fat per serving to your day, and eating, eating, eating, and enjoying. That's my point.

Allergic to milk? Same solution: the nondairy, low-fat brands.

Want only high-quality food? Nondairy, made without chemicals, dyes, flavorings, junk. It's out there, and the choice is yours.

> I'm eating fruit for my snacks instead of candy bars. It fills me up, is better for me, and is cheap! The fruit sticks with me longer than the candy bars used to.
> —*Travis, Quincy, Illinois*

Why does that need to be called anything but common sense? Do we have to do research, spend millions of dollars, and argue for years before we can agree that it's possible to get down to the low fat, the healthy, and the highest quality just by reading the labels and using our brains? Nope.

Not necessary, Davey and the boys. We don't buy that line anymore because it's taking too long for you guys to figure anything out.

Let's just take the "health food" label and chuck it. Get rid of the high- and low-fat, lean, light, low-cholesterol lies and dump that confusion. Blow off the label "healthy" forever. Ladies, how about we start our own labeling.

Common-bloody-sense labeling.

Foods that help your body look and feel good.

High-quality fueling foods.

Prevention foods.

Foods that make your bowel move.

Foods that don't clog . . .

It doesn't have to be proven by the AMA before we start increasing quality and decreasing fat at the same time. Why would you wait for them? We'll all be dead by the time they "prove" that not eating paint thinner, even in minuscule amounts, is a good idea.

There was nothing scientific about what I was figuring out. It all came from the tiger, the tiger in the old car commercial that I think is a figment of my imagination, but I remember it as if it were yesterday.

Ping, ping up the hill?

The tiger talking about motor oil or gasoline?

The higher-quality the fuel, the higher-quality the performance?

Sound familiar to any of you?

Did I make it all up?

Was I the only person in the 70's to see that commercial? Please, if you have a clue about my little figment, write to me. We'll start a tiger fan club, because it's the tiger that got me thinking about higher-quality low-fat fuel.

If one's good—and I knew I was onto something with this low-fat thing—and the other has something to do with being healthy, then combine both? What harm could it do? More important, what good could it do?

Think monk. Think nun. Think cloisters (finally got to the point). When you think monk, you think

Dark, dungeony housing?

Chanting music?

Loads of praying?

Beds of nails?

The most basic clothing, only to cover the sin of the flesh and all?

And food? What do you think of when you think monk food? Or have you ever—why would you, why would anyone, why are you now?

Good questions, and ones that have answers that apparently take chapters to get around to. All the same, there are answers. Because when you think monks or holy men or women and the food they eat, you don't think a big twelve-ounce steak with plenty of steak sauce covering it, potato on the side with tons of sour cream and butter, salad from the bar with loads of Thousand Island dressing. That, my friends, is the high-fat overload that gets you overfat and unhealthy.

And then there's that other version: the low-fat, chemmy-filled kind of food that has nothing real in it. The monks don't eat a low-fat breakfast bar with a diet soda and some packaged low-fat powdered protein supplement for breakfast either.

No matter what, something's wrong with this picture. Suggesting that we all become monks, is that what stage two is all about? Dampening our houses, growing some mold on the walls—is that where we are headed? Cover the sins of our flesh with only the basics, give up fashion forever? What, what, what do you think I'm suggesting here?

Mental, spiritual, physical clarity.

Moments of pure joy.

Different dimension.

The holy guys and gals.

Let's connect it to food because it's all somehow connected. Not completely—wouldn't want to take anything from God and all—but other than the damp walls and praying, these guys include simple, clean food in their spiritually connected way of living. What they eat has something to do with how they are feeling, and you know these guys feel peaceful. (Either that or they are the walking dead, because all you've got to do is have a look at Gandhi's face. Forget about the revolution that was going on around him—and because of him, I might add—he had some big-time peace going on inside him.)

That's it. That's what I was thinking about when I was getting well, feeling better, raising the boys, getting a divorce, trying to scrape my life up off the road after the Mack truck hit me broadside. Doesn't that make a whole lot of sense?

Combining both. The high quality right along with the low fat, right along with eliminating some of the things that just aren't good for us, always making sure the volume is there, keeping those coals in that fire so that you have the energy to get through the day, and always improving the quality.

What did I get: Gandhi? Permission into the convent? A monk's pass to the monastery? Nope.

Just feeling great.

I was feeling great.

What was happening was happening.

I didn't care if I or anyone else understood how it was happening, it just was.

I fixed some brown rice yesterday. Put it in a skillet and heated it with soy sauce and some fresh chives coming up in my herb garden. My daughters loved it.
                                                    —*Karen, Greentown, Indiana*

I'll tell you what. You do it for yourself. Throw in some high-quality whole foods once in a while and watch what happens to your body. Add a brown rice dish to your low-fat, portion-controlled, well-assessed stage-one meal. Experiment with some of the foods mentioned in the next couple of chapters.

What the hell, try a millet casserole. Hey, go berserk and eat some oaty things for breakfast instead of your low-fat Danish. See how you feel, see if it makes any difference in the way your body looks.

Cut back on half of the chemicals you have been eating, probably without even knowing.

More whole, real, from-the-earth, fibery foods? What harm can it do to give your body a break from trying like hell to get rid of foods that sit in your digestive track for up to three days. Talk about a work overload!

Throw in some veggies once in a while.

Something other than preservatives and additives? Is there a soda with less junk in it? After the fifth soda of the day, maybe some bottled water would quench that thirst that just won't quit.

Nothing health nut about that, it's just basic common sense. Easy to apply. No rabbit food, just good food. Hey, it's not going to interfere with your life, it's going to make it better. And you don't have to worry at all about waking up and finding yourself wandering the aisles of some herb store trying to find your way home. Eating foods that support and help your body do the work it's gotta do to get your system digesting, your cells building, your heart pumping, your bowel moving, your body-fat reducing, and your metabolic rate increasing—you want busy and overworked in the worst working conditions possible, just stop for a moment and think about what we put our bodies through!!

Where are the regulations governing, the laws protecting, the unions representing the human bodies?? The FDA sure as hell isn't on the case, because they have no clue about any of this. (I'm slowly but steadily giving up on Dave and his boys ever protecting us from the chemicals, poisons, and diseased dangerous. Can you see it happening right before your eyes? It's sad because it's the beginning of the end, but very exciting because when one door closes another opens.) We're making our own decisions, whether or not the AMA or Dave and his boys have figured it out yet, whether or not there have been a million studies. The holy men and women of the cloisters figured out something a long time ago.

Simple and pure.
Whole and real.

Respecting the body that was so brilliantly designed by God has something to do with the way you look and feel. What's so crazy about that? Eating real food once in a while is crazy, but socially acceptable suicide and heart disease aren't crazy?? PLEASE!! Eating foods that we know clog arteries, destroy our body, and stop it from functioning properly is normal?? I don't think so, and I also don't think that you need ten years, millions of dollars in research, and some panel of whomever telling us it's O.K. What do you think?

It isn't crazy to eat high-quality, real food. Never was and never will be one or the other:

> Suburbia versus the wheat grass people—never.
>
> Medical versus alternative—shouldn't be.
>
> Rabbit-food eaters versus real-food eaters.
>
> Meat eaters versus vegetarians.

How stupid it all is. How about this instead? Human beings taking care of themselves by increasing the quality of the fuel they are putting in their mouths.

There's nothing extreme about suggesting any of this. It's rational. It's sane.

If you want your light to shine brighter, a little more clarity in your life, if the size of your thighs means as much to you as it did to me, then give it a shot. How can anyone say that physiologically giving your body what it needs in the highest quality, with the proper frequency, and without all the crap thrown in doesn't help that happen? Why would we listen to anyone who does say that?

Try it. Live it for a while and see what happens. If your doctor says it's hogwash and has no clue, I suppose we should say a prayer for him or her; isn't that what the monks would do?

Let's voluntarily get off our high horses, throw out old ways of thought, and start looking into this high-quality food thing with open minds and a pure heart, shall we?

HIGH-QUALITY FOODS BY SUSAN POWTER, FOOD P.I.

Having a look at some of the most common high-quality foods, the ones everyone's talking about, the least frightening things that pop out of bulk bins, before you ever step into a health food store will help you walk in with an air of expertise, and I'm sure that's one of your lifelong goals: to walk into a health food store with that air.

This may be a beginning for you, an intro to many a food you've never heard of and have no clue what to do with, but have no fear: It was you and I in your local hyper mart, and it's you and I in the aisles of your local health food store.

GRAINS

Let's do a quick grain test and see where you are in the grain department (sound like you're lost in a health food store already?).

When you think rice you think

> (a) Fried rice.
>
> (b) Stir-fried veggies over rice.
>
> (c) Kung Pao chicken over rice.

When you hear the word bulgur you think

> (a) It's time to get up.
>
> (b) Of the old military days.
>
> (c) Of getting the kids music lessons before it's too late.

Couscous makes you want to

> (a) Grab your camel and get the hell out of town.

Get my meaning? We don't have a clue about grains because we don't eat them. I think it's safe to say that grains are one of the foods we don't have a clue what to do with.

It used to be that you only heard people who hadn't washed their hair in months and lived on beaches year-round talk about grains. Even if you were a curious housewife in the suburbs, a closet grain lover, and tried to find bulgur or couscous a couple of years back—forget about it.

Well, my friend, times have changed, and it isn't because we've all gotten a whole lot more curious or experimental. The availability and social acceptability of grains have much more to do with the death and disease rate than with curiosity.

It's what our old friend Dr. McDougall said way back in stage one (how's that for forgetting where you came from?). Once we realized that modern medicine wasn't going to save us, we had to take responsibility and make some changes: Do our own studying, ask our own questions, and save our own lives.

Grains are not so tough to find anymore. (Why, just the other day I stopped in a grocery store in a very, very small town—while traveling to another very, very small town—to get some food for the road and all but bumped into a bag of bulgur. Imagine that, a bag of bulgur right in front of my nose in the middle of the Midwest.) And you don't have to worry about being looked at like a closet beach liver (as in occupant, not internal organ) when you ask for these very, very 90's foods.

Hip and healthy—that's what the next couple of years are all about. So throw on a pair of Birkenstocks—what the hell, everyone else is, despite my protests (hideous, that's what those things are)—and grab your grain.

Grab your rice, to be more specific, because that's the grain we're starting with—

RICE

Not because it's the best, most nutritious, or greatest grain but because we are all kind of familiar with rice. It's not gonna scare anyone away, staying right with that socially acceptable theme.

Some interesting facts you probably didn't know about rice:

- It is more than half the earth's staple food.

- It was first cultivated (check this out) five thousand years before Christ.

- Archeological digs in China have found sealed jars filled with rice harvested almost seven thousand years ago, and (you won't believe this) other than a bit of mildew, the grain was still edible!! Like a cockroach, rice lives forever!

Rice consumption, you may be asking? Big question on your mind: Who's ahead in this international game?

Burma. The Burmese win hands down. A person in Burma eats five hundred pounds of rice a year, about 1¼ pounds a day. Nothing else to eat, is that the problem?

- Rice is the grain most of the world eats to survive.

- Rice supplies 55 percent of man's daily food requirements.

If it's food energy you're looking for—and we very much are, don't you think?—then listen to this:

- One pound of rice gives you four times the food energy of the same amount of potatoes or pasta.

- There are literally thousands of varieties of rice grown on every continent except Antarctica. (I mean, does anything grow in Antarctica?)

- Forty thousand varieties of rice exist.

Didn't you think it was all white and came in a box?

- The United States exports more rice than it consumes.
- The United States is the twelfth largest rice producer worldwide and the second largest exporter of rice.
- The average American consumes only twenty pounds of rice per year. The Burmese beat the hell out of us in the rice-consuming contest.
- Out of the twenty pounds per year that we consume, four pounds of that can be attributed to the rice used in brewing beer. That's right, we get our rice intake by drinking beer—have you ever?

See what's happening here? We make it. We sell it. We brew some of it. But we're not eating it.

We're eating lots of steak, milk, cheese—look at the foods we are eating and check out the foods we have no clue what to do with and are sending to the Burmese. Isn't it interesting when you just stop for a second and have a look? The foods we are eating are connected with heart disease, obesity, and high cholesterol, just to name a few diseases.

> 2000–3000 B.C.: The Sumerians learned to grow barley, bake bread, and brew beer.

But now that you've got more history on rice than you ever thought there was, you may be thinking nutritional value: What's the nutritional value of this long-living stuff? You might never have thought about the nutritional value of this little kernel, but why not start now? It's perfect; 90 percent of the calories in rice come from complex carbohydrates. This is a good thing. Good fuel stuff here.

Rice is 80 percent starch and 12 percent water.

Water is important.

Rice contains almost no fat.

Touches my heart.

Rice is cholesterol free and low in sodium.

Not a big-concern food for the high-cholesterol watchers.

Rice is a good source of fiber.

Who doesn't need a bowel moved once in a while?

Rice is a fair source of protein, containing all eight essential amino acids.

Good. The aminos are important even though nobody on earth understands much about them. (You will, though; as soon as you've finished with the protein chapter, you will no longer have any amino fear.)

Pretty great stuff, don't you think? Highly nutritious, not that we get any of that nutrition, except of course from our beer. So we're talking low fat, highly nutritious, lots and lots of fiber, and two other things that the rice historians didn't mention but every mom in America needs to know:

Cheap.

Rice is cheap, cheap, cheap.

Versatile.

You can't imagine how much can be done with rice. (Not a sexual reference, I might add. Can you imagine rolling around in bed with someone you love and rice—horrible, like crackers, not good in bed. But you know rice has something to do with fertility. Why do you think we throw it at weddings?)

What is this magical stuff that all the world knows about but us? Let's get to know our rice so that we can at least understand what it is that we are giving away. I know you know white and may be aware of some kind of brown rice. You may have even seen wild rice in some gourmet stores along the way, but any other kinds of the kernel?

> Familiar with them?
> Have a clue what's out there?
> Could care less what's out there?

You never know until you investigate (my new life's motto).
A listing of many different kinds of rice:

Aromatic

Basmati

Black Japonica

Brown

Glutinous

Instant

Italian

Jasmine

Long-grain

Medium-grain

Parboiled or converted

Quick cooking brown

Rice bran

Rizcous

Sushi

Sweet brown

Texmati

Valencia

Wehani

White

Wild

Let's go to the three big ones:

Long-grain

Medium-grain

Short-grain

Brown

White

Noticed something? That's five, not three—pardon me.

Rice seems to be sort of a cultural thing. Our diet doesn't revolve around rice like some other cultures, and so it shouldn't. I like the way things work around here. We've got our problems, but this is it. I mean, where else are you gonna live?

Here's a thought, though: How about including some rice here and there?

Once in a while eat some of this wonderful food other than when you go out for Chinese (which if you lived with me would be often).

Remember portion control? One of the benefits was, and will be if you decide to do it, taking the food that needs to be portion controlled—usually the high-saturated-fat and high-cholesterol stuff, meat and dairy—and placing less emphasis on that and more on another kind of food: a lower-fat, more nutritious, higher-fiber food.

How about rice?

Come on, what else are you gonna use to refocus your portions with—vegetables? Who the hell is gonna be satisfied replacing a big slab of steak with some carrots? Rice may be the answer to getting that meat-and-potatoes kind of guy of yours who's overweight, unfit, and building his cholesterol count by the minute to eat something different. Do you think he's gonna yell when he sits down to a big heaping plate of:

Rice Pilaf

Rice Dumplings

Spanish Rice

Vegetable Rice Soup

Corn and Rice Chowder

Tomato and Rice Soup

Eggplant and Rice Casserole

Stir Fried Rice and Broccoli

Wild Rice Salad

Lentil and Rice Casserole

Rice and Beans with Roasted Chili Peppers

Red Peppers Stuffed with Rice, Spinach, and Garlic

Green Chilies Stuffed with Rice and Tomato Sauce

Meatless Meatloaf with Rice, Lentils, and Oats

Rice with Roasted Garlic

Orange Rice with Raisins

Summer Rice Salad with Mandarin Oranges and Scallions

Tuna and Rice Casserole

Curried Rice

Brown Rice Cooked in Orange Juice and Ginger with Dried Apricots

Wild Rice with Grapes and Toasted Almonds

THOUGHT . . .

This is a perfect opportunity to chop up that portion-controlled beef and put a few cubes into the rice dish the first couple of times.

What does he know? Wean him like a child from a breast or a junkie—wean, wean, wean him slowly, less painfully. All that man of yours wants is to be served. He has to feel full, and he's gotta like the taste. Where's he going? To the TV with his beer. (You must excuse me for making your husbands, boyfriends, fiancés sound like Archie Bunker—I apologize. I have too much respect for you to do that; however, you get my drift, don't you? Understand why I took this artistic liberty in this particular case? You know what I mean?)

Nobody's gonna know the difference, but your body will. Fiber? You may not have had any in years. A whole food? Your bowel won't know what to do with it. You get some fiber. You eat something that has the nutrients you need to be healthy. You cut back on your fat. You increase your options by including high-volume, low-fat, wonderful foods in your daily eating. What do you think is gonna happen to your hips when you eat the high-fiber, low-fat, highly nutritious rice instead of the saturated fat? Come on!

START HERE START NOW

Keep a bowl of cooked rice in the fridge for a quick dinner. Warm it up while you sauté some fresh veggies in no-fat vegetable broth. (You can always use frozen veggies if you're in a hurry.) Top with tamari or soy sauce, and you've got a great Chinese dinner. Toss in a few cooked shrimp or some chicken if you like.

Here are some of my favorite quick, easy "unofficial" rice recipes:

Susan's Unofficial Rice Pilaf

Sauté lots of onions, garlic, and mushrooms in a barely oil-coated nonstick pan. Add a little Tabasco, some thyme, and more of your favorite spices.
Follow the directions for cooking rice but replace the water with your favorite low-fat stock and cook it in the sauteed mixture until the rice is done.

Susan's Unofficial Vegetable Rice Soup

Chop up tons of veggies—carrots, celery, onions, cabbage, tomatoes. Add corn, peas, fresh lima beans, all your favorites. Chop up some garlic and chives. Put into your biggest soup pot and add lots of liquid, either stock or water (if it's water, add extra seasonings).

Load up on the spices, garlic, seasoning, salt, celery seed, bay leaf, pinch of cayenne . . . try some arugula—it's a dark green leaf with a nutty, "horseradishy" flavor. Simmer until vegetables are about half-done, and add about a cup of rice (basmati is good in this soup) and cook until rice is tender.

🎵 Susan's Unofficial Tomato Rice Soup

For the stock, use 2 18-oz cans of low-fat chicken stock, and a 36-oz can of crushed stewed tomatoes. Add loads of basil, fresh garlic (try some fresh chopped fennel bulb, wonderful!) and your favorite Italian seasonings. Simmer, covered, for about an hour. Throw in a couple handfuls of rice and cook until rice is done. Season to taste.

🎵 Susan's Unofficial Stir Fried Rice and Broccoli

Prepare rice according to directions.

While rice is cooking, get out your biggest frying pan or a wok.

Add a touch of sesame oil or any good oil (or a mixture of tamari and water) and saute chopped broccoli, celery, carrots, spring onions. Add to the sauté water chestnuts and snow peas. Add some soy sauce and a little chopped ginger.

Continue to stir fry until veggies are just cooked.

Add some veggie broth and cook a few minutes longer to "marry" the juices.

Remove the veggies and make a thickener by stirring together some apple juice, soy sauce, vinegar, and a little honey with some cornstarch that has been dissolved in water.

Stir until thickened. Return the veggies to the sauce, heat up, and serve over the rice.

BARLEY

Not so exotic. Who doesn't know barley soup? But when is the last time you had some? In the middle of the winter, a heaping bowl of barley-and-vegetable soup will satisfy anyone. When the boys were young, I used to sing them a song by Raffi, the children's singer of all time; this guy can wail about things that fascinate kids like no other:

Oats and beans and barley grow.

Oats and beans and barley grow.

You and I and everyone knows that oats and beans and barley grow.

I sang that song twenty-five thousand times—one hundred times a day for years. I should have known I was going to end up writing a food book and talking about oats and beans and barley growing. What the hell else could I have ended up doing with subliminal messages like that going on in my head? If repetition is the mother of invention, then consider this chapter invented ten years ago when my oldest son was one and his brother was just born. Help me!! Even thinking about those days makes me tired. Boy, was it tough.

We'll get to the oats and the beans, but right now it's the barley part of the song that we're talking about. If you think rice has some history, check out barley. We're talking Stone Age when we talk barley. Yep. What do you think those Stone Age cakes were made of? Wheat and barley baked in the sun, what else!!!

Barley's got a reputation for being one of the toughest grains around, able to withstand drought and floods. It can't leap tall buildings in a single bound, but it's pretty super just the same.

Besides the cave men and women and their little cave kids, the Chinese were some of the earliest barley eaters and from the beginning the world figured out how to grind barley to make flour and malt for the brewskies.

And here's another little secret that's been around a long time: Barley makes it bigger (something you might want to share with the husband). That pot of soup, you want to make it bigger? Add some barley. One cup of dry barley expands up to four times that amount when added to the soup! Barley the bargain grain.

Barley is as nutritious as grains come. Two cups of cooked pearled barley offer the same amount of protein as a glass of milk—without the saturated fat and cholesterol, MILK BOYS. We don't hear that, do we? Where's that slogan? The barley boys don't have the same amount of cash as the milk boys do. All we hear is "milk does a body good." Does it?

Millions and millions of people are searching for a way to cut back on fat and cholesterol but still get the protein they think they desperately need, but do they know they can do it with barley? You get protein, niacin, thiamin, and potassium if you eat barley. This, my friends, is no schleppy grain we're talking about here. It's strong, it's durable, it's nutritious—what more could you want?

Maybe having a clue what to do with it? Coming right up, but if you're gonna get to know your grain, then you need just a bit more information.

Barley, just barley? No, sir.

Hot Barley with Skim Milk and Honey
Barley Pilaf
Barley Risotto
Barley and Vegetable Casserole
Barley, Bean, and Vegetable Casserole

Cabbage Rolls Stuffed with Barley

Stuffed Winter Squash with Barley

Vegetable and Barley Stew

Mushroom and Barley Soup

Krupnick (popular Polish soup with barley, potatoes, and dill)

Barley Salad with Sliced Mushrooms, Tomatoes, Peppers, and Vinaigrette

Hot Steamed Barley

Vegetable and Barley Chowder

Stir Fried Barley

"Unofficial" recipe time again!

Susan's Unofficial Mushroom Barley Soup

Sauté lots of sliced fresh mushrooms, onions, garlic, carrots, and celery in a touch of oil. The mushrooms will reach a point of releasing liquid and will become soft. Continue to cook until pan dries again.

Add enough vegetable broth to make a soup and toss in a handful of barley. Cook, covered, until barley is tender. Add more stock if the barley absorbs too much. Add spices, (sage, parsley), bay leaf, salt, and pepper.

Susan's Unofficial Cabbage Rolls Stuffed with Barley, Eggplant, and Mushrooms

Cook barley according to directions but replace the cooking liquid with low-fat chicken or vegetable broth, and add some fresh oregano, garlic, salt, and pepper. Boil cabbage leaves in water with a little vinegar until leaves are wilted. Drain and set aside.

Next, take sliced mushrooms (portobellos are best) and sliced eggplant, spice with garlic salt and pepper, lay on a slightly oiled baking pan, and put under the broiler until golden brown. Turn over and repeat. Set aside.

Take some of your favorite zesty low-fat tomato sauce and spread a thin layer on the bottom of a casserole.

Lay your cabbage leaves out and put a layer of the mushrooms and eggplant, then a spoonful of the barley, in the center of the leaves. Fold in the edges and roll up. Lay seam side down in the baking dish.

Pour the rest of the sauce over the rolls (if sauce is too thick, thin with some chicken broth). Cover and bake in the oven at 350° until the sauce starts to brown around the sides of the casserole dish.

Susan's Unofficial Stir Fried Vegetables with Barley

Cook barley according to directions and use vegetable broth as the cooking liquid with fresh thyme.

Sauté all the veggies, carrots, celery, onions, garlic, shallots, Chinese cabbage, mushrooms, broccoli (check your veggie bin for more) in a mixture of veggie broth, soy sauce, mirim (an oriental wine), and some chopped fresh ginger.

When veggies are cooked, set aside and make a sauce with the juices and a little cornstarch mixed in cold water.

Return the veggies to the sauce and heat through. Serve over the barley.

OATS

You may have figured out that there is no alphabetical order going on here. I'm just hopping around the whole grain subject, so it's right from barley into oats.

You know oats. Made by the Quaker guy. Probably no need to even cover them because you are already an oat expert!

Oat bran, right.

That life-saving grain you've read about in every newspaper and magazine in the country. The stuff that when added to food saves your life.

The only stuff you need to have a healthy heart and colon.

Hold on. Guess who got their dirty little hands on the oat bran issue and went wild with it? The media. The media jumped all over oat bran a few years back, and everyone immediately manufactured some, hoping to cash in on the new health craze: OAT BRAN . . . EXCELLENT SOURCE OF SOLUBLE FIBER, HELPS LOWER CHOLESTEROL.

Of course so does not eating cholesterol, but forget about that. This was an instant cure, something we could take that would help lower cholesterol without changing our life-style. And if you don't think the media ran with that . . . People were buying oat-bran cereals, oat-bran doughnuts, oat-bran breakfast bars, oat-bran pancakes, oat-bran everything they could get their bowels on.

Sure, oat bran is good for you. Grains are good for you—but you don't see people running out and buying brown rice doughnuts, do you? It could be because they don't exist, but if they did, would you buy them? Adding oat bran to tons of junk food is not gonna make it good for you.

- Whole oats are very good for you. They are loaded with seven B vitamins, vitamin E, and nine other minerals including calcium and iron.

- Oats are fairly high in protein, and the quality of the protein in oats is high compared to the quality of other grains.

  Now let's do the fat formula on some whole oats:
  ⅓ cup of oats has 111 calories and 2 grams of fat so . . .
  2 grams of fat times 9 = 18
  18 divided by 111 = 16 percent

- The American Cancer Institute recommends 20 to 35 grams of fiber daily, and oats are a wonderful source of soluble fiber.

And do you know where most of the oats grown in the United States go—85 percent, to be exact? To the livestock. To feed the livestock so that we can eat the beef and get the saturated fat and cholesterol that cause heart disease. There is some humor in this, even though it's dark. The food that the American Cancer and the American Heart associations say we should eat to be healthy is being raised and used as feed for the foods that are killing us.

A little confused? Very sad. Talk about ass-backwards. This, I'm afraid to say, is a good example of the state of affairs when we're talking about our eating habits. But all of that is changing with the American woman becoming more and more aware of the truth.

And the one good thing about the media's focusing attention on oat bran in the last few years is that now it's not so tough to find. No driving for miles is necessary if it's a few oats you're looking for.

When we're talking oats, we're talking:

> Instant.
>
> Rolled.
>
> Whole and oat groat.

No clue what an oat groat is? Don't worry, neither did I when I first picked them up in some dusty bag in some dusty health food store years ago. Remember I told you when I wanted more and more of that clarity (that I never found a better word for) stuff, I thought just something whole once in a while? Well, when it comes to breakfast, what better than a whole oat, and if it's real oats you want, then it's oat groats you have to get to know.

So I bought them and boiled them. Horrible? Like white glop. That's what my first batch of oat groats looked like. Never got to the tasting part, because as willing as I was to drink the fungusy stuff or get whole foods into my life, nothing would have made me taste what was looking up at me from the pot when I attempted to cook oat groats.

Now the kids and I have it down. I cook 'em up, pour on the maple syrup, mix them with brown rice and granola (my low-fat version, of course), add some fresh fruit, and breakfast? The best hot whole cereal you've ever tasted!!

O.K., O.K., you've twisted my arm. I'll give you my oat groat breakfast cereal recipe when we've finished getting to know our grains. Doesn't take much, does it?

Want more oats in your life? What can you do with an oat? Here are a few suggestions:

Oatbread.

Oat bran muffins.

Oatmeal with skim milk and honey; with chopped dried fruit, cinnamon, and raw sugar; cooked in fruit juice with cinnamon and vanilla.

Oat groats pilaf with toasted sunflower seeds.

Thicken soups with groats.

Substitute half the beef in meatloaf with oats.

Oat pancakes.

Oat burgers.

Scottish stew (cabbage, oats, squash, and spices).

Oats and applesauce muffins.

Golden oat biscuits.

Oatcake.

Cobblers with crunchy oat crust.

Oat porridge.

Here's that "unofficial" breakfast oat groat recipe I promised you . . .

Susan's Unofficial Breakfast Oat Groats

Cook oat groats. (I'll tell how on a chart in just a minute.)
Throw in leftover plain rice. (Brown rice is best.)
Sprinkle with low-fat granola and top with maple syrup.
Done!

MILLET

Have you ever? Everybody knows the name, but talk about a food that stumps everyone every time! Millet. What is it and what the hell do you do with it?

The stuff that looks like birdseed. Little yellow round kernels of millet. A very, very good balance of essential amino acids, this millet has, and it is good, good, good for your body.

I have a millet story for you—surprised? When don't I have a story? Way back trying to figure all this stuff out, I found a recipe for millet mashed potatoes. You see, coming from the Australian lamb-and-mint sauce kind of family, with mashed potatoes being a big part of the complete meal, you don't mess with mashed potatoes. "They have to be smooth and creamy" I'm thinking to myself while I'm mashing the millet. "It's never gonna happen with this birdseed stuff." Well, mash I did, and amazed I was. Does it taste good? Well, you mash and you tell me.

Millet Mashed Potatoes

I found this recipe years ago in Mary Estella's cookbook, *The Natural Foods Cookbook: Vegetarian Dairy-Free Cuisine* and decided to give it a try.

Peel and dice 4 or more potatoes into ½-inch cubes. Place in a pot. Wash 1 cup of millet until water runs clear; drain. Pour millet over potatoes and add 2 tsp. caraway seeds, ½ tsp. sea salt, and 3 to 3½ cups water. Slowly bring to a boil over medium flame. Lower flame and simmer 20 to 30 minutes until water is absorbed. Stir before serving; add chopped parsley for garnish.

Variations

Mash potatoes in a mixer. Add a little soy milk (or skim milk if you like . . . now this is my idea, not Mary's) or ¼ cup of water mixed with 2 Tbsp. of tahini (check your local health store if you're not familiar with tahini). Mix until blended. Substitute cauliflower for potatoes. Omit caraway (that's a seed) and add your favorite herb or spice. I made the recipe using the variation for mashed potatoes . . . DELICIOUS!

My friend Suzi said she made them the other day with rice milk and soy sour cream for her daughter, who's allergic to dairy and said the whole family loved it. She took the leftovers and sliced thin wedges out of the bowl (it had gotten firm in the fridge overnight) and fried them in a nonstick pan that she wiped with a little oil. They came out like potato pancakes. A big, big hit with the kids! She was even going to shape some of it into little balls and drop them in her veggie soup tonight . . . what a great idea, Suzi!

There are hundreds of grains and hundreds of ways to cook them. Let's get down to a few easy-to-cook, basic grains so you can get down to some great low-fat, high-volume eating.

Rice

Per ½ Cup Uncooked

	LIQUID (Cups)	COOKING TIMES	YIELD (Cups)
Brown, long-grain	1	25 to 30 minutes	1½
Brown, short-grain	1	40 minutes	1½
Brown, instant	½	5 minutes	¾
Brown, quick	¾	10 minutes	1
White, long-grain	1	20 minutes	1¾
White, instant	½	5 minutes, let stand 5 minutes	1
Converted	1⅓	31 minutes	2
Arborio	¾	15 minutes	1½
Basmati, white	½	15 minutes	2
Jasmine	1	15 to 20 minutes	1¾
Texmati, long-grain, brown	1 (plus 2 tbs.)	40 minutes	2
Texmati, long-grain, white	¾ (plus 2 tbs.)	15 minutes	1¼
Wehani	1	40 minutes	1¼
Wild	2	50 minutes	2
Wild Pecan	1	20 minutes	1½

Barley

Per ½ Cup Uncooked

	LIQUID (Cups)	COOKING TIMES	YIELD (Cups)
Hulled	2	1 hour, 40 minutes	1¼
Pearl	1½	55 minutes	2
Quick	1	10 to 12 minutes (let stand 5 minutes)	1½
Grits	⅓	Let stand 2 to 3 minutes	⅓
Flakes	1½	30 minutes	1

Millet

Per ½ Cup Uncooked

	LIQUID (Cups)	COOKING TIME	YIELD (Cups)
	1½	15 minutes	2½

Oats

Per ½ Cup Uncooked

	LIQUID (Cups)	COOKING TIMES	YIELD (Cups)
Groats	1	6 minutes, let stand 45 minutes	1¼
Steel-cut Oats	2	20 minutes	1
Old-fashioned Rolled Oats	1	5 minutes	1
Rolled Oats, quick	1	1 minute, let stand 3 to 5 minutes	1
Oat Bran	1	6 minutes	1

Quinoa*

Per ½ Cup Uncooked

LIQUID (Cups)	COOKING TIME	YIELD (Cups)
1	15 minutes	2

* Quinoa should be rinsed to remove any powdery residue.

Wheat

Per ½ Cup Uncooked

	LIQUID (Cups)	COOKING TIMES	YIELD (Cups)
Whole Berries	1½	1 hour, 10 minutes	1¼
Cracked Wheat	1	15 minutes	1
Bulgur	1	15 minutes	1½
Wheat Flakes	2	53 minutes	1

BEANS

Can't talk whole, can't talk real, can't talk high quality without talking beans. Beans, beans, good for your heart. The more you eat the more you . . . well, I think everyone knows the rest of that rhyme . . . but what else do you know about this incredible food? Did you know that beans are

- an excellent source of protein
- low in fat and calories
- loaded with fiber
- a good source of calcium
- a great source of iron
- high in B-vitamins

Not only are they good for you, they are versatile, cheap, cheap, cheap, easy to store, and variety, don't ask!

What more could you want from a food?

When you're talking beans you're talking

> Mung beans
> Chick-peas
> Black-eyed peas
> Navy beans
> Red beans
> Pink beans
> Black beans
> Lentils of all types
> Split peas
> Asuki beans
> Anasazi beans
> Kidney beans
> Lima beans
> Pinto beans
> White beans

And when you're talking cooking beans, here's what you're talking about . . .

Bean Cooking Chart

½ CUP UNCOOKED

	LIQUID (CUPS)	COOKING TIME	YIELD (CUPS)
Azuki Beans	2	40 minutes	1½
Black Beans	2	1 hour 20 min.	1⅓
Black-eyed Peas	2	1 hour	1½
Cannellini Beans	1½	1 hour 35 min.	1½
Chickpeas	2	1 hour 5 min.	1½
Cranberry Beans	2	1 hour 5 min.	1½
Fava Beans	2	30 to 40 minutes	1
Flageolet Beans	2	1 hour 10 min.	1½
Great Northern Beans	2	1 hour	1½
Kidney Beans	2	55 minutes	1½
Lentils, green (whole)	1½	35 minutes	1½
Lentils, orange (whole)	1½	20 minutes	1⅓
Lima Beans	2⅔	45 minutes	1⅓
Mung Beans	2	35 to 45 minutes	2
Navy Beans	2	1 hour	1½
Pinto Beans	2	1 hour	1½
Red Beans	1½	45 minutes	1½
Soybeans	2	2 hours 25 min.	1⅓
Split Peas	2	30 to 35 min.	1

Pick a few beans, cook 'em up and try these "unofficial" bean recipes.

Susan's Unofficial Bean Dip/Spread/Filling

Take a couple cans of non-fat or low-fat refried beans, heat up with a couple of spoonfuls of your favorite hot sauce, some cumin, garlic, chopped onions, cilantro, tomatoes, and a package of frozen corn kernels.

Heat well and serve with chips or stuffed in a taco shell or rolled in a flour tortilla or spread onto a tostado shell, and topped with taco fixings.

Susan's Unofficial Hummus

Take a bag of garbanzo beans (chickpeas) and follow the cooking directions on the back or use canned beans. Either way, drain the beans and blend until creamy, adding lots of chopped garlic, parsley, oregano, fresh lemon juice, salt, and pepper. Serve with chips, on a dry crusty bread, use as a sandwich spread, or stuff in a pita pocket with freshly sliced tomatoes, lettuce, and shredded carrots.

Susan's Unofficial Spice Chili Beans

Take a large can of crushed tomatoes, couple cans of pinto beans, and your favorite packet of chili spices.

Put everything together in a pot and simmer.

Garnish with chopped onions, nonfat cheddar cheese, jalapenos, baked corn chips.

START HERE START NOW

Instead of loading my Chinese food with sweet-and-sour sauce at 35 calories and 2 grams of fat per tablespoon, I use rice wine vinegar mixed with grated ginger, hot chili sauce, or one of my favorite concoctions of soy sauce mixed with lemon and garlic.

P.S. I always order extra steamed rice to mix with whatever I'm eating. More volume, less fat. I love it!

O.K., onward. Gotta get to veggies . . .

VEGETABLES

NOTHING TO BE SAID ABOUT THEM AT ALL.
Basically, who cares? Sure we get:

  A bit of fiber
  Vitamins
  Minerals

Lots of versatility:

  Sautéeing
  Steaming
  Pureeing (YUCK)
  Boiling
  Juicing
  Frying (oops, sorry, we're cutting back or eliminating that)
  Grilling

Or, as on the cover of the book, skewering. Do what you want with them.
  Here's my motto: Try to eat something green once in a while. Think veg-

gies. Eat the ones you like. Don't touch the ones you hate. Experiment. Place them all over the husband's body and go to town—who knows? Just get some into your body once in a while and eat, eat, eat, eat, eat, eat.

I've got some interesting "unofficial" veggie recipes—check 'em out:

∅ Susan's Unofficial Veggie Sub Sandwich

Toss some shredded lettuce with some balsamic vinegar or freshly squeezed lemon juice and some seasoned salt and pepper.
Load up on some or all of these:

> Thinly sliced purple onions
> Jalapenos (if you're daring)
> Fresh tomatoes
> Vegetarian lunch meats (check the labels)
> Non-fat cheese or soy cheese
> Pickles
> Capers
> Sliced artichoke hearts
> Sliced radishes
> Cucumbers
> Leftover veggies from last night's dinner

Pile it all on a fresh French Roll.

∅ Susan's Unofficial Quick Cream of Potato Soup with Peas (kids love this one)

Peel and dice baking potatoes. Boil them in water until potatoes are falling apart.
Pour out two-thirds of the water and replace half of the amount with skim milk.
Turn the heat down. Heat through. Take out two-thirds of the soup, blend, and return to pot or mash it right in the pot.
Add salt and pepper.
Add a package of frozen peas. Cover and turn off heat. Delicious!

∅ Susan's Unofficial Veggie Pizza

Buy a low-fat ready-made pizza crust or make your own.
Cover the crust with your favorite spaghetti or pizza sauce (check labels) and pile on:

Pineapple and bell peppers and onions
Roasted chilis and sun-dried tomatoes
Tons of grilled vegetables, onions, mushrooms, peppers, tomatoes;
   add capers and spices
Artichoke hearts with tons of sliced onions
Fresh basil with marinated tomatoes in oil-free vinaigrette

Bake in oven.

Just a few suggestions.

Just a few ideas.

Just a few recipes.

Just a step—a stage 2 step—into some foods you may never have thought about.

Surprise the family, surprise yourself, surprise everybody with a great veggie soup, a fabulous rice pilaf.

Try some whole, high-quality foods once in a while.

Enjoy.

CHAPTER 8

PROTEIN

*I*f you cut back on the beef, the chicken, and then the dairy because you want to cut back on the saturated fat, eliminate some of the highest-fat foods in your life so that you get leaner, faster and forever, and maybe cut back just a bit on cholesterol, don't you also take away all the protein? Aren't the very foods that will make you leaner and healthier if you cut way, way back on them also the only foods that you get protein from? At least the real protein? The complete protein? The best source being the beef, chicken, and dairy?

> Real men eat beef.
> Isn't it "complete" in some way?

The athletes can't build muscle and won't have energy without it, right? Isn't it a complicated amino-acid sort of thing? Surely you have to be a doctor or dietitian to figure this out, don't you?

Protein confusion. We all suffer from it. Nobody is immune because we all received the same training and information from the start. Years ago, fat and feeling out of control, I thought you had to be a doctor, dietitian, or at least a scientific genius to understand protein. Visions of seventh grade science class (which I must admit I avoided at all costs—all those molecules connecting amino acids that looked like an Etch-a-Sketch drawing) and the whole protein-connection thing turned me off forever.

What I did know was that not getting enough protein made me too weak to function. Any physical activity was impossible. My hair and nails wouldn't grow. I'd be sallow, weak, and malnourished, and because everything I ever read seemed so confusing and complicated, I just accepted what I was taught from the day I can remember first hearing about protein: You can't live without it, and not getting enough is deadly.

One of the big reasons so many of us don't make changes in our life-style is fear—fear that if we do something wrong we'll . . .

Die.

Not feel good.

Create some permanent physical problem.

Get jellyfish muscles because of lack of protein.

Turn toothless at thirty-five because we tried some crazy thing and cut too far back on protein.

. . . so we keep doing what we've been doing, which is killing us in record numbers. Make sense? If you want to learn about protein, you've got to go back in time and unlearn.

Back to the basic four food groups.

Back to the classroom.

Back to the food charts.

Dairy and meat being two out of the four. The dairy and meat are where you and I are going to get most of what our bodies needed to grow—that's all I knew.

When you see that protein is responsible for muscle and bone growth, well, even in the second grade I could figure that muscle and bone growth is kind of important if we're talking about a healthy, happy human being. So that was that. I put food into my body every day, without question, based on the advice of a second grade teacher.

As the teacher says, let's review what we've learned, starting with one of the two big "complete" protein boys.

MEAT

In our society, meat equals protein. It's easiest to lump them both into one chapter and discuss them together. Makes for a better discussion, much more feisty, and gets it all cleared up in one fell swoop.

What we know now is that Sister Mary lied. (Sister Mary was the nun who taught me in kindergarten.) Now I'm not suggesting that she did it deliberately—because in the Catholic religion it's an automatic pass through the gates of hell if you even suggest a nun lies. Nevertheless, Sister Mary lied. Norman lied, Sister Mary lied, they all lied.

Learning the truth about protein has sent me flying back to the therapist's couch.

"If Sister Mary lied about protein, what else in my life is a lie?"

"Where does the truth begin and the lies end?"

We now know that meat is very high in saturated fat and cholesterol. We know for sure that diets high in what used to be called the "best" foods are directly connected with heart disease, many forms of cancer, and many other diseases. We also know, because many of you are living with this one, that a high total daily fat intake is directly connected with obesity; fat makes you fat and all, so it would only figure that if the top-of-the-mountain boys on the food chart are high in fat, and they are, they wouldn't be very good for you.

How they got their reputation as "the best" foods on the food chart is a very interesting story and one that we'll be getting into, but for now, getting leaner is our goal, throw in healthier here and there, and if it's fat you want to talk about and get out of your life without dying of protein deficiency, then you can't talk protein without talking meat, without talking the truth.

My foundation was rocked and yours is about to be, and we can blame it on the nutritional experts of yesteryear. The charts, the basic four, the meat/milk theory—all wrong. The concept that you can get quality protein only from two of the basic four—wrong. All wrong.

The numbers . . . WRONG!

The amounts needed to sustain that healthy muscle-building body of yours . . . WRONG, ALL WRONG.

And the most amazing part concerns who is feeding this info to Sister Mary, which in a sense forces her to lie to all the schoolchildren. (Now, I know that if I get a gate pass to hell for suggesting that a nun lies, the person who is feeding her the information and making every word that comes out of her mouth about protein a lie is the devil's right-hand man. So here it is straight from the mouth of Susan Powter, Food P.I.: You guys are guaranteed to go to hell.)

THE MEAT AND DAIRY INDUSTRIES ARE GOING TO HELL IN A HAND BASKET.

Can you imagine being my publisher, Simon and Schuster—both of them have a hell of a lot of nerve, don't you think? That's probably what you think right now, but once we unravel the protein issue, you'll find that the truth is common knowledge among thousands of physicians, dietitians, and nutritionists, and all the top organizations that govern the food industries in this country. Study after study, both international and domestic, has proven it to be true. The only ones who haven't known about a subject that affects our health so drastically are you and I. Like the cheated wife, we are the last to know.

Guess who's selling us the high-protein theory. The products that they are selling are some of the highest fat around—so we have a couple of problems: obesity, disease, and way, way too much protein. Yep, you heard it right. We don't have a problem getting enough protein. The problem is that we're getting way too much—and getting way too much fat. Fat. Fat. Fat. That's what you want less of in your life, and less of it is going to make you leaner, leaner, leaner.

Remember, ladies, no fear necessary. Big subject. No requirements, no rules in this book, just information that you can base your own decisions on for you and your family. I say this now because the minute you start talking protein and meat, half the country throws the book into the fire and assumes that the only alternative to eating meat is "living like a rabbit on that lettuce stuff."

Well, fellow Food P.I.'s, not true. The first order of business in getting leaner and healthier is sorting out all the junk that's been thrown at us all these years—that's what this protein/meat chapter is about—and then making better choices that work for you and your family. Not mine and not your doctor's family, yours.

So sort it out we must, and it's right back to the classroom for you and me.

> The stuffed peppers are just as good (or better) without the ground meat.
> —*Jane, Athens, Alabama*

PROTEIN

Yes, you do have to have protein. According to the World Health Organization, the Food and Nutrition Board of the National Academy of Sciences, the National Research Council, and thousands of physicians, dietitians, and nutritionists all over the world, you need the stuff.

Protein is a very essential nutrient. It helps build, maintain, and repair just about every part of our bodies.

If it's good hair you want, get yourself some protein.

Nails and skin? The big P.

Cartilage and tendons? That's right.

Protein, protein, he's my man.

Consider protein the building blocks in your body. Haven't you heard that a million times and had no clue what it meant?

Protein is one of the big three fuels—along with fat and carbohydrates—although (we may as well start smashing myths right away) very rarely is it used as energy. Only in extreme diets—remember those stupid high-protein diets we all did where you'd go into ketosis? (You know, when you used litmus paper for the first time since science class to determine whether you'd sent your body into this abnormal condition? Ask me how much I love the diet industry. Please, those idiots . . .) Anyway, extreme conditions such as that diet and starvation are the only times protein is broken down and used as energy; otherwise your body uses fats and carbohydrates to fuel that fire and get you going.

Didn't you think protein was the "fuel"?

Didn't you think it was stored in muscles?

Haven't you heard those muscleheads talk about beefing up with lots of protein, eating meat left, right, and center, having twelve eggs for breakfast, and making sure they get enough protein by sucking down those protein shakes?

Haven't you heard it a million times? Isn't that what you associate protein with? The other day I heard the commentator on a local radio show telling people to make sure they get enough protein, eat plenty of chicken and eggs, and go ahead and take a protein supplement if they feel they need one, especially when they are pumping hard. Frightening. It's as if people like this are living under rocks. Don't they read? Haven't they seen all the studies done on this subject? Bad information like that will continue, so it's up to us to get the facts and make the right decisions, because there will always be people who choose to stay under rocks.

Getting tons of protein isn't about building muscle. Getting enough protein is about your body having the building blocks it needs to function properly, but what's "enough" is the big question. How much do you need, and what are the best sources?

Protein is formed from building blocks called amino acids. There are approximately twenty-two different kinds of amino acids that form billions—yes, billions—of varieties of proteins. But forget about going into all those billions, because billions is too many to research, even for Susan Powter, Food P.I. But out of those billions there are twenty-two that we need to be aware of.

Out of those twenty-two there are eight—nine in babies—that our bodies do not manufacture. They're called the essential amino acids. That's what you've heard over and over again. Do you want to know what they are?

Get to know your essential aminos:

> Valine
>
> Leucine
>
> Isoleucine
>
> Lysine
>
> Tryptophan
>
> Methionine
>
> Phenylalanine
>
> Histadine

So who cares? Means nothing to us, right? Right. It does mean nothing except that the myth that meat and dairy are the best source of these essential amino acids, and that without them you are never going to have any energy or be able to build a respectable muscle, has been based on the notion of complete and incomplete proteins.

"Complete" means (at the time they were discovered and still today, according to the rock people) proteins that contain all eight, nine in children, essential amino acids. (Proteins and amino acids are very much connected, something we are going to jump into later on and come out feeling like the geniuses we are, because they're not so complicated.)

But then "complete" started meaning

> Better than
>
> Real
>
> Solid
>
> All you need
>
> The most important

And "incomplete"—the foods that didn't contain all the essential amino acids in the right proportions—started meaning

> Less than
>
> Not quite as good as
>
> Weenie

Complicated

Inferior

That's probably all they're ever going to mean to you, because you, like me, will never want to know the names of the eight amino acids again as long as you live since—as you'll soon see—there's nothing to making sure you get them all and getting your body what it needs to be healthy.

But there's one small obstacle in your way to the truth about protein: the protein pushers and the relatives they've brainwashed.

Here's what the protein pushers want you to believe:

- You can't get enough.

- You can't get them unless you eat meat.

- They're impossible to get without the big beef unless you get a degree in chemistry and do nothing all day but food combine.

- And God forbid you try any of this without a dietitian living in, because if you do, you'll shrivel up and die.

Now, for the sake of information and information alone, unbiased, objective as they come, and in all fairness, what a load of crap that is. How in the hell have you guys been feeding us all this junk for so long without being questioned?

I know how: loads of cash, great ad campaigns, and fear. That's how you got us believing this nonsense. You guys have us all so afraid that we'll never be able to eat as many plant-based foods and find the right combo of aminos, and that we'll die, or at least shrivel up slowly and painfully.

So it's easy, so very easy, just to eat some beef and not think about it. Convenient. Just eat the beef and get the amino acids you need. But safe it's not, because of all the other things you're getting along with your slab of steak. And once you know the facts, you'll see that you don't have to compromise your health just because you can't figure out the right combo of plant foods to eat to get what your body needs.

I'm trying to convert my husband from a "slab and spud" freak to a healthy eater. . . . If I can make veggies and grains look and smell appetizing, he'll eat them. We both like red beans and rice quite a bit.

—*Barbara, Frankfort, Kentucky*

The problem begins with the amounts that have been suggested in the past. We just don't need as much as we've been told we need—by guess who?

Yeah, you need protein, but how much?

John McDougall says:

"There is no question that meat, dairy products, and eggs are high in protein. But the average American consumes 90 to 120 grams of protein a day, while the ideal intake for a human being is 20–40 grams per day. Most Americans today are worried about getting enough protein, but in fact are eating far more than necessary and far more than is healthy."

There's a big difference in these numbers—90 to 120. Let's take the low end of this "must have to be healthy" number that's been presented by the beef and dairy boys—90—and compare it to the high-end number that everyone else seems to be talking about.

John Robbins says that according to the World Health Organization, the Food and Nutrition Board of the International Academy of Sciences, and the National Research Council, the maximum total daily protein intake we need is 8 percent of our total daily calories.

"Human mother's milk [the finest food in the land—pardon me for breaking into a quote, but it is] provides 5 percent of its calories as protein. Nature seems to be telling us that little babies, whose bodies are growing the fastest they will ever grow in their lives and whose protein needs are maximum, are best served when 5 percent of their food calories come as protein."

Time to stop, get away from the great quotes for a moment, and chat. Talk about a concept and one that ties right into what I've been saying all along about man versus nature. Mother Nature's plan is being screwed up by us. If ever I had an example to use, it is this. Great thought, John Robbins. (Not that this thought was his alone. Every expert in the field of nutrition has been talking about the protein requirement for babies and their growth versus adults' needs for a long, long time. It's just that we haven't heard it because we've been too busy being yelled at by the beef boys—real food and all. If you think beef is real food, try some breast milk. Now there's a food . . .)

There it is, the greatest point you can make about the protein issue. Never, ever in your life will you be developing and growing as you grow when you are a baby. Muscle growth, bone growth, brain growth, teeth, nails, hair, every cell and muscle in our bodies growing at the speed of light. If you need protein to grow (remember, you're never gonna do that kind of growing again), then doesn't it make sense that *that's* when you need the most protein?

As important as all bodybuilders in the country think they are, they ain't growing as fast or as brilliantly as a newborn baby. And if it's the protein requirements of a bodybuilder you want to know about, why not ask the best? Arnold Schwarzenegger—yeah, that's right, Mr. Terminator himself—has some opinions on protein. The muscleheads ought to listen to him; after all, he's got what they want so bad—quite a few hit movies.

> "Kids nowadays tend to go overboard on protein, something I believe to be totally unnecessary. I state my formula for basic good eating: Eat about 1 gram of protein for every two pounds of body weight."

And if you want to know what it takes to meet Arnold's protein requirements, just ask John Robbins. You'd do fine without meat, dairy products, or eggs. If you ate only broccoli, you'd get three times the quota that Schwarzenegger suggests for protein.

O.K., so there's a big discrepancy in numbers here, but there isn't any discrepancy in whether too much protein is harmful for our health. That's kind of been decided.

> Too much?
>
> What do we need?
>
> Where do we get it from?

Questions, questions, questions.

Look at what some of the experts have to say about eating too much protein.

> "A long-term high-protein diet can cause heart disease (because of the saturated fats) and kidney problems (because of the difficulty of disposing of urea, a waste product of protein metabolism and excess sodium)."
> —*The Complete Guide to Health and Nutrition* by Gary Null

> "In addition to the general workload on the entire digestive system, protein metabolism especially taxes the liver and kidneys."
> —*Natural Health, Natural Medicine* by Andrew Weil, M.D.

> "A high-protein diet also results in phosphorus deficiency."
> —*The Complete Guide to Health and Nutrition* by Gary Null

"The diuretic effect of high protein intake leaches minerals out of the body, including calcium. Loss of calcium from bones can produce osteoporosis. . . . "
        —*Natural Health, Natural Medicine* by Andrew Weil, M.D.

"I believe that high-protein diets can irritate the immune system in some people, aggravating allergies and autoimmune disease (such as rheumatoid arthritis and lupus, in which the immune system mistakenly attacks the body's own tissues)."
        —*Natural Health, Natural Medicine* by Andrew Weil, M.D.

"Animal foods are also dangerously high in protein, which contributes to kidney damage, kidney stones, and osteoporosis."
        —*The McDougall Program for Maximum Weight Loss* by John A. McDougall, M.D.

"High-protein diets impose a workload on the digestive system and may contribute to feelings of fatigue and lack of energy."
        —*Natural Health, Natural Medicine* by Andrew Weil, M.D.

I now eat vast quantities of low-fat food (instead of keeping McDonald's in the black!).

        —*Kelly, Manchester, New Hampshire*

Let's talk about getting protein from plants. First we have to find out how, if it's as good, and what the deal is with plant protein versus beef protein. And we will. But what we don't need to confirm, because we already know it, is that with plant foods (other than a very, very few exceptions) you don't have to worry about saturated fat, and you never have to worry about cholesterol in the plant world. That much we do know, and that much needs to be said so that we can sum up all the advantages, get the story, and make up our own minds.

So, Doc John, tell us about plant-based proteins, aminos, and all there is to know about them.

"Proteins are abundant in foods derived from both plants and animals. The eight essential and fourteen nonessential amino acids are all found in plants in generous amounts. Protein deficiency is almost unknown in humans worldwide, but protein excess is a real problem in developed societies. When protein content of the diet exceeds 15 percent of calories consumed, the body's liver and kidneys are burdened with the task of removing the excess amounts of proteins."

What would it take to get 15 percent of your total calories from plant-based protein?

"Virtually all unrefined foods are loaded with proteins. Rice is 8 percent protein. Oranges are 8 percent. Potatoes 11 percent. Beans 26 percent."

Hey, doesn't that just about say it all? Not quite. You should hear what Dr. Dean Ornish, author of *Reversing Heart Disease,* says:

"In the United States most people (rich or poor) eat too much protein, at least twice as much as they need. It is very difficult to eat too little protein."

The amino acids that come from plant foods are exactly the same as the amino acids that come from animal foods. You don't have to be a scientist or a nutritionist to combine foods properly. It's as easy as eating any grain and any legume one time during the same day. Examples:

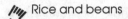 Rice and beans

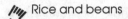 Tacos with beans

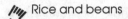 Tofu with rice

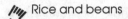 Whole wheat pasta and beans

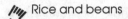 Pea soup and cornbread

Wow, pretty clear, don't you think? And it doesn't end there, because John Robbins has more to say on the subject of amino acids and plant-based foods:

"A clinical study reported in the *Journal of the American Dietetic Association* compared the intake of the essential amino acids for meat-eaters, lacto-ovo vegetarians (those consuming dairy products and eggs), and pure vegetarians (no eggs or dairy products). This study" was uncompromising in that it "raised the protein requirements for each amino acid to a height that would cover even the needs of pregnant women and growing children. The researchers found, however, that not only did all three diets provide sufficient protein, they were all well over sufficient. Each group exceeded twice its requirements for every essential amino acid and surpassed this amount by large amounts for most of them."

How hard is it to get your protein from plant-based foods? John's got some food and protein stats that will amaze you:

Wheat, 16 percent protein

Oatmeal, 15 percent protein

Pumpkin, 12 percent protein

Doesn't sound too difficult to me; how about you? Less worried now about shriveling up and dying if you decided to cut back on meats, dairy, and eggs? Sounds to me as though it's much easier to cut back on the stuff that's killing us and making us fat, and not worry about the nutritional problems we thought would plague us, than it is to eat the other stuff and try to stay lean and healthy. I don't know about you, but simplicity is my deal. I want it to be simple and effective and make me look good; that's my motto for living. How's that for enlightened!!

In 1955, the first McDonald's, operated by Ray Kroc, opened in Des Plaines, Illinois.

If you think it ends there, you're wrong. There's a whole lot more where that came from. There are experts a-plenty in this department.

Frances Moore Lappé, who wrote *Diet for a Small Planet* years ago, used to talk about food combining, and now, years later, in a new updated addition to a wonderful book, sums up the protein issue in one sentence.

"If people are getting enough calories, they are virtually certain of getting enough protein."

"Americans consume an average of 160 grams of protein daily or about 8 times what we need."
                    —*The McDougall Program for Maximum Weight Loss*
                    by John A. McDougall, M.D.

"Individuals can and do, if they can afford it, consume two to three times their estimated protein requirement."
                    —Nevin Scrimshaw, Ph.D., Head of Department of Nutrition
                    and Food at the Massachusetts Institute of Technology

By the way, I hate the phrase "plant foods." Who'd want to eat anything that sounds like that? You gotta admit that part of the reason plant foods haven't been able to hold their own is the name alone. Standing next to a name like BEEF, it just doesn't hold up. PLANT . . . BEEF. The beef's got it in the name department, and in the saturated fat, cholesterol, antibiotics, and every other kind of department.

Let's find a different name.

I know: Root Man Foods. But what if it doesn't have a root?

The Seed Weed—a little too science fictiony.

Dig 'Em Up Foods—too sing-songy.

The kids and I are still working on it. If you have any suggestions, send them to Simon and Schuster. We'll have a contest. I'm sure they'll appreciate that!!!!! In the meantime, we'll just have to stick to plants, and we'll refer to them as the "other" kind of foods. There it is: I've taken something that had a name, a weak one but one nonetheless, and I've stripped it of its name and made it a no-name category.

Back to aminos. The aminos in the "other" food category are exactly the same. Nothing to worry about, and no food combining necessary. How did it all get so crazy? If you really want to know, we've got to get a little history here. Beef history.

The Cattlemen's Association.

Fair enough, what else would you expect a cattleman to say but eat beef?

McDonald's. Big supporter of beef. This is kind of an obvious link. They make billions of dollars off _____. (Fill in the blank; you know the answer.) So it's a given that they would promote it. How far they go in their promotion is another story—don't get me started on the connection between the children, advertising, and foods. I'm doing so well at being the objective, fair reporter. We'll get into the children, but right now it's full steam ahead with who's telling us to eat this stuff.

The Beef Council. Again, what would you expect them to say? Here's a bunch of big guys—you know they are big and fat because they eat their own product, and you know they are guys because no self-respecting Beef Council man is going to allow a little lady to help make the decisions. The ladies in these guys' lives are all at home pounding their flesh (pardon the phrase) and tenderizing the big piece of steak that their big beefy councilmen are coming home to.

Frank Perdue is a big advocate of meat/chicken eating. Before we discuss the millions of dollars that Frankie puts into advertising his product, may I ask a question that's been bugging me for about a year now? Are Frank Perdue and Ross Perot cousins? Those ears, that voice, that squinchy little face—can that be anything other than a family resemblance? Maybe they are one of those separated-at-birth stories and can now, after the publishing of this food book, find each other and live happily ever after.

Oh, one more person we all know well is, or was, a big advocate of beef eating: James Garner. He used to think real people ate beef until he had quintuple bypass heart surgery. I wonder what he thinks now.

Other than a few back bush (an Australian term kinda meaning hillbilly) doctors and nutritionists, nobody can say eat beef without concern for saturated fat, cholesterol, and excessive protein without making it really clear that he or she hasn't read a thing about food and health in the last five years.

Who's saying be aware, cut back, don't eat it, be healthier, and leaner, live longer, and have a better quality of life?

Dr. Michael Klaper, one of the world's leading authorities on nutrition.

Dr. Dean Ornish, author of *Reversing Heart Disease* and *Eat More, Weigh Less*.

Dr. John McDougall, author of *The McDougall Program* and *The McDougall Plan,* to name a couple of his books.

Dr. William C. Roberts, editor in chief of *American Journal of Cardiology.* Who would argue with a title like that, Ronald McDonald?

Who else—any research done lately?

The China-Oxford-Cornell Project on Nutrition.

Thousands of articles published in the *New England Journal of Medicine.* The next time your doctor says there is no connection between what you are putting in your mouth and how you are feeling, ask him if he's read his *Journal* lately and then run out the door.

Hey, how about *American Journal of Clinical Nutrition, Journal of the American Medical Association,* and *Lancet?*

Fair enough if your doctor or nutritionist hasn't read *Lancet,* a journal written by the Brits, but every other journal he or she reads has made it very clear that if you want to look and feel better, cutting way, way back or eliminating meat consumption altogether is a damn good idea. The leading authorities in medicine, nutrition, and health say it; the journals say it; and so does almost every organization in the world that has a connection with human health:

> U.S. Surgeon General
> Senate Select Committee on Nutritional and Human Needs
> National Research Council
> National Cancer Institute
> American Heart Association
> National Academy of Sciences
> Food and Nutrition Board
> World Health Organization
> United Nations Food and Agriculture Program

It's time to take a breath, a moment to think about something. All of these physicians and experts, all the journals, and all the organizations I just listed don't have the same power or influence on us as one person—not even a person, a clown, and a bad one at that—Ronald McDonald. The most powerful clown on earth. More powerful than all the health organizations? He convinces us with that goofy smile of his, his oh-so-happy disposition, and his tiny plastic toys that it's not only O.K. to eat what he sells, but it's fun, convenient, and sooooooo good.

The real question here is the Ronald question: Does this clown have unearthly powers? Has he put a spell on us all? Does anyone know the history of this guy? Let's find out. And if he is not the demonic clown he appears to be, let's elect him president. He has the ability to make millions of us do what he says without questioning. His word has weight against every authority in the world who says otherwise, and he does it all with a smile. What more could we want? Ronald McDonald for president—after his background check, that is!

> In 1597, John Gerard wrote his monumental book, *Herball,* in London, in which he describes hundreds of food plants, many for the first time.

If you want to know how to get your new and improved 20–40 grams a day of protein without the saturated fat and cholesterol, it's easy to do. Check out some of these ideas:

MEATLESS ENTREES

Veggie Burgers

Meatless Hot Dogs

Bean Burrito

Vegetable Lasagna

Macaroni and Non-fat Cheese

Vegetable Pizza

Stuffed Peppers with Rice

Lentil and Rice Loaf

Stuffed Tomatoes with Spinach/Scallions/Orzo Pasta

Pasta Primavera

Minestrone Soup

Enchiladas Filled with Low-fat Cheese

Stuffed Baked Potatoes

Steamed Veggies over Mashed Potatoes with Brown Mushroom Gravy

Grilled Vegetable Fajitas

Veggie and Bean Tacos

Lentil Meatloaf

Vegetable Kabobs over Rice

Whole Wheat Pita Pockets Filled with Grilled Veggies, Yogurt Dill Sauce

Soups, Soups, Soups . . .

   Stews, Stews, Stews . . .

      Pasta, Pasta, Pasta . . . Anything

Still think the only way to get your protein is your meat? Look again:

● ●

Non-Animal Protein Options

Item (1 cup portions)	Protein (g)	Saturated Fat (g)	Cholesterol (mg)
Small-shell pasta	5	0.11	0
Oatmeal	6	0.42	0
Orange (medium)	1	0.02	0
String Beans	2	0.08	0
Broccoli	3	0.05	0
Whole Wheat Bagel (2 oz)	6	0.12	0
Seedless Raisins (packed)	5	0.25	0
Corn	5	0.32	0
Wheat Bread (1 slice)	2	0.23	0
Blackeyed peas	5	0.16	0
Corn Tortilla (1)	2	0.10	0
Black Beans	15	0.24	0
Brown Rice	5	0.35	0
Whole Wheat Pita Pocket	4	0.19	0
Sweet Cherries	3	0.08	0
Banana	1	0.21	0
Carrots	2	0.05	0

● ●

Protein . . . important to your health? You bet.

Gotta eat your weight in beef and beef products to get enough? No way.

Most of us—I know I was—were raised in a meat mentality world where the beef boys were king and we were taught the only way to grow strong and healthy was by eating two or more servings of meat products daily.

You lied to me fellas! Yes, our bodies do need it, but there are some great sources other than beef that just might do a body better. . . .

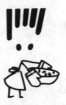

CHAPTER 9
SUGAR

Sweet, sweet sugar. One of the biggest soothers in the food department for sure. Talk about connected to our heartstrings. It's never a baked potato you think about eating when you're hurting, is it? How about a bowl of stir-fried veggies (no oil, of course) just before you snuggle into bed? NOT. It's the cookies, the ice cream, the cakes, the chocolaty snacks that we dive into. And understandably so.

> Sweet tastes good.
> Sweet feels good.
> Sweet is good.

It's at the very core of the emotional connections we have with the food we eat.

Romance? Box of chocolates.

Broken heart? Box of chocolates. (I had to put the two together because in my experience romance and broken heart are connected like the twins I saw on "Maury" recently.)

Reward? You don't get a bowl of brown rice when you've been good, do you?

Treat? When you sit down for that afternoon "break" in your day (yeah, reality for most of us?), what is it you sit with?

a) Whole wheat pita and veggie sandwich

b) Snickers Bar

It's an emotional thing. Association city. And as you and I have already discussed at length while you were "bearing with me," in stage one changing our associations is part of changing our lives. And let me tell you that making the connection between sugar, disease, and dietary imbalance is as tough as getting the message across that eating saturated fat and cholesterol contributes to heart disease. It ain't easy when you're talking about something people like—and boy oh boy, do people like sugar. No question about that.

A pleasure, a luxury, one of the best taste sensations out there . . . but there's just one little problem with sugary sweet. We've got the same problem with sugar as we do with fat.

Nothing wrong with it.

Your body's gotta have it to function properly. About two teaspoons a day, to be exact, to do its job.

Your body breaking it down? No problem. Everything's fine with the digestion and fuel utilization of the stuff once it's inside our bodies. Our bodies know just what to do with the cake you eat, but there is still something terribly wrong. Very much off balance. And that is (here's where the similarities between fat and sugar come in) the amount we eat.

Don't you see something that keeps appearing over and over again? A very interesting pattern in the way food is connected to how we feel?

Too much fat . . . overfat.

Too much saturated fat and cholesterol . . . heart disease.

Too much caffeine . . . all kinds of problems.

Too much alcohol . . . you know what that does.

Too much sugar and . . . what?

What's the problem with eating 100 to 110 pounds a year per person? Yes, that's right. If you are an average American, and we all are, and you're eating the average American diet, and we all have been because we didn't know any better and we've been told for years that what we put in our mouths has nothing to do with how we feel, then you are consuming a whole heaping load of sugar in your daily food intake.

According to the government, the pounds and pounds of sugar each of us eats a year boils down to about **thirty-one teaspoons of sugar per day** for every man, woman, and child in this country. Just a touch more than the two teaspoons we need to get what our bodies need, wouldn't you say? If you're a teenager, you're consuming more than the rest of us, up to 150 pounds a year. Excessive? What do you think?

Whether the experts agree on the exact amount that we average Americans are eating or not (some say 110 pounds a year, some say only 95 pounds a year) or whether there is conclusive evidence, satisfactory to physicians, linking our out-of-control sugar consumption to certain disease, wouldn't you say we are taking in a bit too much?

We've got some big, big problems connected to sugar. Excess sugar consumption can interrupt normal metabolism, send your insulin levels through the roof, create havoc in the pancreas, and screw up your whole system pretty easily. Excessive sugar consumption can

> Make you fat.
>
> Sap your energy.
>
> Contribute to diseases like heart disease and obesity.

Sugar and heart disease—connected.

Rise in triglycerides—yep, connected to our sugar intake.

Hypertension and excessive sugar intake—joined at the hip.

Diabetes? Sure, according to Nobel Prizewinner Dr. Frederick G. Banting, the Canadian physician who discovered the hormone insulin:

> "In the U.S. the incidence of diabetes has increased proportionately with the per capita consumption of sugar."

Don't you think it is safe to say that taking in this much of anything would have some side effects? Any at all? Sure it does.

But can you believe that this is hard for some people to admit? And guess who's having the hardest time admitting that we have some major problems with the amount of sugar we take in daily? The sugar manufacturers who pour the sugar into the food we eat.

The problem is that instead of talking about these problems, everybody is busy arguing about:

> Which sugar is better.
>
> Which kind is more nutritious.
>
> Which digests fastest.
>
> Which kind causes the problems.
>
> Whether raw is better than refined.

Nobody is getting to the bottom line and getting you the simple facts about this simple/complex food: the amount we are eating and how it's affecting our lives. So I figured while everybody's arguing, we'd get some basic facts and break them down, and you take it from there. See what you think.

Best of all, I have no ice cream or chocolate cravings (two of my biggest desires) at all because we are now eating healthier.

—*Christine, Greentown, Pennsylvania*

I'm sure you know about the instant energy you get when you eat sugar and then the big lack of it you have to live with hours later. For the last twenty years everyone has known about the sugar highs and lows that are guaranteed; we just don't have a clue about anything else. If those 110 pounds of sugar we've been eating a year have anything, and we mean anything, to do with how we are looking and feeling, then we want to know about it.

NOW. NO MORE SUGAR-COATED INFO. JUST TELL US WHAT'S GOING ON.

Here it is, the simple, sweet, bottom-line truth about sugar: Sucrose. Table sugar. The chemical name for sugar is sucrose.

Sugar is a simple carbohydrate with a nutritional value of nothing. None. Nada. Once it's refined, there's nothing left.

Sugar is highly caloric, meaning that you get a lot of calories for a small amount of no-nutritional-value-at-all food. Fine if you burn those calories off, but most Americans don't. Fact is, unless you are a marathon runner, you can't burn them up as fast as you are eating them. If you are a healthy person, fit, with a healthy percentage of body fat and lots of lean muscle mass, then you might not have to worry so much about taking in a bit too much sugar once in a while. But if you are unfit, overfat, with not much lean muscle mass, and you're eating as much sugar as many people are—you've got some real problems with sugar.

YOUR BODY AND SUGAR

Before it is used for energy, sugar is broken down by your body as glucose or blood sugar. It's the speed of breakdown that makes one kind of sugar better or worse than another, according to the experts.

You get hungry, your blood sugar drops, you eat, your blood sugar rises— food will do that every time. As your body is digesting the food, your blood sugar begins to rise, and your pancreas responds by sending out the insulin telling your body, "Yo, we've got blood sugar to deal with."

Your fabulous body does different things with the sugar that the old pancreas is doing its thing with. Cells will pull the glucose from your blood and use it for some good immediate energy. Fat cells break it apart and use it to build more fat cells—just what we want happening inside our bodies. How about that—let's eat more sugar and hand our fat cells the ability to make more and more of themselves. Sounds crazy to me.

Your muscle and liver cells use glucose in a different way. Glucose is the selfish fuel that your muscles can store and use as their very own fuel source. Mr. Muscle can synthesize it and create long chains, otherwise known as glycogen. You've heard that term used by muscleheads, haven't you? (I've heard so many of them repeat it so often; it's sometimes the only technical term they know.)

Muscles use sugar differently from cells; fat cells use it differently from muscles; and all in all your body does just fine with it. Unless of course you're eating 110 pounds of it a year.

SUGAR—WHAT IS IT?

What we start with, before we process the hell out of it, has some value. What we end up with after all the processing, on the other hand, is very, very different; interesting theme, don't you think?

Once the food manufacturers get their hands on it and refine it:

According to *Understanding Nutrition* by Eleanor N. Whitney and Sharon R. Rolfes, "A refined food is a food from which the coarse parts have been removed. . . . Refined foods may have lost many nutrients during processing. . . ." That bowl of sugar sitting on your kitchen table has been so chemically processed that about 90 percent of the natural plant has been stripped away . . . and just what was in the 90 percent? Fiber, protein . . . you know, the good-for-your-body stuff!

Yeah, you might say that table sugar you've been eating has lost just a few nutrients. . . .

Let's talk about eating a sugary snack, like the one you may have had seconds ago (to eat 110 pounds a year, we've got to be constantly eating this). Your body gets an immediate dose of simple sugar and dumps loads of glucose into your system. Your pancreas has to respond fast and with a large dose of insulin; after all, you just dumped a big load in. What happens then was clearly explained by Gary Null, one of the nutritional experts we love the most, in his great book, *The Complete Guide to Health and Nutrition:*

> "The excessive insulin causes all of the glucose to be drawn from the blood at once, leaving the body more deficient in energy than before and encouraging one to repeat the cycle."

It's almost as if we cause the whole system to go haywire because we are dumping in more than the old pancreas and insulin levels can deal with, so our wonderful body has to respond by throwing out more, and then that fabulous insulin does its job, all too well—and we get stuck in a cycle.

The best "helper" was comparing my daily Snickers bar to all the tasty and fulfilling food I could consume instead. Every time I reach for a cookie I stop now and think: I could eat carrots, rice, pasta, and/or grapes until they come out my ears and still be leaner and stronger. . . . Know what? I skip the cookie.

—*Karen, IRB, Florida*

But you don't eat that much sugar, you say. You've cut back a lot in the last few years on those **SUGARY SNACKY THINGS IN THE MIDDLE OF THE AFTERNOON.**

Once in a while you'll have a candy bar.

Just a couple of sodas a day.

You've gone from loopy things every morning to a whole-wheaty kind of cereal.

The sugar-coated doughnut isn't the first thing you reach for anymore, and you don't eat chocolate-coated individual snacks, whether they melt in your mouth or hand—at least not every day.

You've gone from ice cream to yogurt—a healthier snack?

You're making a big effort—where have I heard that before? You've made that conscious effort and are cutting back. So you think you're better than the average Joe who hasn't put two and two together yet and figured out that Wheaties are better for you than a Danish in the morning for breakfast? You, after all, are a woman of the 90's. Maybe you've even gone as far as including more carbs such as grains in your diet, so surely this sugar chapter doesn't apply to you. You are not one of those 110-pounds-a-year sugar eaters. After all, where would it be coming from?

But guess what, you're up against those lying labels again:

Old-Fashioned Natural Fruit Grape Jelly

INGREDIENTS: GRAPE JUICE (WATER, GRAPE JUICE CONCENTRATE), CORN SYRUP, HIGH FRUCTOSE CORN SYRUP, SUGAR, FRUIT PECTIN, CITRIC ACID.

Non-fat Caramel Sundae Syrup

INGREDIENTS: HIGH FRUCTOSE CORN SYRUP, CORN SYRUP, NONFAT MILK, FRUCTOSE, STABILIZER (WHEY, PROTEIN, HYDROLYZED OAT FLOUR), FOOD STARCH-MODIFIED, SALT, POTASSIUM SORBATE ADDED AS PRESERVATIVE, NATURAL AND ARTIFICIAL FLAVORS, XANTHAN GUM, DISODIUM PHOSPHATE, SODIUM CITRATE, ARTIFICIAL COLORS (YELLOW 6, RED 40).

Peanut Butter Granola Bars

INGREDIENTS: GRANOLA (ROLLED OATS, ROLLED WHOLE WHEAT, SUGAR, PARTIALLY HYDROGENATED SOY-BEAN AND/OR COTTONSEED OIL, SKIM MILK, HONEY), SUGAR, CORN SYRUP, ENRICHED WHEAT FLOUR (CON-TAINS NIACIN, REDUCED IRON, THIAMINE MONONITRATE [VITAMIN B₁], RIBOFLAVIN [VITAMIN B₂]) INVERT SUGAR, VEGETABLE SHORTENING (PARTIALLY HYDROGENATED SOYBEAN AND COTTONSEED OILS), RICE FLOUR, CORN SYRUP SOLIDS, PEANUT FLAVORED DROPS (SUGAR, PARTIALLY HYDROGENATED SOYBEAN AND COTTONSEED OIL, PARTIALLY DEFATTED PEANUT FLOUR, SKIM MILK, SOY LECITHIN [EMULSIFIER]. SALT, AR-TIFICIAL FLAVOR), ROLLED OATS, GLYCERIN, SALT, NATURAL AND ARTIFICIAL FLAVOR, MALT SYRUP, HIGH FRUCTOSE CORN SYRUP, EGGS, LEAVENING (BAKING SODA, CALCIUM PHOSPHATE), BHA (TO PRESERVE FRESHNESS), CITRIC ACID.

Fat Free Whole Wheat Fruit Cobbler Cookies

INGREDIENTS: MIXED FRUIT FILLING (SUGAR, CORN SYRUP, DEHYDRATED APPLES, MODIFIED FOOD STARCH, WATER, CHERRIES, STRAWBERRIES, NATURAL FLAVORS, PECTIN, CITRIC ACID, LOCUST BEAN GUM, SODIUM BENZOATE [PRESERVATIVE], ARTIFICIAL COLOR [RED #40, BLUE #1]), WHOLE WHEAT FLOUR, CORN SYRUP, EN-RICHED WHEAT FLOUR, (WHEAT FLOUR, NIACIN, REDUCED IRON, THIAMINE MONONITRATE (VITAMIN B1), RI-BOFLAVIN (VITAMIN B2), SUGAR, HIGH FRUCTOSE CORN SYRUP, BROWN SUGAR SYRUP, EXTRACT OF MALTED BARLEY AND CORN, CORN SYRUP, GLYCERIN, DAIRY WHEY, LEAVENING (SODIUM BICARBONATE, MONOCAL-CIUM PHOSPHATE), CARAMEL COLOR, SALT, SOYBEAN LECITHIN (AN EMULSIFIER), SPICE, EGG WHITES.

Strawberry Flavored Cereal Bars

INGREDIENTS: STRAWBERRY FRUIT FILLING (SUGAR, STRAWBERRIES, HIGH FRUCTOSE CORN SYRUP, CORN SYRUP, DRIED APPLES PRESERVED WITH SULFUR DIOXIDE, MODIFIED FOOD STARCH, DEXTROSE, NATURAL FLAVORS, CITRIC ACID, PECTIN, SALT, LOCUST BEAN GUM, SODIUM BENZOATE [TO PRESERVE FRESHNESS], ARTIFICIAL COLOR [CONTAINS RED 40 AND BLUE 1], ENRICHED WHEAT FLOUR (CONTAINS NIACIN, REDUCED IRON, THIAMINE MONONITRATE [VITAMIN B1], RIBOFLAVIN [VITAMIN B2], SUGAR, WHOLE WHEAT FLOUR, RAISINS, CORN SYRUP, HIGH FRUCTOSE CORN SYRUP, GLYCERIN, SKIM MILK, LEAVENING (BAKING SODA, CAL-CIUM PHOSPHATE), SOY LECITHIN (EMULSIFIER), SALT, EGG WHITES, ARTIFICIAL FLAVOR.

HIDDEN SUGAR

. . . just like the hidden fat that's killing us. Hidden sugars are just as big, and both are connected to our being overfat and unhealthy.

The studies say that 20 percent to 25 percent of our calories come from sugar. Carbohydrates are a great source of energy; you know you need them. You are just beginning to understand them: brown rice, potatoes,

apples

asparagus

barley

beans

> blackberries
>
> carrots
>
> corn
>
> grapes
>
> oatmeal
>
> pastas
>
> sweet potatoes
>
> tomatoes
>
> whole wheat breads
>
> yams
>
> just to name a few carbohydrates.

But did you know that in the average American diet over half of our carbo-hydrate caloric intake is in the form of sugar? Simple sugars that we are eat-ing by the ton? Help me. That's not what every food expert in the country means by suggesting we increase our consumption of carbohydrates and de-crease our protein and fat intake.

Big numbers adding up, coming in by the truckload in the prepackaged food we buy. You probably didn't know you were taking in one-half of your carbohydrate intake by eating simple sugars even though you read labels, health-conscious consumer that you are. You know sugar when you see it. And you do, but when you don't see the word sugar and have no clue how many different words there are that mean the same thing, what you don't see still adds up to sugar in the food you are eating.

THE LABEL LIE

You want abuse? "No cholesterol" on every label we read these days doesn't come close to the label lies about sugar or "sugar free"—and they've been around a lot longer, we love the stuff, and the guys that make them have this deception down.

But no matter how much the food manufacturers want to keep playing the big sugar cover-up, the fact is that we are getting tons of the stuff, and it ain't just coming from the sugar bowl in the middle of your table. (Does anyone have a sugar bowl in the middle of their table anymore?)

Up to 70 percent of the sugar you've been taking in comes in the form of an additive to the prepared foods you are buying and eating. That's why sugar is known as the most common food additive (although preservatives are creeping up fast as number one). There are so many different ways to talk about it, so many places to hide it, that it could take you one hundred years to get the answers.

The food manufacturers have all these names to play around with:

Corn Syrup

Fructose

Galactose

Glucose

Fruit juice concentrate

Honey

Lactose

Maltose

Maple syrup

Molasses

Saccharin

Sucrose

Nothing like twenty names for the same thing. See how easy it is to confuse the hell out of everyone, make it a complicated mess, continue arguing, and never get down to the nitty-gritty?

So making the effort isn't enough. Trust isn't part of getting your life healthy and your body functioning properly—it's your getting the information you need to make different decisions. That's what it's all about, and when it comes to sugar and the amount we are all taking in, starting with the hidden sugar is a good idea.

THOUGHT . . .

Taking in loads of a certain kind of fuel that has no nutritional value, no fiber, no proteins, and no essential fats, vitamins or minerals is fine once in a while—nobody's perfect—and eating something that has no nutritional value once in a while couldn't hurt you, so who cares? But eating that non-nutritional, totally empty calorie stuff as half of our very important carb fuel requirement—is that O.K.?

There doesn't need to be some big scientific research done on that question. It's pretty easy to understand.

WHAT'S GOOD, WHAT'S BAD

It's the speed of breakdown, the absorption rate, and the lack of or inclusion of any nutrients that define good sugars versus bad—although as far as your body is concerned, sugar is sugar, with very few exceptions.

Unsulfured molasses supplies some B vitamins and minerals. That's good because at least you get some nutritional value for your money. That's why molasses has such a good name. But who uses it other than your 120-year-old grandmother? When is the last time you cooked, baked, or dipped your finger in molasses? Never in my thirty-six years is my answer to that question. Now that I understand the difference in sugars, and since I'm someone who always wants more nutritional value for my money, I'm going to try using it once in a while. Who knows, maybe I'll become a molasses expert, maybe there'll be a molasses book. It's something new for sure, but so was the low-fat stuff until recently, and that worked out well.

Sucrose, as in your common ordinary white table sugar, has no nutritional value, no fiber or anything else left after we refine it. Funny how "refine" has always implied making perfect. But does it?

> Take the rough edges and clean it all up.
>
> The nuns tried to refine me.
>
> My mom worked hard on it.
>
> The guidance counselors tried their best.
>
> My home ec teacher really, really tried, but it didn't work.

The rough edges are still there, and based on what I keep reading, taking the original and refining it, you also lose something in the process of cleaning it up. The original form may be rough, but at least when you're talking about sugar and me, it sounds like refining it makes it useless.

Refining sugar takes away all its value and leaves you with nice, shiny white nothing. It's hard to tell whether this little story I just told about refining and me means a damn thing, but when it comes to sugar, there are cold, hard facts about what you're left with.

> Nothing.
>
> Low-quality fuel at its best.

You've got your people out there who think it makes no difference at all whether you eat this useless stuff or have a bit of molasses. And there are others who think:

[Our bodies] "react differently with varying degrees of sensitivity, and a higher-quality sweetener will produce a smoother response in blood sugar."

I tend to agree with Gary Null because he knows what he's talking about, and it makes perfect sense to me that people react differently. We all know that every "body" is different. Varying degrees of sensitivity makes a whole lot of sense. Some people are allergic to some things, and some aren't. This isn't taking a very big stand, it's pretty basic.

As for the higher-quality sweetener producing a smoother response in blood sugar—well, I guess the experts can argue all they want. But it seems to me that if your body has something to digest—a B vitamin here or there, an ounce of fiber, minerals, something—then it would do so. After all, that's what your body does, and that would take a bit more time than what your body needs to do to digest some white, shiny, useless stuff with nothing at all in it going through the old digestive tract. Call me simpleminded or call me Mr. Gump, but doesn't that just make sense?

Something that the big boys can't seem to say. It's like the word "marriage" or "commitment" for some men; they just can't get the words out, no matter how hard they try. Yes, sugar is nnnooooooot sssoooooo ggggooood for you. We should cccuuuuuut bbbaaaaacckkkkk jjjjuuuuust a bit.

But right from Null's mouth, the truth: at 99.5–99.9 percent pure sucrose, white sugar is "one of the purest chemicals manufactured." Powdered sugar is nothing but "pulverized table sugar."

Brown sugar? "Crystallized sugar with molasses added back to it for color and flavor."

Turbinado sugar? "Highly refined sugar." Highly refined sugar is highly refined sugar, no matter how you look at it. Your body doesn't know the difference between bleached white table sugar that we all grew up on and turbinado sugar, which people are buying in bulk thinking it's better for them than bleached white. Why? Because it isn't white? Because the health food people say it is? Because it's "natural"? But where's the cane? (That would be "natural" sugar.) Turbinado sugar doesn't grow the way you buy it; they have to process it to get it into your bulk bin at your local health food store. Maybe they refine and process it with sandals and cotton clothing on, but they refine it all the same.

Brown rice syrup—ever heard of it? "Derived from grains and still maintains a percentage of complex carbohydrates." The absorption rate is longer than it is for white table sugar, and because of that you minimize the roller-coaster effect of high and then low energy levels.

See . . . see . . . see . . . it absorbs differently, as in more slowly, because it has something different in it.

Barley malt. Same thing.

Molasses. Just look at the list of nutrients in one tablespoon of molasses:

Thiamin-B1	.008 mg
Niacin-B	.919 mg
Vitamin B	.137 mg
Folate	.09 mcg
Pantothenic	.165 mg
Calcium	42 mg
Copper	.1 mg
Iron	.969 mg
Magnesium	49.6 mg
Phosphorus	6.38 mg
Potassium	300 mg
Selenium	13.3 mcg
Sodium	7.56 mg
Zinc	.059 mg
Water	5.31 mg
Calories	54.5
Carbohydrates	14.1 mg
Total Fat	.021 g
Complex Carbs	2.83 g
Sugars	11.3 g

You could hardly say molasses has no nutrients in it!

These are slower absorbers. Think food. More fuel in these sweeteners for your body to grab hold of.

But if you want to know more about the processed and the refined, the bad and the good, the war of the sugars, you've also got to know about sweeteners such as:

Concentrated fruit juice. Everywhere these days. Used by the food manufacturers because they think that you and I are going to be fooled into believing that because it has the word fruit, we will buy it without thought. But you see, they don't know us. We want the facts, and these are the facts: Fruit juice sweeteners are highly refined, at 68 percent. How much fructose or glucose or sucrose depends on the fruit. Nobody knows if concentrated fruit juice is better for you than white table sugar, but too much of it is too much, no matter how you break it down.

Refined is refined. It originally came from fruit? So what. Bleached white originally came from the cane, but by the time you and I eat about fifty pounds of it (before the calendar year's even half over), that isn't what our bodies are getting.

Fructose. Fruit sugar. Good when you're eating the apple, because when you're eating the whole fruit, you're getting everything else it has to offer—such as fiber and nutrients. But this stuff is refined, most of the time from corn starch.

Fructose is sweeter than sweet—15 percent to 80 percent sweeter than sucrose (white table sugar). Some people say it's absorbed more slowly than glucose, and some don't. The jury is still out on fructose, except that the health food industries are using it in everything, suggesting that it's better for you than white table sugar. But sugars are all absorbed the same inside your body. Refined is refined. Too much is too much—that's the sugar chant (can't get away from that chanting, can I?).

I haven't wanted ice cream in so long. Not even frozen yogurt. . . . Why? Not because it's bad, but because I just don't want the sugar or the NutraSweet without the vitamins and nutrition.

—*Susanne, Larkspur, Colorado*

MORE ON SWEET . . . ARTIFICIAL, THAT IS

Artificial Sweeteners: In these modern times you can't even think about talking about sweet without including artificial sweeteners. But you can't talk about them in the same breath that you talk about sugar—because they aren't sugar.

Saccharin is not a sugar, and it is not a food. "It is a non-nutritive artificial sweetener made from coal tar." Saccharin's been around for a very long time—it was discovered in 1879. It's a petroleum product, is non-caloric, and is three hundred times sweeter than sugar. Would you say that our sweet tooth is out of control?

If you want confusion, massive confusion, then all you've got to do is step into the sweet and low controversy about saccharin. You're gonna find every argument under the sun.

*//// "As bad as sugar is, it's still better for you than artificial sweeteners," says the Center for Science in the Public Interest.

*//// Everyone and their mother says that saccharin is a possible human carcinogenic, suspected of increasing risk of bladder cancer.

⚡ But according to a recent study at the University of Nebraska Medical Center, "While there is still a little room for caution, the evidence seems convincing that saccharin does not cause cancer in humans, nor do humans possess the same alpha 2U globulin that rats do."

What the hell is a 2U globulin? And what does it have to do with me and saccharin?

You've got the FDA banning it in 1977 and the federal law requiring warning labels on anything that contains saccharin:

Use of this product may be hazardous to your health. This product contains saccharin which has been determined to cause cancer in laboratory animals.

But it isn't just saccharin that's being used in our chewing gum, puddings, yogurt, sodas, and thousands of other products. Now there are artificial sweeteners like aspartame.

NutraSweet and Equal—ever heard of them? Then you've heard of aspartame. Ye olde aspartame was introduced in 1981 and is considered the most popular artificial sweetener in history. Quite a title, wouldn't you say? That's one hell of a billing. Aspartame is only 180 times sweeter than sugar. Wonder why it won the most popular title when saccharin is so much sweeter, and they're both artificial?

It could be because aspartame has been given a "clean bill of health" by the Center for Disease Control, the American Medical Association's Council on Scientific Affairs, and the FDA. These are the guys you can trust. HUH? They've done some of the worse policing of all times when it comes to our safety and the foods we eat. We know that. The AMA—they've done such a good job putting together disease and the foods we eat?? HELLLLLLLLLLP me with this, could you?

They have done some work on the subject of aspartame, and they all agree there is an acceptable daily intake. Hey, hey, our "acceptable" daily intake of 50 milligrams per kilogram of body weight equals, for a 120-pound woman:

> 15 cans of aspartame-sweetened soda
>
> 14 cups of gelatin
>
> 22 cups of yogurt
>
> 55 six-ounce servings of hot cocoa.

So the Center for Disease Control has given aspartame a clean bill of health, but there is one warning required on labels: "Phenylketonurics: Contains Phenylalanine." And the possible side effects of that are:

Rashes

Mild depression

Headaches

Nausea

Ringing ears

Vertigo

Insomnia

Loss of motor control

Loss or change of taste

Slurred speech

Memory loss

Blurred vision

Blindness

Suicidal depression

Seizures

The FDA says we can have fifty-five six-ounce servings of hot cocoa a before we have to worry about this particular artificial sweetener. But the Burton Goldberg Group says there are numerous side effects, "a result of either sensitivity to aspartame or changes it brings about in brain chemistry."

So, surprise—there's controversy when you sit down at the table to talk about artificial sweeteners. What we know is that we've got saccharin, aspartame, acesulfame-K, and all kinds of other sweeter-than-sugar-could-ever-be artificial sweeteners floating around in our dry beverage mixes, instant coffees and teas, nondairy creamers, and in more foods than you can list—unless, of course, you were writing a book on lists of artificially sweetened foods, but we are not. (Notice that suddenly the author of my book is now "we.")

Whether or not they are good for you still has not been decided. If it took twenty-five years for the people doing the deciding to decide that eating saturated fat causes some problems, then it may take one hundred years for them to figure out that anything artificial in these huge amounts may also cause some problems—and we are taking in a boatload of artificial sweeteners in all the foods we are eating.

I don't know about you, but I'm not waiting on them to decide anymore. Here's my opinion about these things. I've said it before, and I'll say it again: Any food with a warning label on the side isn't for me. I really believe the same rule applies to these artificial sweeteners. If you have a healthy, fit body that is doing its job efficiently with the help of lean muscle mass, healthy internal organs, and some kind of a balance in your daily food intake, and you eat some artificial sweeteners once in a while, you probably don't have to worry too much about it. But that's not what's happening. We are taking in tons of it. There isn't a balance in so many people's daily food intake, and when you add this to the list of other things sending us into the pendulum swing that so many of us live in, then it's got to cause some problems. And over and over again it's been proven that the boys in the government and the AMA say something is safe and then—ten, fifteen, twenty-five years later—come back and say **NEVER MIND** . . .

Are you willing to take the chance?

Do you need them?

Can you increase the quality of the foods you're eating to the point of cutting way, way back on stuff like this?

Can you eliminate the risk by eliminating the artificial sweeteners?

Do you want your kids eating this stuff when the jury is still out on whether or not it causes cancer?

See how much of it you're eating. Is it imbalanced?

Are you and your children taking in more than you ever thought you were, and is that O.K. with you?

The only thing to do when it comes to the artificial sweetener argument is to read, read, read, question, question, question, and make your own decisions. I did. I have. My children and I don't eat the stuff. Hey, you decide.

In 1886, Dr. John Pemberton, an Atlanta druggist, invented a soothing cough syrup. An employee put some in carbonated water, and Coca-Cola was born.

SO WHAT DO YOU DO?

Never eat sugar again? Who can even think about that? Worry every time we put something sweet in our mouths that it's refined to the point of instant, insulin-releasing, pancreas-panicking, a-million-teaspoons-of-no-nutritional-value junk? Avoid artificial sweeteners like the plague? Please, spare me that—it ain't gonna happen. But is there is a solution to 110 pounds of sugar a year and all the havoc it creates in our bodies? Can you live without artificial sweeteners and not be a social outcast?

THOUGHT . . .

Moderation? Not that I came up with it; there's nothing original about most of this. We are just dealing with common sense, figuring out a way to live our lives without getting sick from the foods we are eating, and trying to make our bodies look a bit better.

So think about this:

*If each soft drink you are drinking has approximately six teaspoons of sugar—and it does—maybe you can have a glass of water instead once in a while.

*If it's sugar you're craving, how about trying a piece of fruit instead of a candy bar? Again, once in a while.

*Or if you really want to go crazy, how about snacking on a complex carbohydrate before you reach for the sugar?

Grab a:

> bagel
> bean burrito
> ear of corn
> potato
> slice of whole wheat bread
> tortilla

Have a bowl of rice, some pasta, a bowl of veggies, some minestrone soup. With an ounce of planning, carrying some food with you, learning more and more about the foods you are putting in your mouth and how they may affect your body, you may just find yourself having an alternative to snacky, sugary things. You see, it's a whole different way of eating: thinking before you grab that handful of whatever.

> M&M-y things
> Mr. Good for you or bad for you bars
> Snickery things
> Chocolate chippy things
> Almond or any kind of joy bars
> Ice creamy things
> Jellybeany things
> Ding Dongy things
> 3 or more Musketeer bars
> Cups o'peanutty butter

Cupcakey things
Fudgey, toffee, caramely things
Full o'sugar soda pops
Twinky dinky things
and on . . . and on . . . and on . . .

By planning just a bit, it won't be the candy bar you'll find yourself eating when your body is screaming for instant fuel.

I'll tell you what I've done that has changed my body and has, I think, done wonders for my health: I became much more conscious of what I was putting in my mouth. Yes, it started with the fat, but soon I was noticing the sugary, snacky stuff.

Remember the clarity.
Remember the nuns.
Remember the monks.
Remember that extra inch of whatever that fell off.

Without thinking twice, I found that just a little bit of thought and some different food here and there made all the difference in the world. Higher quality does make a difference, no matter what the FDA says.

Choose your sugar battles by being aware of the truth.

CHAPTER 10
CHICKEN

Chicken.

The saving grace to a meal with substance?
The last "healthy" meat we can eat?
The only thing left to put into a sandwich?

The "proven to be better for you than beef kind of meat." The stage-one alternative to beef in terms of lower fat, because it is—if you're counting your total fat intake—lower in total saturated fat than beef.

Chicken is the cool stuff. It's the kind of meat everyone is choosing these days, easily seen in the increased buying over the last few years.

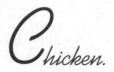 In 1990, Americans ate more than 90 pounds of chicken per person—double the amount eaten in 1970.

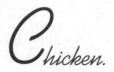 The poultry industry has grown from 2.1 billion birds in 1964 to more than 6 billion in 1990.

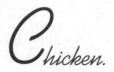 Automated chicken slaughtering houses process 21 million chickens a day—at speeds up to ninety-one birds a minute.

Chicken—when you think about it, all that probably needs to be said is to skin it, broil it, and cut back on your daily fat intake by eating it. No need for a whole chapter on the bird.

But that would only do for the average Joe. Food P.I.'s need more, look deeper, and want the whole bird story. And if you really want the lowdown, then we've got to dig a bit—you know that by now. Enter stage two and our discussion about chicken.

Nothing screams cuteness like a tiny baby chick, the little fuzzy-headed, pink-eyed creature poking slowly through the egg. So sweet, fuzzy, vulnerable, so very, very cute. Isn't that what you think of when you think chicken hatching? Can't you just see the newborn fuzzy-headed creature growing up in the henhouse, producing its eggs for us to eat for breakfast, hanging out with its henhouse friends, and eventually ending up in the farmer family's, or our, pot for dinner? A normal evolution for the henhouse chicken.

The little chickadee's day begins with the proud rooster (probably its dad) calling in the dawn. Some nights may end with a visit from the fox. All the little chickens fighting for their lives, flocking together, feathers and dust everywhere, and finally after a typical day on the farm, where roosters can be roosters and hens can be hens, they settle down for a good night's sleep. There it is, a day on the chicken farm in the mind of Susan Powter, Food P.I.

Tainted by the cartoons of my earlier years? Foghorn, leghorn fantasy beyond your wildest dreams? Absolutely. All of us have the cartoon version of the henhouse in our minds. There isn't a person in this country whose image of farms, henhouses, and fox visits hasn't been clouded by cartoons and prime-time television. The Waltons made me want to give up city life, throw on a slightly worn but well-pressed floral dress, and run to the Blue Ridge Mountains, toward the good life. My floral dress would have turned into overalls within minutes, and given my disposition, I would have been the one adolescent whom the mountain's magic just couldn't do anything about. But in my dreams I always thought there was something to that farm stuff that could teach us all a lesson or two about humanity, love, togetherness, and all the other important things in life. So I watched and dreamed, and my vision of farm life was firmly planted in my mind—until now, twenty-some years later. Until I started writing this book.

Our vision of the American farmer and his farm, the fertile soil, the family value system isn't just about our feeling warm, it's where our food comes from, the stuff we eat and live on:

> Food.
> The title of this book.
> Food, one of the things we just can't do without.

Food. The American farm. Connected in a big, big way.

The morning milking of old Bessie.

The henhouse and those farm-fresh chickens.

The sausage being cured, the jelly being jammed, the eggs being sold
farm fresh and all.

Well, not anymore. That picture you have in your mind about where
your food is coming from and the natural order of things, even if it's a little
closer to reality than my twisted foghorn vision, it's not even close to what's
going on.

La Cuisinière Bourgeoisie by Menon, a four-hundred-page cookbook for
the lower middle class with recipes for cooking inferior cuts of meat and
other hints on how to eat well inexpensively, appeared in 1746. It became
a best-seller as the masses scrambled to learn how to cook.

Let's talk chicken:

The henhouse

The hatching

The growing of the chicken that ends up on your plate is important to your
health because what's involved, how it's done, what's been added or taken
away, all affect the quality of the food you are eating and therefore affect your
life.

Your body getting what it needs isn't just about the nutrients you put into
it, just like getting rid of fat isn't only about chowing down on low fat without quality anymore. How about cleanliness—mean anything to you? When
you're talking about chicken you gotta ask about cleanliness. The way something's handled before it hits your boiling pot, what's been added to it, what's
going on in the henhouse? Do they have anything to do with you and your
body? Let's take a look.

So you go to the store and pick up some chicken that's nicely wrapped in
plastic. You feel safe, secure, confident that the food you are about to feed
your family has been inspected, is clean, and is what it says it is.

You skin, broil, add lemon to, and get the protein you need. Live your life.
What's wrong with that? Millions and millions of people are doing it. Tons
and tons of chicken are being eaten every year.

The first thing we've got to do is tie in what we already know about labeling with the chick you have just bought.

Inspected?

98 percent fat free?

You know only too well at this point what believing the labels will get you: fat, unhealthy, and half dead, because the snack makers, the lunch-meat makers, and the chicky manufacturers are all motivated by the same thing.

YOUR HEALTH?

NO, NO, NO.

PROFIT.

Caution applies to all labels forever. That's a given, Food P.I.'s.

Unless you've been living in the mountains without any electricity for the last ten years, you've seen those reports that every news show in the country has done "behind the scenes at the butcher counter and in the henhouse." You've seen the rotten meat being flipped over to look good under the plastic. Heard the hidden microphone conversations of the managers showing the new employees how to get the most out of meat, rotten or not.

We've all seen reporters inside the meat factories with those god-awful hidden cameras in their hats that make you seasick watching the story—the improper handling, lack of inspection, and gross things going on with our meat and chicken before they even get to the trucks, on the butcher shelves, and into our mouths.

We've all lived through the massive advertising campaigns that follow a story like this from the food chain or the food manufacturer that got slammed and the government agency that didn't do the job. And then it all dies down until the next "one in a million" incident.

So you know that caution is necessary and that something isn't quite right. But again, the boys uncovering the cover-up didn't say enough or didn't give us the information that would give us a clue about what it is we are supposed to do.

Watch out for what?

Go where when we think we've been eating bad meat?

Do what to solve the problem?

And the most important thing: What does any of this info have to do with us? Our lives? Our family's health? The way we feel? Our bodies? Why should we care that once in a while some bad meat passes through the system?

I bet I can tell you what you're thinking while you're watching these programs.

"I've been eating chicken for twenty years and never got sick!! Why should I be concerned because a couple of people in the Midwest got tainted chicken?"

Right? Did I hit the nail on the head?

"What does it have to do with any of us?"

Good, good question.

"Does the lying butcher affect our health?"

Brilliant!!! The American public is very smart and isn't going to get all up in arms unless there's something to get all up in arms about. Unless it affects us directly, who cares?

That's the way most of us think. Fair enough.

Hey, news shows: Why are you showing us this one-in-a-million case and then leaving us with no answers or connection to our lives?

The top news shows may not have been able to get you the answers, but believe me, when Susan Powter, Food P.I., goes undercover to the henhouse, she gets the answers to what's going on and how it affects our lives.

So let's go to the farm. Off to the henhouse.

THE HENHOUSE

Sad news. Try as we might, you ain't gonna find a henhouse anymore with a big red rooster. (I'm not talking chewing gum—what was the big red rooster product from our childhood?) The henhouse is gone. It has turned into a chicken factory that processes thousands and thousands of chickens at a time.

These things are huge. They house up to eighty thousand chickens in one plant. Old Farmer Joe isn't feeding his chicks early anymore in the morning from the grain sack; he is not bonding with his birds. The henhouses of today have unbelievably sophisticated feeding, watering, and temperature-controlled systems to do what Old Farmer Joe used to do so lovingly. (Do you think this opinion is slightly tainted? So far Old Farmer Joe is Saint Farmer Joe lovingly tending the chickens, and the henhouse of the 90's is as cold as they come. I know every farmer in the country wasn't Old Saint Farmer Joe, but let me retain my simpleminded version of the farm, please.)

Let's get off the fairy-tale version of the chickens and get down to why we have poultry factories. There are a lot of people to feed in this country. As sad as it may be for my nostalgic brain, eventually we had to modernize the system and make it more efficient. As hard as it may be for all of us to understand, there was surely a reason for wiping out the American farm and using massive warehouses to raise our chickens.

We'll talk about it, understand a bit more about it than we do right now.

But before we get to that, I've got to warn you that our henhouse tour is going to bring up a couple of issues that we need to get out in the open.

Such as animal cruelty, which with all due respect I'm not interested in, but it does go on in the henhouse. (Better clarify that before I'm written up as the meanest woman alive by those animal righters. I am concerned with cruelty, whether it's a chicken or a child, although to be quite honest I do find it hard to believe, with the children of our country dying left, right, and center, that anyone could really expect us to care about the dogs and cats. However, someone's got to stand up for the little buggers, and we really shouldn't be experimenting with, harming, doing bad things to God's creatures.)

A very complicated issue, for sure.

Tell you what: The animal people can protect the animals, and the children people can protect the children—or maybe we can join together, do both, and talk about the real issue behind the problem: the fact that we, as human beings, think we have the right to do whatever we want in the name of industrialization, profit, and experimentation. We don't. When the big judgment comes, all of us will have to do a whole lot of answering about this abuse-the-world-and-all-its-creatures-because-we-think-we-are-so-superior thing.

(Sometimes I wonder if it's because I have such a great platform, my book, or because I have always been somebody who speaks her mind, but I can't seem to keep myself from going off on these tangents. Consider these spurts of Susan's opinions a roundtable conversation smashed between the covers of a food book—and again, pardon me.)

Back to the henhouse.

Other than my tangents, this isn't a book about animal rights, which is what I meant when I said I didn't care. It is a book about you, your health, how you look and feel, and what affects that, so I'm not going to get off on the living conditions in the chicken factories or the inhumane treatment of the chicks unless it affects your food—because that's what we are talking about right now. Later, when we are more evolved and healthy as horses (pardon the animal reference), maybe we'll talk about animal rights. There it is, the next book:

The Abused Chick by Susan Powter
The Chicken Without a Home by Susan Powter
The Homeless Chickens of America . . .

For now, the fact that the henhouse has turned into a hellhouse for any chicken born to breed eggs or end up on our plates for dinner isn't my focus. You'll read, and as usual you'll decide.

> I was a big steak and pork chop fan. Now I'm down to chicken (maybe) and
> beans instead. I do feel a lot better, and I can see a waistline coming.
> —*Barbara, San Bernardino, California*

The chicken that's in your sandwich is mass-produced. The henhouse has
been totally industrialized with one thing in mind: profit and efficiency.
Those are two things, but when you are talking big business, they can safely
be lumped together as one, because that's what it usually boils down to.

The current chicken factory system has very little regard for your or your
family's health and certainly none for the animal, but as promised we won't
go into that.

With up to eighty thousand birds packed into one warehouse, five birds in
a 16-by-18-inch cage, without ever seeing the light of day and being sub-
jected to the most unnatural living conditions, there are bound to be consequences. And there are.

In all fairness to the chicken manufacturers, you can't have eighty thousand of anything in one big room without disease. I mean, it's inevitable.

Open sores

Pus

Infections

Hormone imbalances

Crazy chicks . . . yeah, they get a little nuts. Never seeing the light of day
(that's to keep them producing) and never moving around (get them fat
fast)—wouldn't you get a little crazy if that's the way you lived? Animal rights
aside, you still gotta feel a little sorry for the birds. They may be chickens, but
they are God's creatures, like you and me, and they have a good natural plan
that this warehouse thing totally screws up—so it's a problem.

With these manufacturing houses pumping out **more than six billion
birds in 1990,** with automated chicken slaughtering houses processing up
to **21 million chickens a day** (that's **more than 14,583 birds a minute,**
in case you care), then we first have to have a look at, go right to, begin immediately with what must be the best inspection system in the country before we can sit down and feel truly safe.

After all, it seems to me that the beginning is where the system would be
at its best. Make sure that all these birds being processed through the manufacturing farms of today are checked properly so that we can be assured of
what we are eating, and it will be easy to get the answers to the rest.

Inspection. If everything's set up right, then if there are any problems, they can be caught in time and we'll be safe.

///y The food the chickies are eating? Sure, something to think about.

///y Living conditions? Only if they affect our health.

///y Animal cruelty? Save for the next book, but disease and the policing of it are a must, because now that we know how really big these places are, you can't expect that nothing would ever get diseased or screwed up.

> I gave up red meat (makes me lethargic and so tired) and ate more chicken and turkey.
>
> —*Linda, Accokeek, Mississippi*

INSPECTION

If you've got birds, apparently you've got bacteria. I understand that, who wouldn't? And if you've got bacteria in poultry, you have two basic types that everyone seems to talking about.

Salmonella. You've heard of it. That's the one the news stories keep talking about:

> Wipe your counter well.
>
> Wash your bird properly.
>
> Make sure you don't get it.

That one.

And then there's *campylobacter*. This is that one-in-a-million bacteria that some poor person somewhere else gets, the stuff that makes other people sick and gives chicken a bad name.

Funny. That's what I thought until I got the facts. Here's the bacteria truth:

"Salmonella and campylobacter are responsible for four million cases of food poisoning a year." That's what the National Academy of Sciences says.

Hey, hey, hey. That's not one in a million or some unlucky bugger somewhere in Kansas. That's a lot of people sick from food poisoning!!

"In 1985 the Department of Agriculture said that 35 percent of all chicken carcasses were contaminated with salmonella."

Just a minute. That's 1985, and that's the Department of Agriculture. Two things wrong here.

First, chicken consumption has gone way up since that time, so this number has to have gone up. And second, you're talking the Department of Agriculture here—what are they gonna 'fess up to, the whole truth? I don't think so. They're responsible for those statistics. Something's up here, my private dick nose can smell it.

In 1989, testing of five processing plants in the Southeast (the country's leading poultry-producing region) found **"SALMONELLA LEVELS OF 57.5 PERCENT." MORE THAN HALF!!**

What are you talking about, one in a million chance? This stuff doesn't affect us?? Come on!!!!!

"Two thousand Americans die of salmonella poisoning each year, mainly the very old, the immuno-compromised, and the very young."

Hold on!! The very old, the sick, and the very young! Why don't we just call it like it is: the most innocent, the weakest, the ones who need nutrition and cleanness most. Why don't we just say that? It's the truth.

Surely with this information things have gotten better in the last five years. But the contamination levels of chickens have risen in the last few years.

> During the late 1960's = 29 percent
> 1985 = 35 percent
> 1990 = 50 to 75 percent

Yo, inspectors, what's up? Seems to me that whatever it is you're doing isn't working too well. Department of Agriculture, where are you boys? Investigate the system. It's time.

My husband, who was a steak-and-potato (with extra butter) kind of man, is now a pasta, rice, chicken, and shrimp man.

—*Laura, Troutdale, Oregon*

The system. The Streamlined Inspection System. SIS. That's what it's called. The boys who have a look at our chicks before they are shipped to the hypermarts.

Here's what the SIS, implemented in 1986 (what in the hell did they do before then?), is required to do. The health inspectors for our chickens, the police department for bacteria, the guards of grossness, the cleanness patrol have to

1. Get a sample of ten birds per line, twice per eight-hour shift. That's ten out of fifteen thousand birds in one large plant.

   Ten out of fifteen thousand? Is it any wonder something can slip past that kind of efficiency?

2. The birds must have three or more sores, three or more abscesses, or one cancer tumor before they are pulled.

   YUUUCCKKKKK. Let me get this straight: These guys are seeing only ten out of fifteen thousand birds, and out of the ten they look at, only the ones with three or more sores or abscesses get pulled? Get out of here!!

   I WANT A BIRD PULLED IF IT'S GOT ONE ABSCESS.

   If the damn chicken even looks like it's developing a sore, I want it pulled and taken off the ready-to-eat line.

   What are you talking about, three sores?
   Who was the moron who said we'd accept that standard?

3. When the birds with the three or more sores or one cancer tumor are pulled, the sores or tumor must be trimmed off, then the birds go right back on the streamline.

So I'm assuming that these inspectors are surgeons. You'd have to be to know for sure that you've gotten all the cancer.

The cancer specialist surgeons who inspect our chickens are allowed to pass ten out of fifteen thousand, and **PUS AROUND THE LUNGS IS O.K. AS LONG AS IT'S NOT TOO ADVANCED.**
EXCUUUUUUUUUSE me?
Who decides what is not too advanced when it comes to pus around the lungs?
I want to meet this specialist.
This is getting sickening, pardon that pun!!!
You think I'm making this up, don't you? There's no way you're gonna believe that this is what's allowed in the U.S.A. to protect you and your family from infection, disease, open sores, pus, and bad meat. You think I'm exaggerating? I'm not. This is the truth. You can't argue with the Depart-

ment of Agriculture. *Scientific American* and the people who have known what's been going on have been trying to tell us for a long time. But there's a whole lot that we don't want to hear because we want to sit down and drive through and feel protected. That's reasonable and the way it should be, but with our current system of inspecting and growing and warehousing our chicks, we can't. What's going on is ridiculous. Don't you agree?

I mean, first, let's get this inspection system organized. Who designed this piece of crap! You boys need to create a much, much better system than the one you've got going now to protect us, Dave. Get off the TV shows, forget about the labels—don't you think this is just a bit more pressing than designing expensive little labels that still don't tell us what we need to know? Davey, what the hell is the matter with you? Help us get through to the Department of Agriculture, Dave, we need you.

We're talking diseased food here. Now that we know how much disease we're talking about, I see the need for antibiotics. Who wouldn't? Talk about creating your own demand. Shove thousands and thousands of chickens into one place, subject them to the most unnatural living conditions on earth, and you are absolutely going to find some disease. So what's the deal with the antibiotics, and where are they coming from? You can't give eighty thousand birds injections, can you?

FEED

So it all goes back to feed—what the chicky is eating becomes part of what we eat. That's why we're talking feed, because if we are what we eat, then the chicken is what it eats, and on and on it goes. You didn't think that made any sense, did ya? Reread it and you'll see that it makes a whole lot of sense and is a heck of an intro to . . . FEED.

Way back when, the chickens on the farm were eating grain. (There's Old Saint Farmer Joe again with that burlap sack on his hip, throwing chicken feed out to the free-range, roaming-wherever-the-heck-they-want-to-roam chickens.) We didn't have to think much about what chickens were eating then. That's a big part of why we can all sit down at the dinner table or drive through the drive-through, eat, and enjoy in trust our Thanksgiving dinner, our chicken cacciatore. (I threw that in because I watched a Robert De Niro film last night—strong, Italian, the brotherhood thing, even if they were all gangsters. So romantic. So thrilling. I think I'm in love with him. Call my husband and tell him I'm in love with Robert De Niro, would you, 'cause from now on it's Robert and me.) Chicken any way you like it. You sit, you eat, you trust that what you are eating is clean, edible, and that you and your family have been protected by inspection and that the feed that the chicken is eating is clean and good and that the chicken you end up with on your plate is clean.

But that's not what's happening with our chickens anymore. You're not eating a grain-fed, roaming-around-the-henhouse kind of bird that was raised by Saint Farmer Joe. Mass production doesn't allow for much roaming at all. As a matter of fact, eighty thousand birds roaming ain't gonna happen ever again.

You'd have to have a mighty big sack of grain, a whole lot of farmers, and a farm the size of the Walton mountain to accommodate that many birds. Common sense tells you with that many birds you've got to come up with another way of feeding them all. And we can't expect that to happen without knowing that the old profit point is going to raise its necessary little head. You and I have to think profit because that's what the chicky manufacturers are thinking, and they're thinking it big-time when it comes to what the chicken is eating.

The feed that your dinner is eating is not designed with the chicken's nutritional needs in mind. It's about two things: Make them fat fast (a plump bird is a better bird) and medicate the hell out of the food so that maybe the manufacturer can fight some of the dozen or so diseases that are the consequences of the living conditions that the warehouse system establishes for mass marketing the birds.

According to *Scientific American* and John Robbins in *Diet for a New America,*

"The modern fowl thrives on a diet almost totally foreign to any food it ever found in nature."

Gary Null says,

"Meat is the most chemical-ridden food in the U.S. diet. Currently some twenty to thirty thousand different drugs are administered to animals."

You see, your chickies get shots out the wazoo to prevent certain diseases, but a lot of the drugs that the animals we eat are getting, administered through the feed, are being given by the ton to counteract the diseases that the living conditions create. They receive chemical-laced feed; that's very different from what was in Saint Farmer Joe's hip sack.

My husband loves the whole plan and is especially in favor of two meatless days per week.

—*Vicky, Arlington Heights, Illinois*

O.K. Chemicals a-plenty. Drugs, drugs, drugs. So what, *Scientific American*, Gary, and John!! That drug-laced food is helping the chicken guys get eighty thousand birds fed at once, laying eggs, getting fat for eating, and making sure we are getting the food we need to feed our families. So what if the food comes from a laboratory and the chick has no idea what nature has to offer? A few drugs here and there—is that such a big deal?? The chicken probably has never been free, so if it's all he/she/it knows, then who cares? (I'm playing the devil's advocate on the printed page, and *Scientific American* answers back. If the fact that I'm having a conversation with a report and they are answering back concerns you, call it my style, call it whatever you want, because it's the way this chapter seems to be going.)

"Virtually all chickens raised in the United States today are fed a diet laced with antibiotics from their first day to their last. Without antibiotics, the industry could not maintain the intensive farming practices."

The chicken manufacturing industries answer back:

"An awful lot of them die anyway, before we can get our profit out of them. Without antibiotics, why we'd be back to the backward practices of yesteryear."

Fair enough, although I don't like the whole thing about how "an awful lot of them die anyway before we can get our profit out of them." But we are free to concentrate on the antibiotics.

Do the antibiotics fed to the chickens affect us?

What are "an awful lot of them" dying of?

Why the need for antibiotics at all?

Is "going backward to the practices of yesteryear" a bad thing for the chicken manufacturers or us?

When was there more disease?

Which system was better?

Does it make a damn bit of difference?

Let's find out.

If you're on the food P.I. hunt for antibiotics, and we are, then all you have to do is head back to the birdie's feed, because when it comes to "feed drugs," antibiotics are considered one of the most widely used. They started using them back in 1949, and by 1954, **490,000 pounds** were being used on the chickens of America. In the 60's when feed drugs were really popular, **1.2**

million pounds were used. Today—when it's hugs, not drugs—is the number down? Has it gotten better? How about **9 million pounds per year** used on our meat?

That's just one example of what happens when the consumer demand rises. Everybody thinks chicken is so much healthier than beef. Consumer demand goes up, and our new system of warehousing gazillions of birds so that we can be more efficient in manufacturing them goes into place. Bingo, you've got two really good reasons why the need for antibiotics has risen in the last ten to fifteen years.

But there's still a question. It seems like a lot of stuff being used. The system doesn't sound too efficient when it comes to preventing disease, the inspection thing is way, way off, but the antibiotics? What's the deal? Should we be concerned?

"These high levels of antibiotics have numerous side effects on the people who eat these drug-ridden animals."

Yuck!!

"After a while bacteria become resistant to antibiotics. The antibiotics themselves are in the animal flesh after it has been slaughtered and are passed onto the consumer. These drugs do build up in your own body and can also make your body resistant to antibiotics when you really need them."

Now that's what I keep hearing from the news shows. I don't want to be resistant to antibiotics just because the chicky manufacturers want to produce trillions of birds at once and get rich. We're not getting rich, just sick. This doesn't sound right to me.

"People who are allergic or sensitive to antibiotics [count me in, I'm allergic to penicillin] may suffer very serious adverse reactions when eating meats full of drug residues."

O.K., Mr. Null. Makes sense. I'm a little concerned about myself and really, really concerned about our children getting the antibiotics and everything else that goes with them in the chickens we are eating. By the way, what else is mixed up in this mixed-up system?? I asked, and I found out.

The chicken feed that our friends the chickies (I'm warming up to the animals a bit, now that I understand a little more about what's happening to them; this may end up being an animal rights book after all. Call Simon and Schuster. Contact Bob Asahina and let him know that the *Food* book will have to wait; that advance they gave me is for a book on animal rights!!) are living on is loaded with sulfa drugs, hormones, nitrofurans, and arsenic compounds. Wow. What is a nitrofuran and an arsenic compound? Hey, I tried like hell to understand antibiotic, disease and all, but all this other stuff that's ending up in our meat? What's going on?

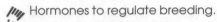 Hormones to regulate breeding.

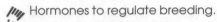 Tranquilizers to promote weight gain.

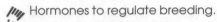 Estrogen.

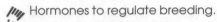 DES, a hormone that was banned from human use in 1960 but was still used on animals until 1979.

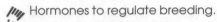 Lutalyse, a prostaglandin, so that all the animals will ovulate at the same time. This drug can affect the menstrual cycles of women and can cause pregnant women to miscarry.

 Pesticides like Vapona. It's in the nerve gas family—the same chemical that's in No Pest Strips.

 In 1940 it took four months to grow a three-pound chicken. In 1990 it takes six weeks. Wonder what changed? Do you think after fifty years of doing this, the birds just genetically altered their bodies so that they could accommodate our need to manufacture chickens faster? It must be some mighty powerful drug treatment that shortens the process of "growing a bird" to six weeks, don't you think?

If you're talking feed, you're also talking vitamin deficiencies:

"Vitamin deficiencies common in poultry factories result in a variety of conditions including retarded growth, eye damage, blindness, lethargy, kidney damage, disturbed sexual development, bone and muscle weakness, brain damage, paralysis, internal bleeding, anemia, and deformed beaks and joints. Dietary deficiencies and other factory conditions can cause a variety of bodily deformities in poultry. Fragile bones, slipped tendons, twisted lower legs, and swollen joints are among the symptoms of mineral deficiencies. Some poultry disease can leave birds with malformed backbones, twisted necks, and inflamed joints."

Thank you, Jim Mason, author of *Animal Factories*.

All right. There's a reason for all this! Is it being done to keep the chickens healthy so we end up with cleaner, healthier birds?

WE ARE NOT ENDING UP WITH CLEANER BIRDS.

Surely these drug-induced chickens are better for our health?

NOT AT ALL BETTER FOR OUR HEALTH.

This must be a protective thing that the boys in the government have going on with the American public. Well, my friends, this is dangerous thinking, dangerous for a couple of reasons. Number one, because it ain't true, and number two, because this type of thinking is what's keeping disease, unhealthy living conditions, cruelty (O.K., I had to throw that in), drug-filled meat, and all the consequences that we live or die with alive in the manufacturing of the meat we are eating.

The only thing that must change is us. We've got to change our "head in the sand" attitude about things that are so easy to cartoon and that we believe aren't happening with our food into a "head out of the sand" so that our bodies don't end up dealing with the consequences of what is going on and has been going on for a long time.

You see, here's the thing: We have been giving these guys the green light to do whatever they want to do with our food by not questioning the facts. You've heard this stuff, just as I have. We watch the news reports and then forget about them, but now it's time to make some changes. Not big drastic changes—who could even suggest that after such good stage-one transitional suggestions—just a few small changes here and there that can make a big, big difference in our health.

> I've given up chicken and meat—I don't want it. I want the vegetables, potatoes, lentil loaf, beans (a new food)—the food that makes me stop dreaming of ice cream and cheesecake. I have so much more energy in my exercising now.
>
> —*Susanne, Larkspur, Colorado*

Did I say health?

Are we talking the inside and the outside now?

Can we consider ourselves fully evolved and mature enough to admit that the quality of what we put into our bodies affects not only how we are feeling and looking but the end result—how we may or may not go ten feet under?

Heart disease?

Cancer?

Connected at all to the junk we are putting in?

Why don't we just have a look at what's going on and start making different decisions about one of the things that directly influences the type of life we live—healthy, unhealthy, high-quality, low-quality, diseased or not diseased: our food. Maybe if we have a look, talk about it, come up with possible solutions, we will have the answer to the "why me" questions that we are all going to have to deal with sooner or later.

> Why me and this cancer?
>
> Why me and this heart disease?
>
> Why has my body forsaken me?
>
> Why am I so sick?
>
> Why don't my joints work anymore?
>
> Why am I so depressed?
>
> Why am I so fat?
>
> Why don't I have any energy?
>
> Why, why, why do I feel like crap all the time?

Nobody can say anymore that the way we live, the way we look and feel, is not directly connected to what we are eating. I've interviewed the folks who want to swim with the whales, the ones who spray-paint on every fur coat they see. I've chatted with the best of the conservatives who believe that any mention of the meat industry's irresponsibility is nothing but a liberal attack on all that's good in our country. But no matter what extreme I talk to, ain't nobody gonna deny this connection anymore.

Does the condition of the bird you buy and cook have anything to do with your health and that of your family? Absolutely.

Is it all so big and out of control that there's nothing we can do to change it? No.

No, no, no. You have all the power, and this has nothing to do with your political point of view or religion. (Unless, of course, you eat meat on Friday, then you go to hell; or has the Catholic Church changed that, too? Who knows? When I was growing up, if you ate meat on Friday, you were right there, standing at the gates of hell, waiting to get in.) You see, you guys (generic reference, of course) have all the power and control over your families' health.

> You buy the stuff, don't you?
>
> You are the consumers, aren't you?

You buy it and you make your own decisions about what goes into you and your families' bodies. So it's wonderful news!!!!!

Does this mean you can never touch chicken again? No, not at all. There are alternatives to infected, uninspected, hellhouse-raised birds. Here's a thought: Grain fed. Organic. Free range. And there's less chicken. Instead of four times a week, eat it twice a week—less chance of disease—lower those risks. You have alternatives.

If you're at a restaurant with friends and the only thing to eat is chicken, have it.

If the bucket is placed in front of you and you haven't eaten in hours, eat it.

The picnic basket's opened and all there is is steak or chicken, eat the chicken.

But if it's every night at the restaurant, don't eat it.

If the only thing you've had in weeks is the bucket o' fried chicken, don't eat it.

If the picnic basket is yours to pack, pack something else.

There's nothing wrong with a bit of chicken once in a while. The quality may need to increase a bit. Portion control is very important . . . the quantity may have to be decreased a bit. Easy to do. You may have to make a stand or two; not buying poisoned food is not a very radical stand when you think about it, it just makes sense and is the best thing to do for you and your family. And increasing our awareness can do nothing but good. Nothing is to be feared, only understood. I have no clue who said that, but it's a good point.

> Awareness.
>
> Decision making.
>
> Changing what's acceptable and unacceptable.

This process of empowerment—who would ever have figured that it might all begin with a chapter on chicken in a book about food? Life's blessings come in strange ways! Don't you agree?

Grain fed, organic, free range . . . does this mean healthy? Well, maybe, maybe not. This is where you're going to need to put on your detective hat and do some research. All these things sound good, but the bottom line is you're going to have to find out for yourself about the company you are buying your chicken from. While it's generally accepted that free-range chickens are allowed to roam freely without being packed into crowded warehouses, there is no legal definition for "free-range" and there is no organization to certify that your chicken is actually raised free—it can mean free to roam an inch or a mile—so when you see these labels you're gonna need to make some calls to the chicken guys, to the grocery store manager, talk to your butcher. Find out how they define "free range," "organic," or "grain fed" and take it from there.

If you're interested in more info about your chook—here are some numbers to call to get the safest, cleanest, lowest-fat birds for your family.

ORGANIC POULTRY SOURCE LIST

Diamond Organics	800/922-2396
Sheltons	909/623-4361
Nokomis Farms	414/642-9665
Organic Mail Order Directory Guide	916/756-8518
Roseland Farms	616/445-8987
Walnut Acres	800/433-3998
Welsh's Family Farms	319/535-7318

Here are some organizations to contact.

ORGANIC PRODUCE AND PRODUCTS

Allergy Resources, Inc.
P.O. Box 888
Palmer Lake, CO 80133
(800) USE-FLAX 873-3529

Walnut Acres Organic Farms
Walnut Acres
Penns Creek, PA 17862
(800) 433-3998

Mountain Ark Trading Co.
P.O. Box 3170
Pump Station Road
Fayetteville, AR 72701
(501) 442-7191
(800) 643-8909

Diamond Organics
P.O. Box 2159
Freedom, CA 95019
(800) 922-2396

Sheltons
204 N. Lorrane
Pomona, CA 91767
(909) 623-4361

Nokomis Farms
W. 2495 County Road ES
East Troy, WI 53120
(414) 642-9665

National Organic Directory
P.O. Box 464
Davis, CA 95617
(916) 756-8518
(800) 852-3832

Roseland Farms
27427 M60 West
Cassopolis, MI 49031
(616) 445-8987

Welsh Organic Family Farms
1509 Dry Ridge Drive
Lansing, IA 52151
(319) 535-7318

Fresh Life Food Shoppe
2300 East 3rd St.
Williamsport, PA 17701
(717) 322-8280

CHAPTER 11
MILK

*A*s all-American as you get. What more needs to be said for this bone-strengthening, disease-preventing, makes-your-hair-and-nails-strong-and-beautiful stuff. It's what we leave for Santa on Christmas Eve. It's what every one of us heats up for the good-night tonic. It's the partner to the cookies when we need a friend (although I always ate the box of cookies and used the glass of milk to dunk them in; nothing like a whole box of dunked-in-milk chocolate chip cookies at 4 A.M. when you feel horrible).

And it is, without a doubt, the connection to that fresh, perfect complexion on that perfect, all-American-looking woman we all strive to be. Even Barbie looked trashy next to the perfect-boned, milk-drinking, healthy girl we saw and continue to see in every ad for milk.

Now I've been known in my day to step out of line, speak when I'm not spoken to, and rock a few boats. But when it comes to milk—rock what? Something this solid isn't rockable. There's nothing to worry about when you're talking about a nice, big, tall glass of creamy white milk. So let's talk about it:

Milk, milk, milk.

Like the chicky's life-style on the farm, things have changed a lot for old Bessie as well. Bessie isn't out in the barn waiting to be milked by Old Farmer Joe at 5 A.M. anymore; that's about as far from reality as the henhouse. Bessie's herded into milking slots and crowded together with thousands of other cows.

Your milk isn't lovingly pumped from the udders of the cow by Old Farmer Joe or his kids who are learning the joys of early-morning rising and milk pumping. We're talking thousands of electrical pumps attached to those thousands of cows in their thousands of stalls, sucking the milk from old Bessie—that's really how your milk's going from the udder to your table.

Times have changed; nothing wrong with that—thank God for technology and those thousands of pumps. More milk for the children, better bones, and a healthier body? Unfortunately, it's not the stall versus the barn, the hand pumping versus the electrical pumping, or the little farm children who will never know the joy of beating the rooster to its crow that is the issue—at least not in this book. It's the food that we are eating.

And when it comes to milk, here's an opening line for you.

The opening line in the *Wellness Encyclopedia:*

"Milk is a highly nutritious food that provides nearly all the substances essential for good health in people of all ages."

That's where the controversy starts. After this glowing report, the *Wellness Encyclopedia* does add that milk has some drawbacks:

"Whole milk contains a considerable amount of saturated fat and cholesterol, which can be harmful to the cardiovascular system. After the age of two years it is advisable to switch to low-fat or skim milk."

In 1666, cheddar cheese was invented in Cheddar, England.

Well, which is it? Once you start looking into this milk-drinking issue, it's hard to stop. It's fascinating, absolutely fascinating, because even from the beginning it didn't make much sense.

Let's start with the fact that we are the only animal on earth that drinks milk after infancy. Even though we think we are better than every animal on earth, the others have a system designed by God that works pretty well. We, on the other hand, have proven over and over again that the minute we take things into our own hands, we pretty much screw it up.

You are born. You are breast-fed (unless, of course, you were born during the last thirty years, because breast-feeding has only recently come back into fashion; yeah, mothers' groups have fought hard to get the word out about how perfect breast milk is, how important it is to breast-feed your child, the benefits both physical and emotional of nursing your baby). And you—unlike every animal on earth—keep drinking gallons and gallons of milk that come from another animal that is compositionally quite a bit different from us.

At 260 pounds, in the depths of depression, the difference between me and Bessie out on the field grazing wasn't so great, but basically the cow is physically a whole lot different from any human being I've ever seen.

Why are we the only animal on earth that continues to drink milk after infancy, and why are we drinking the milk of another animal?

To suggest that nature knows more than we do is heresy to the guys who are selling us this concept of "milk for life," but in my experience (I'll say it again) when we try to restructure or make anything that nature has designed better—go against the grain, if you will (pardon the nature and grain pun)—you can pretty much guarantee that we'll bugger it up every time.

So let's talk milk, and when we talk milk, we gotta talk lactose.

LACTOSE

Lactose, according to Webster's, is a white, crystalline sugar found in milk and prepared by the evaporation of whey and the subsequent crystallization of the sugar. Whatever, Mr. Webster!!

Lactose is what we are talking about because it's the lactose in the milk we are drinking that causes a lot of problems for a lot of people. We can't digest it. All mammals, including us, are born able to digest lactose. Good. As babies we drink and drink and drink. Our bodies are capable of digesting—not a problem in the world except when we get older. Lactose intolerance: It's a term that's come up only in the last couple of years. Until recently we never, ever heard about it.

As we get older we produce less and less lactase in our intestines, and slowly we lose the ability to digest milk. So by the time you're what, forty, fifty, you figure that you're having a little trouble with your tummy and can't digest the milk.

Nope. The problem doesn't start when you're fifty. Try four. That's right. By the time you are four you start to lose the ability to digest milk. In order to figure out what "lactose intolerance" means, we gotta know a little bit about what's involved in digesting lactose.

> "Lactose intolerance is a normal physical reaction because humans stop producing the lactase enzyme once they are weaned from their mother's milk or formula."

Normal physical reaction, this intolerance for lactose? What are you talking about?

Yep, the inability to digest milk begins with the enzyme lactase, which breaks down the milk's lactose in your intestines. This stuff is produced in smaller and smaller quantities in all of us after infancy, and the difficulty or inability to digest milk occurs because it isn't there. The stuff's just not there to help you digest milk—unless, of course, you're an infant, which is when you're supposed to be drinking the milk.

Makes a lot of sense if you are following nature's plan. After infancy you stop drinking milk, just when your body can no longer digest it. Our bodies have been designed that way, and it sounds good to me.

But that's not what happens. We follow the American Dairy Association's plan instead. It's almost illegal to suggest that a child stop drinking milk. Pregnant women not drinking milk? AGGGHHHHH!!

What are you, nuts?

Screw nature, we know that you can't stop drinking milk because if you do, you'll die, or at the very least live an extremely unhealthy life. You and I both know that we have to have milk. I mean, if we didn't, we'd have all kinds of health problems:

Rickets—whatever the hell that is.

Osteoporosis left, right, and center.

Skin, hair, bones, teeth, and eyes—without milk, useless for the rest of your life.

Children can't live without it, adults require it as a supplement to good health, and all in all this is nature's wonder food. This lactose thing, who ever heard of it anyway? And if it's true, why doesn't everyone stop drinking milk? It's crazy to even suggest such a thing.

> I'm discovering the wonderful way grains can be fixed and am enjoying them much more than the cheeseburgers I used to stuff down my throat.
> —*Kathy, Salt Lake City, Utah*

Well, should you or shouldn't you drink milk? What's the real deal behind this perfect white drink? What's the problem? Why can't we get the info that we need to truly make an educated decision about what we are drinking and eating?

Here's the problem: It's the right-to-choose thing again. Drink milk or not drink milk—whatever you choose is your deal, but in order to make the right choice for you and your family, you have to have the facts, and we don't. A lot of people have been suffering for years and years as a result of lactose intolerance, but there is very, very little attention, focus, or information about it. Why?

Well, the dairy boys don't want us to talk about it. How they keep this under the covers is something that should be studied in every college in the country. The dairy industry has its hands right up the cow's udder—my dairy equivalent to the old "hand in the cookie jar" saying (doesn't quite translate that well, does it?).

It took years and years for it to be socially acceptable to say you were cutting back on red meat without people staring at you in disbelief. "You don't eat meat?" The sickest-looking-family-on-the-block prize was sure to be awarded to you and yours within weeks of cutting back on—or, God forbid, eliminating—red meat, knowing full well that your family wasn't getting the protein it needed to live.

Well, you've probably done it. Everyone in the country has done it, because the facts speak for themselves. There is no such thing as lean red meat—contradiction in terms. Beef is high in fat, saturated fat. Cholesterol comes from animal products, beef is an animal product, and there's nothing difficult or depriving about using other foods for your entree. It's easy, cheaper, and better for your health. So simple: Cut back or cut out, it's your decision.

The same goes for dairy. It's just a lot harder to get the facts, because these boys are slick. You wouldn't believe how powerful the dairy lobby in our country is and how many udders these guys have their hands on.

And they start the brainwashing when we are very young.

In the classroom.

In the cafeteria.

School lunches: the federal government controls the dairy menu for school lunches.

The United Dairy Industry Association doubled its advertising budget in the United States from 1990 to 1991. They were spending $44 million a year on getting that fresh-faced message out to us all; now they expect to spend $110 million per year.

Let's say that you and I decided to spend $110 million a year to convince people that slugs are an important part of our daily nutrition. For a moment let's pretend that slugs are a good source of one or two things. What do you think? Calcium? Throw it in out of nowhere: Slugs are high in calcium, and we are going to spend $110 million, get the best production, the best media time, the most powerful advertising to convince everyone that they are something we can't live without. Do you think we could do it?

If it was packaged right.

Presented properly.

Sold to the children and the moms.

Our campaign could involve:

Distributing free recipes on how to prepare slugs.

Sponsoring food fairs all over the country that have the biggest and brightest slug presentation.

Having doctors, nutritionists, counselors, and teachers all spouting just what they've been told in the brochures, medical studies, and pamphlets about slugs that we—the slug organization—handed out.

SLUGS—THE BEST SOURCE OF CALCIUM AROUND.

SLUGS DO A BODY RIGHT.

I'M FROM THE SLUG GENERATION, THAT'S WHY I'M SO PERFECT.

SLUGS—FOR THOSE SPECIAL TIMES BETWEEN YOU AND YOUR BABY.

SO YOU CAN KNOW ALL'S WELL . . . IT'S SLUGS AND YOUR BABY.

Before long we'd have half the country believing that slugs are something none of us can live without, and after a while the other half would join in because they would be so afraid that they were missing something and that something could hurt the health of the people they love the most—their family—if they didn't eat slugs.

We could do the same thing with doody if we spent that much money, time, and advertising on it.

Meanwhile, the milk campaign marches on, and it's very well planned, designed, and targeted. And who are the suckers that they target directly because they can tie right into their emotional bond with family, health, and the well-being of their children? The women. New moms and babies. All you gotta do is have a look at the new target of the calcium issue. They're targeting the women. They're targeting us.

Ladies, we are being hit hard with a message that causes great confusion, guilt, and fear. Without milk you can't survive, and you increase your and your family's chances of being so nutritionally deficient that you'll be lucky to be alive if you even think about giving up milk.

I felt a little stupid when I first found out that that isn't the truth at all and that there is so much more to the story of milk in our lives. I kinda felt like a sheep being led. Without question I did what I was told and drank milk. Fed it to my children until it almost killed them (lactose intolerance being a big issue in my home) and really believed it was a very important part of our daily nutrition.

But after doing research to find the answer for my kids and then for this book, and speaking to all the experts I've had the privilege to speak with, I realized that there's nothing to be embarrassed about, because even the U.S. Department of Agriculture is not immune to the power of the dairy boys.

When the Department of Agriculture unveiled its "Eating Right Pyramid," it called for people to eat less dairy because they are high in saturated fat and cholesterol. Well, the chart was quickly kept from national distribution after an "outcry" from the dairy industry. So it's not an easy thing to get to the bottom of—even the Department of Agriculture, big weenies that they are, back down when the dairy industry has an "outcry."

Throw out the guilt, tie up the shame, forget the fear of falling to pieces without your glass of milk for a moment, and let's find out about these guys who are crying out loud, holding back charts, and painting these pretty pictures for us at a cost of $110 million a year. Let's get to know them a bit better if we are going to talk about 'em.

THE DAIRY INDUSTRY

The National Dairy Council, founded in 1915, is the largest and most important provider of nutritional education in the country. Tooting their own horn. Hand in the biggest cookie jar around.

We already know they spend millions a year to promote dairy consumption. Like all big organizations, the National Dairy Council has a board of directors, and it is made up of milk producers, milk processors, manufacturers, jobbers, and equipment distributors in the dairy industry. Objective? What do you think? How often do you think they would vote for, implement, or suggest anything that would tarnish the industry that they are processing, manufacturing equipment, or jobbing for? (What in hell is a jobber in the dairy industry?) How do you think they are going to vote? For or against the increase of dairy products? No matter what the health risks?

Big profit involved here, remember. You can pretty much bet that their profits are the deciding factor and that this is not the most fair or best representation of the American family and their health that you've ever seen. I mean, if it's objective and fair you want, let's get a bunch of truckers, accountants, bank tellers, housewives, and moms on the board of the National Dairy Council. Don't you think we'd have a better chance for objectivity, the truth, the facts?

So, guys, my friends at the National Dairy Council, let's do it. I'd be glad to volunteer. We'll get some nutrition experts on the panel—this is going to be big fun—and get down to the nitty-gritty about this milk-drinking thing once and for all. Why not? Sounds perfectly rational to me, fair, and pretty much the solution to this one-sided panel.

But they don't have to let us on the board, because this thing is big and powerful. Yeah, they've got something on us, all right, but we've got something much more powerful on them: The women of America are smart as hell. We pay for the groceries, and what do they think their product is? Nothing more than one of the many groceries we buy every week for our families. We want what's best for our families, and we are not afraid of you or your slickness, dairy boys. We need to get the facts and make our own decisions.

The women and the dairy issue is not at all the dairy guys have on their minds. In 1993, the California Dairy Industry was looking to invest $23 million in partnerships with cookie and cereal manufacturers to target the sales of chocolate milk, cereals, brownies—you know, kids' foods—in its advertising promotion. Who's gonna say no to $23 million and riding the tail of the dairy industry's advertising campaigns? Nobody. Milk is being forced down our kids' throats by law because federal law requires that whole milk be served to kids through the National School Lunch programs. Schools can offer low-fat milk, but whole milk is required. Oh, and guess what? With this program, butter is given to the schools for free.

Free?

I was raised Catholic, so I truly understand calling something what it ain't more than most people. Annulment—meaning what? The marriage never existed? Confession—you mean all I gotta do is say fifty eight Hail Marys and it's wiped clean, like I never did it at all? Hitting me with a ruler isn't a beating? What would you call it?

But this petting your own horse is like nothing I've ever seen. Do you know how broke some of our schools are? Do you know what many of us would do for free butter, if you know what I mean? All we must do to get free butter, by law, is serve whole milk to our 11 million obese children. So what if it's saturated fat. So what if it's high in cholesterol. So what if heart disease starts at an early age. So what . . . We get free butter if we make sure their product is being served, and they are all doing it.

> **START HERE START NOW**
> *In a hurry? You can always prepare boxed stuffing and rice mixes with skim milk and leave out the butter. They still taste fabulous.*

Besides the saturated fat, the cholesterol, the dairy industry's control, and our lack of complete information about this food that we consume 280 million glasses of, there are other very important health considerations (forget about lactose intolerance) that should be discussed when you're talking milk.

ENRICHMENT

Adding vitamin D to our milk supply was intended to prevent rickets in children. Again I ask, what is rickets? Maybe I can ask that question and have no clue what it is thanks to the American Dairy Council and the addition of vitamin D in our milk. Who knows about the rickets problem?

Here's what we do know about vitamin D. Rickets may be gone, but calcium deposits are in. Adding vitamin D to our milk supply encourages calcium deposits because the regulations are not so good, and we are getting way, way too much vitamin D from our fortified milk.

A couple of years ago Boston University researchers found the amount of vitamin D in the milk and what was on the label were "nowhere" near the same. They told the dairy industry, and the "dairy industry promised to do better." But according to *Health Magazine:*

> "The problem seems only to have gotten worse. Recently the scientists took to the aisles again, evaluating seventy-nine milk samples from ten states. Eighty percent contained 20 percent more or less vitamin D than labels indicated."

How far off are they sometimes?

> "One jug of milk contained 914 percent more than it should have. That could be dangerous: Over the long haul too much vitamin D can cause problems like malfunctioning kidneys."

Surprise, surprise. What you are reading on your label and what's actually happening aren't the same thing? Hold on, boys. Even forgetting the saturated fat, cholesterol, and that little problem of lactose intolerance after infancy, you want us to accept the fact that you can basically do what you want adding vitamin D to our milk, and you, in turn, will "try and do better"?

No. That's not right. We need more facts—the truth about this creamy white stuff.

Study after study (of course none that we hear about), has shown that added vitamin D has been identified as a factor in:

> Injury of the cardiovascular system.
>
> Calcification of the kidneys.

The lack of control over the addition of vitamin D to our milk supply is only one of the connections between milk and disease. But if you think those dairy guys don't want you to know about the saturated fat and cholesterol associated with their product, can you imagine how crazy they get and how far they'll go to make sure we don't get the info on the "haphazardly fortified" vitamin D in our milk supply?

Milk as a food has been connected with many diseases—such as some forms of cancer. You guys know about the connection between a diet high in saturated fat and cholesterol and cancer. Well, don't apply that info just to your beef; remember that cholesterol and saturated fat equal animal products, and milk is very much an animal product.

Study-a-plenty shows us what *The Lancet*, the British medical journal, so clearly says:

> "Women who regularly consume yogurt, cottage cheese, and other cultured dairy foods have an increased risk of developing ovarian cancer."

Dr. Daniel W. Cramer from Brigham and Women's Hospital in Boston found:

> "Women who ate dairy products are 70% more likely to develop ovarian cancer."

Milk was never very popular among the American Indians, who for centuries had no domesticated milk-bearing animals. When the Spaniards introduced milk to the New World in the fifteenth century, the Indians found the drink disgusting; they viewed it as an animal's excretory waste.

It doesn't end with too much vitamin D, kidney problems, or ovarian cancer. Our daily dairy intake has been linked to atherosclerosis, heart attacks, strokes, and osteoporosis.

There is a definite link between osteoporosis and milk—not in its prevention but in the cause of it. This one's going to blow your mind a bit, but hear out the facts, then decide. According to everything we've been told (check out who's doing the telling—it's those dairy boys again), milk is one of the surefire ways to avoid osteoporosis, that dreaded disease, that back breaker and killer of women.

A couple of issues here. We'll get to osteoporosis, but first let's talk about the theme we keep seeing when it comes to information that we stake our health on and who's feeding it (pardon that one) to us.

When the industry that profits from increasing our intake of their product is the one telling us that it's a lifesaving thing to do, they've got us right where they want us—afraid. You'll be doubled over with osteoporosis if you don't drink milk, because there is a problem with calcium deficiency, and milk has calcium in it. That's all we know, and we are doing what we are told based on that information and that information alone.

CALCIUM

Well, what about calcium? Is there no other place on earth to get it but milk? How much do we get? How much is enough? What are our choices? I mean, after all, if we are allergic to milk—as many of us apparently are—what do we do? Are we destined to be brittle-boned and die? What about the saturated fat and cholesterol? I know, it's a point I seem to be harping on. (Again, can you blame me? You know the old saying, fat makes you fat. It's my thing. I was 260 pounds, so I'm a little sensitive about the fat issue, pardon the hell out of me.) But if we do want to cut back on high-fat food so that we get leaner, feel better, and get healthier—which even the dairy boys and that $110 million advertising budget they have to work with can't dispute—and milk is one of the foods that we choose to cut back on or eliminate altogether, are we doomed?

Well, if it's calcium you're worried about, lets see if there's **any other source** besides milk.

• •

Calcium Sources

100 mg (3½-ounce) edible portions

Food	Calcium in Milligrams
Sardines	443
Almonds	233
Amaranth Grain	222
Hazelnuts	209
Parsley	203
Turnip Green	191
Brazil Nuts	186
Sunflower Seeds	174
Garbanzo Beans	150
Black Beans	135
Pistachios	135
Pinto Beans	135
Kale	134
Collard Greens	117
Sesame Seeds	110
Chinese Cabbage	106
Tofu	100
Walnuts	99
Okra	82
Brown Rice	33

From sardines to brown rice and all the other stuff in between—who would have ever thought there were so many other sources of calcium. Seems to me you can get calcium without the saturated fat and cholesterol.

• •

FOOD ALLERGIES

Food allergies affect millions and millions of people in our country. And guess what food leads the pack? Dairy. Dairy products are the leading cause of food allergies in this country. Dairy products contain more than twenty-five different proteins that may induce an allergic reaction, some of which are gastrointestinal, respiratory, and skin problems; behavioral problems; blood problems; colic in infants; runny noses and respiratory infections; ear, nose, and throat infections.

Here's where I have to tell what I've been promising for chapters—the saddest food story of my life. If it's food allergies we're talking about, then you have to hear what happened to my son.

Like his brother after him, my son was the cutest, most brilliant child in the land (of course I knew that when he was just hours old). Perfect in every way except that he started to die on me at around six or seven months old. I swear. I couldn't even talk about any of this until very recently because the thought of it made me cry.

When I tell you my son didn't sleep for more than a couple of hours in a row for the first couple of years of his life, I'm not kidding. He cried. You think colic is tough; this child was colicky beyond colicky. All he did was cry. Cried all day and cried all night. Cried loud, cried softly. Cried till he turned blue. Cried everywhere we went (obviously we didn't go many places with him). Cried, cried, cried, cried nonstop.

No doctor knew what to do with him. Every diagnosis under the sun was given.

> Failure to thrive
>
> Colic
>
> Spoiled child (what a load of crap that is)
>
> Intestinal problems

The diagnosing continued until he got sick enough to end up in the hospital. Months in the hospital, my marriage breaking up, pregnant with the second child—I don't think I need to explain what kind of pressure that was.

However many experts later, a diagnosis was made: My son had diabetes insipidus, a disease of the pituitary gland that has nothing to do with sugar diabetes and required medication for the rest of his life.

The agony of watching my son get sicker and sicker, his hair falling out, his beautiful complexion turning translucent. Getting thinner and thinner, no matter how much he ate. IV. Heart monitors. CAT scans. Medications left, right, and center. Seizures. Grand mal seizures. If you want to understand the true meaning of fear, all you have to experience (and I pray to God nobody reading this ever does) is a child not breathing, turning blue, dying right in front of your eyes. Your child. Nothing can compare. Nobody can explain the feeling except someone who's been there.

Seven physicians later, Nic, Grandma, Grandpa, uncles, aunts, brothers, and sisters, all very, very concerned about my son's health and convinced that medications and hospitals were the way to go. Everyone but me.

You see, the more I questioned the info I learned about diabetes insipidus, the more I became convinced that it wasn't what was wrong with my child. But even suggesting that or questioning any of the experts on the case got me strange looks, got me an appointment with the staff psychiatrist (not one I asked for—we're talking "assigned" here), got me labeled an interfering mother (what was I supposed to do? Sit back and not think when my son was wasting away in front of our eyes?) and told over and over again that I should leave this to the experts and just listen.

Well, I didn't. And I'm thrilled that I didn't, and so is everyone else in my family, Nic's family, and everybody connected to this horrible time in our family's life. It turned out my son didn't and never will have diabetes insipidus. He has severe food allergies. Dairy. Severely allergic to dairy. Chemicals, colorings, junk, poison—allergic, allergic, allergic as they come.

How do we know this? Because he was taken off all the foods he was allergic to, and he was fine. (By the way, just in case anyone is interested in the genetic connection, Nic's family has more allergies and allergic reactions than I've ever seen. Tomatoes—everyone's lips swell, itch, get redder than the tomato they ate. Stomach cramps every time they eat dairy. Sneeze, sneeze, sneeze at everything they look at. In my life I've never seen so many reactions to so many foods, which was one of the things that got me thinking about whether his son might have the same problem.)

This child went from not being able to sit still and crying all the time to playing for hours with his little toys on his little blankie. (I found out that was normal, but it wasn't something we were familiar with.) He was calm, his hair grew back, and there have been no more seizures, eleven years later. The greatest, calmest, most wonderful child you've ever met is my son.

Now. What did we do? Some magic formula? Something from an ancient culture? Witch doctor? Nope. Just took him off all the foods that he was, is, and always will be allergic to. Foods don't affect the way we feel? I don't think so anymore, do you?

The reason this story is in the middle of the milk chapter is that milk was the biggie when my son was so sick, in such pain, and going through so much. To this day when he has anything with milk in it, the stomach cramps, the bowel contractions, the pain he is in is beyond anything you can imagine.

Between the list of allergic reactions possible with milk and my son's story, it's safe to say that this perfect food ain't so perfect. There are a lot of things in this world that aren't perfect which we all still choose to do, and downing gallons of milk may be one of them. Bravo! Do what you want, but don't down it under the false impression that you are gulping down the all-American dream, the untarnished, completely-good-for-you food, because you aren't. And the most important factor here is being able to make your own decision without feeling that you're sending your family to the ashes-for-bones institution for all those poor souls who don't drink milk.

START HERE START NOW

Wanna save yourself about 24 grams of fat while eating dessert?
Substitute a cup of sorbet for that cup of premium ice cream you're
used to eating.

Let's continue in our milk discussion by jumping right into:

BOVINE GROWTH HORMONE

Ever heard of it? Do you have a clue what I'm talking about? Did you know that people all over this country are dumping milk into the street in protest? Bovine Growth Hormone, BGH, added to our milk supply, helping make a not-so-perfect food less perfect, and increasing our milk production.

Do we need increased milk production? Are the children not getting enough? Is there a shortage of milk in this country of ours? If so, then bring on anything that's going to help us solve the problem. The babies need milk, don't they? So maybe these companies are just trying to solve a problem by adding BGH to their bottles. Is that the case? We need to find out what's going on here.

Do the babies need more milk? No. Not at all. More milk is produced in the United States than is consumed. We produce 146 million gallons of milk a year.

What is Bovine Growth Hormone? BGH is a genetically engineered hormone that when given to cows increases milk production by 15 percent. Wonderful for the sake of increased milk production, but what does it mean for you and me?

BGH was a natural protein found in cows until we figured out how to synthetically manufacture it. Not so bad, and it surely has a place. Like anything new, there's bound to be controversy, some group screaming and yelling about the problems with this particular new addition to our food chain. True, true. BGH certainly has its share of controversy, and you don't have to look too far to find the questions or the answers.

Here's the Food P.I. fact sheet on BGH, the bottom line on BGH, the skinny on the hormone:

Name: Bovine Somatotropin, otherwise known as BST
Aliases: Bovine Growth Hormone, otherwise known as BGH
Trade name: Posilac
Manufactured by: Monsanto
Current sales: Brisk sales with new product
Estimated worldwide market: $1 billion a year

One billion a year—that's a lot of hormone, boys. Big profit expected, and all for the good of the people, because according to the folks that manufacture this synthetic hormone, "milk from BGH-treated cows is indistinguishable from ordinary milk."

And then there's David Kessler, the commissioner of the FDA. You remember Dave. When interviewed about the new label laws last year, Davey boy said they were "one of the most important public health landmarks" that his agency has ever engaged in, because Dave himself had "no idea whether 6 grams of fat was high, low, or medium." The man who heads the agency that is supposed to protect us did not have much of an idea about fat until very recently. If he thinks figuring out fat percentages is a thrill, can you imagine how much fun doing something about the chemicals, toxins, deadly poisons, and synthetic hormones in our food is going to be? Dave, we've got something very exciting for you. I'm a little concerned about what old Dave knows about BGH. I wrote him about the label laws and his updated knowledge about fat, but he never got back to me. Rude, don't you think? Oh, well, maybe he'll write after this book's published, because he's all over this food issue.

Dave has been asked about BGH—not that night in my hotel suite (sounds like we're lovers, doesn't it?) but in almost every article I've read about this stuff. Here's big Dave's answer:

"There's virtually no difference between treated and untreated cows."

"Virtually"? What, Dave, what does that mean? Kinda no difference? Almost no difference?

Dave, what do you mean by "virtually"? This BGH stuff, Dave, what's the deal?

Well, up until biotech figured out how to produce this stuff, the only source of BGH was from the pituitary glands of butchered cows, but now we don't even need those butchered cows, we can produce it by gene splicing. AGGGHHHHHIIIIIIIHH!!!!! So they have added BGH to our milk supply because Dave said that it was O.K. Did we even know it was happening? Well, it's done.

This is America, and technology is good. It's brought us far, so a little BGH to increase the milk production—what's the problem? Let's do it, see if it works, and let the consumer decide. You can buy your basic BGH-injected milk and see if there are any side effects, distinguishable differences, or "virtually" anything wrong, or you can get milk without BGH—right?

WRONG. Very, very wrong, because they—Dave's boys—are not labeling the BGH-injected milk.

Why not? What's the point of that?

Why would anyone take away our choice to decide whether or not our children are getting BGH-injected milk? Isn't that against the Constitution? As un-American as it comes??!!

Who's decided not to label? What could the motive possibly be to do something so absolutely un-American? Ask and you shall receive—one of those solid biblical principles again. It's the biotech industry, the guys who produce BGH, who have fought very, very hard not to have labels on milk products that contain BGH. They are afraid that you will get scared off and not buy their products. That's why they haven't labeled it. Better you don't know.

Well, I'm afraid, too, guys. Afraid of the possible consequences of drinking a synthetic chemical, afraid of not having a choice in the matter, and really, really afraid of your power to do that to us.

I asked a couple of questions and got a couple of answers that certainly confirm the need to be afraid, cautious, worried, concerned, whatever you want to call it. Check this out:

There are some problems with BGH milk other than the fact that we've lost our right to know if it's in our food supply. One of the big problems is infection. Udder infections increase in the cows treated with BGH. Besides the fact that this is painful for the cow (again, animal rights will have to wait on this one, though between the chickens and the cows, I'm starting to get a little animal rightsy here), these infected udders affect us directly, because in order to treat the infection, large amounts of powerful antibiotics have to be used. And where do you think the antibiotics go? From the milk supply right into our bodies.

We've already got the antibiotics coming in from the chickies. Now let's pour some more into our bodies, because the FDA decided to add BGH to cows' milk to increase milk supply (profit raising its ugly but very familiar head at this point in our food awareness investigation), and we're getting extra antibiotics because of the extra infections due to BGH.

O.K., I'm getting a little confused here. Aren't we adding to an already existing problem and causing more problems in the name of profit and production again and again and again? When do we stop and look at all the symptoms we are creating? Dave, this does affect us.

First, I gotta say, Davey boy, we do deserve the right to choose, to make the choice that's best for our families. As many shows as you've been on lately, and as big as your title is, Dave, you can't argue with that—it's been fairly well established in something called the Constitution of the United States of America. So why don't you just label the stuff and give us back our right to choose? What's the deal?

Wow. It's a wonder you and I get any information at all with all the deciding being done for us by the guys who are supposed to protect us. There are so many organizations fighting like hell to get the truth out to you and me about what's been added to our food, and one of them, Jeremy Rifkin, of the Washington-based Foundation on Economic Trends was important enough to be mentioned in a small blurb in *Time* magazine:

"Brave New World of Milk," *Time* magazine, February 14, 1994:

". . . cows treated with BGH are more susceptible to udder infections and they [Rifkin's Foundation on Economic Trends] are worried that unless milk is rigorously inspected, antibiotics used to treat the cows for these infections could find their way into the milk supply. While there is a germ of truth to their [the Foundation's] argument, their tactics—and their rhetoric—go overboard."

Well, well, well, Jeremy. Overreacting, they say. Hey, Jeremy, are you? Let's get the facts straight from your Foundation.
Just a few health facts from a Consumer Warning flyer from Rifkin's Foundation on Economic Trends:

Let's get the facts straight.

"Genetically engineered hormones could be in your milk and dairy products."

"rBGH is like 'crack' for cows. It 'revs' their systems and forces them to produce a lot more milk—but it also makes them sick."

"Even the FDA admits that cows injected with rBGH could suffer from increased udder infections (mastitis), severe reproductive problems, digestive disorder, foot and leg ailments, and persistent sores and lacerations."

"The powerful antibiotics and other drugs used to fight increased disease in rBGH-injected cows may lead to greater antibiotic and chemical contamination of milk and dangerous resistance to antibiotics."

"The FDA has released studies that milk from rBGH-treated cows could have more saturated fat and less protein than regular milk."

"Both the U.S. General Accounting Office (GAO) and the Consumer's Union, publisher of *Consumer Reports* magazine, have warned of the

potential hazards to human health caused by consuming products derived from rBGH-treated cows."

"The FDA has also refused to require labeling of milk and other dairy
products derived from use of the genetically engineered hormone, even
though more than 90 percent of consumers favor labeling of rBGH products so they can avoid buying them."

"The Food and Drug Administration (FDA) admits that the use of rBGH
in cows may lead to increased amounts of pus and bacteria in milk."

WAIT A MINUTE, BOYS. PUS, DID YOU SAY PUS? Dave, you admit that
pus is in my milk, but you won't give me the right to know which milk has
the "potential" pus in it? Is this part of your "virtually no difference" thing,
David? (That's what I call him when I'm upset with him.)

The FDA has released studies showing that milk from BGH-treated cows
could have more saturated fat and less protein. (Just what the average American needs—and the children, yeah, let's give them more saturated fat in their
milk. Maybe we could win the world record for heart disease! Jump right
ahead of the Finns.)

If you think for a minute that this pus with extra antibiotics comes cheap,
think again. It's costing us lots of cash, our no-right-to-know Bovine Growth
Hormone.

"According to the federal Office of Management and Budget, BGH use
will cost the taxpayer between $300 million and $500 million over the
next five years in increased price supports for milk."

Now David, I've just about had it with you and your boys. I gotta pay more
and still not have the right to know if this infection-causing pusy stuff is in
my milk? No, Dave, that ain't right. Even Lenny in *Of Mice and Men* could figure that one out; surely the commissioner of the FDA can understand it.

And what about Bessie? I know I promised we'd leave the animal cruelty
thing out of the whole food picture, but I got to tell you that when old Bessie
gets BGH, it's like crack to her system. It "revs" her up, forcing her to produce more milk, and makes her sick.

Who cares about the animals and all? But there's a point to all of this. All
these facts, and it's not just Jeremy and his group talking. If you want to know
who's talking about BGH in your milk supply, then all you've got to do is
read.

U.S.A. Today—you know, one of the biggest newspapers in the country—February 14, 1994. Big heading:

> This Stuff is Dangerous.
> Consumers need to be alerted.
> Genetically engineered hormone is a serious potential health threat.

Richard Kressler, executive director of the New York State Consumer Protection Board, wrote the FDA demanding that the agency "immediately suspend approval" of the hormone because of "significant health and safety concerns":

> "It is more likely that milk from treated cows will be of lower quality, containing more pus and bacteria."

YUUUCCKKKKK, there's that pus stuff again.
Then there's The New York Times, *no small newspaper:*

> The FDA's chief spokesman said the agency was considering the requests, but he declined to discuss what the FDA was considering or when any guidance documents would be issued.

The National Institute of Health and the American Medical Association have said the genetically engineered hormone is safe. The Food and Drug Administration has said that milk produced with the genetically engineered hormone is indistinguishable from milk that is not.
New York Newsday:

> Last year, Food and Drug Administration Commissioner David Kessler [there he is again with the photo; as I said, not the most attractive but definitely the boy next door] approved rBST [BGH], the synthetic version of a cow's naturally produced growth hormone. . . . Short-term studies show no direct danger from the hormone. But long-term research is still needed on rBST's indirect effects (infection and antibiotic residues in milk).

In an experiment, one thousand cows were treated with BGH. The FDA allowed researchers to sell the treated milk without labels on the market, yet no follow-up tests were done to track those who drank the treated milk. Why not? By now such tests might have shown more conclusive evidence. God help the people who drank the milk without even knowing if we do find any evidence of danger associated with drinking BGH-injected milk.

At this point, especially after this chapter, you guys can't say that you haven't been warned—about the ice cream and infant formula from treated cows that are "laced with genetically altered, artificial hormones" and "large amounts of pus."

All right. Now I'm tired—something I don't say often, believe me, but this has made me tired. The issue, the controversy, the confusion about this milk thing is tiring. I've been involved in this for a long time because my children are both lactose intolerant (along with most other kids past four years old, according to old mother nature, but what does she know?).

There are advantages to writing a food book—being able to talk to the experts and sorting out all this junk. That is more than most of you guys reading this have had, but I'm telling you that even with all these advantages, it's tiring as hell.

Making changes is tough. Learning that what we thought was true and the best thing for our families isn't is scary, but the wonderful thing about networking, supporting one another in our life-style changes, and living in the U.S. of A. is that we can, if we look hard enough, get the answers and then make our own decisions.

If after having a look at all the information in this chapter, hearing the pros and cons, and learning more about that glass of milk than you probably ever wanted to know, you decide it's best for you and your family to cut way, way back on or eliminate milk altogether, then you can—without fear, without guilt, and knowing full well that you are not harming yourself or the people you love. Then my job is done, and the chapter on milk is finished.

This is a personal decision. What isn't, when you think about it? How far you want to go with this is your decision, and if you want more information on this subject or anything else in this book, I'd be glad to give you the references, organizations, information that I read, asked about, and investigated so you can do your own investigation. After all, you, like me, are fast becoming Food P.I.'s.

If you are interested in cutting back on your milk intake, then, you've got to do what you did to cut back on fat and cholesterol: you've got to read labels.

Look for milk.
Look for milk solids.

Check for cheese.

Read, read, read.

Learn, learn, learn.

I've spent the last eleven years learning about milk substitutes—both boys allergic to dairy will do it every time. Here's what I've found:

Three most popular nondairy substitutes

Soy milk: Made from soybeans and water. You can dilute soy milk with water.

Rice milk: Made from cooked fresh fermented brown rice. Rice milk is lower in fat than soy milk and has a lighter, sweeter taste.

Almond milk: Made from brown rice syrup, almonds, salt, water, and flavorings.

Remember always to read the nutritional labels, do the fat formula, and make the best choice.

You can get calcium from other sources. You get more from your calcium intake. You can live with less of it or none at all and be healthy, have strong bones, and cut back on your total fat intake.

Hey, Jeremy, where can we reach your organization for more info?— 800/253-0681.

CHAPTER 12
BEAR WITH ME

I've felt this stuff. Known it, lived it, but never put it together the way John Robbins did so beautifully on the phone with me this morning. And guys, this is a biggie. This will help you with your transition. A totally different life from anything you ever could have imagined. Do you think I'm nuts?

Have I flown off the deep end right in front of your eyes? Well, I haven't. That's why I'm going to parallel what happened to me, what happened to John, and what's gonna happen to you. Watch, read, you'll see.

As far as I'm concerned it's another day, another perk. You know how I felt about having the pleasure of interviewing Dr. John McDougall. Well you can't imagine what was going on inside my head when I knew I was going to interview John Robbins, author of *May All Be Fed* and *Diet for a New America,* only one of my favorite authorities on food and wellness ever!! Only the man who has so many wonderful things to say that everyone who reads his stuff walks away with loads and loads of information, insight, and truth. Just got off the phone with him, and I can't wait to share what we talked about with you. But just before we chat, I gotta ask you: When I say John Robbins, do you know who this man is? Robbins. Name sound familiar?

> We're talking Robbins.
> As in Baskin and.
> The 31 Flavors!!!

Baskin-Robbins Ice Cream. As all-American as you get. The biggest ice-cream parlor in the land. Mr. Ice Cream. What you and I grew up with. Before John's

Dad, Mr. Robbins, and his uncle, Uncle Baskin (can you imagine having an uncle with the name Baskin, half of the ice-cream fortune; that's like having an uncle named Ford—big stuff!) gave us flavors with names such as Rocky Road, Cookies and Cream, Daiquiri Ice, Pralines and Cream, and the famous flavor-of-the-month category, ice cream was just ice cream. Uncle Baskin and John's Dad, Mr. Robbins, revolutionized ice cream and changed forever our expectations of one of America's favorite pastimes—licking an ice-cream cone on a lazy Sunday afternoon.

Like father, like son. Revolutionizing. Making enormous changes in society. Increasing awareness. Giving us more options and increasing our expectations. You'd expect it to run in the family. So what do you think John's been working on for the last couple of years?

A thirty-second flavor around the bend?

Bigger, better ice-cream stores?

Beyond the cone?

What? What? What is the son of Mr. Robbins up to? Where has he been all these years, and why has he allowed Baskin-Robbins Ice Cream stores to slip into second, third, or fourth place, letting the yogurt boys take over? Not believing it's yogurt is a national pastime now. They've grown like weeds around what was the king. Hundreds of stores, and yogurt flavors of the month clamoring to dethrone the king. Ice cream.

The competition is fierce, and the heir to the fortune—and folks, it is a fortune that was made from those 31 flavors—has been very, very busy. John's been traveling all over the world, speaking, writing, documenting, fighting. Protecting, caring for, and standing up for ice cream?

He's traveling the world all right, increasing awareness, giving options, but not for the flavor of the month—for the animals, the human beings, every living thing. You see, the heir to the family isn't the heir. He gave it up. All of it. Mr. Robbins's son turned away from the family fortune and headed in a very different direction.

Do you understand how much cash this man walked away from? We are talking millions and millions of dollars. When I found out that he left the family business far, far behind and went to find his own way, I thought to myself:

Animals are important, absolutely.

Cruelty is wrong, no doubt about it.

But this is millions and millions of dollars we're talking about. Couldn't we (notice how easily I stepped into heirdom) take the millions and then work on saving the animals?

Here's a thought: How about using all that cash to hire somebody to save the animals and the humans for you? Build a big forest and give the native cultures a place to live? When you're talking that kind of cash, you can probably teach them to protest, raise cash, lobby the government, and let them stand up for themselves. That's what I would have been thinking about if I were Uncle Baskin's nephew. I mean, before you made the big decision to give up the loot, wouldn't you?

You and I maybe, but not John Robbins. Straight from the horse's mouth, here's what he was thinking.

"There is a sweeter and deeper American dream than the one I turned down. It is the dream of a success in which all beings share because it is founded on a reverence for life. A dream of a society at peace with its conscience because it respects and lives in harmony with all life forms. A dream of a people living in accord with the laws of creation, cherishing and caring for the natural environment, observing nature instead of destroying it. A dream of a society that is truly healthy, practicing a wise and compassionate stewardship of a balanced ecosystem."

John, you turned down millions to balance the ecosystem? So now we have a million (pardon the cash pun) questions about the dream, the calling, the ecosystem, all the stuff you're talking about.

Is the dream really sweeter than the cash? How close are we to balancing things? What's the deal with all living things living in stewardship? And John, what the hell are you talking about? These are all questions on my mind when I had the privilege of interviewing Mr. John Robbins, author and human being extraordinaire, about change, transition, moving forward in our life-style changes.

> It was the easiest thing in the world for me to get into this new life-style. . . . Now I don't have to deprive myself any longer, and it feels wonderful.
> —*Laura, Troutdale, Oregon*

"Once a human being makes a decision to make any change, no matter how small, that decision sets in motion the movement toward the change."

All right, John, there are millions of Americans who want to make a change in their life-styles; they don't really want to go the noncruelty, save-the-penguins route but do very much want to look and feel better. What do we do, John?

Step one on the John Robbins plan.

"Start with cutting back on the highest fat meats. Pork, for instance—you can live without bacon, nothing difficult about it and it's a great step in the right direction."

No saving the whales? What about the ecosystem? Do I have to jump right into or off that as I'm changing my diet? Nope, not according to someone who's made the change in a big way. From ice-cream heir, growing up on the all-American diet, to a six-foot-one, 150-pound, lean-as-they-come forty-six-year-old marathon runner, a triathlete, having nothing to do with the ice-cream business in any way, shape, or form, married for twenty years, and with a fabulous son. (When I asked John about his wife, he said, "I honor her every day of my life." Now, ladies, are you dying over that one? Honor her! I went right to my husband, who was outside doing some work, and repeated Mr. John Robbins's words verbatim. You guys know how much good that does, repeating the words of an evolved man to your husband because that's the sort of thing you want him to say to you! Real effective, isn't it?)

And how do I know John's son is wonderful? Because I asked him. You figure that when you've got a father who's walked away from the family fortune, you end up with a kid who's a money-hungry, commercially success-ful entrepreneur who hates animals?

SON OF WHALE SAVER GOES ON A BANK ROBBING SPREE . . .

SON OF NON-MEAT-EATER EATS RAW FLESH . . .

Yeah, the *Enquirer* would love it. But that's not how it is. The son of the ex-ice-cream heir is a wonderful human being who started, funds, and works in his own environmental organization—Youth for Environmental Safety. The *Enquirer* may not find that newsworthy, but any parent would!

Back to the question I asked about the changes we need to make.

"There is enough support in our culture to get the beef out of your diet, so it's an easier change to make. Dairy is still considered sacred in this country, but cutting back on beef is socially acceptable these days. So you see, one of the reasons it's more difficult to get rid of the dairy in your diet is the social pressure."

This you and I understand. Call someone you love and who loves you. During the course of the conversation mention that you've decided to change your eating habits. Tell him or her that you want a healthier, more vital, higher-energy life and that you are going to start by getting rid of red meat.

Your someone who loves you will probably respond by saying, "That's wonderful. You know too much red meat is bad for you. Great, cutting back on saturated fat and cholesterol. Good move, you know that red meat is high in fat . . . " (Have you noticed all these responses sound as if Mr. Milquetoast, Ken—you know, Barbie's boyfriend—is your best friend? Sorry about the all-American-upper-middle-class-Milquetoasty answer, but I'm trying to prove a point, and what better way than with Babs's boyfriend?)

Now, do the same thing with a different someone who loves you. Tell him or her that you are making a life-style change so that you can have a healthier blah, blah, blah life—and say that you and the family are giving up dairy. Check out the response you'll get on this one:

> Give up dairy!!! As in no more milk?
>
> And cheese, what about cheese? How do you live without cheese? What do you eat?
>
> Don't be silly. People can't live without dairy.

If you stick to your guns, insisting on your life-style change of no dairy, within minutes the threats will start:

> Where are you going to get your calcium from?
>
> The children will have no chance for a healthy future!
>
> Ever heard of brittle bones, Miss Nutritional Expert?
>
> Have you lost your mind? The human body must have dairy to survive!

And it continues until you start questioning your own sanity, no matter how much you know, no matter how many facts you have that prove the people who love you are wrong. It is tough, just like John Robbins says: Transition does have something to do with social acceptability. Dr. Micozzi made that clear. You know that from back in stage one. If you didn't know it before, you'll know it after this.

I love the new, energetic, and ambitious person that I'm becoming. Not only have I changed eating habits (and many other things), our life-style has transformed into a healthy one.

—*Brenda, Burlington, Ontario, Canada*

We need to spend a little more time on this concept of social pressure being a part of your life-style transition and change. Right along with portion control, assessment, respect for you and your family's tastes and needs should be the discussion of social pressure. I wish someone had been talking about it when I was trying to explain to everyone that dairy was hurting my kids, and they were getting all the calcium they needed to grow from other sources!!!

John understands because he went through one hell of a transition. So the most logical question to ask would be: What's his transition been like? (Notice that I get a little info in about food and transition, the subject at hand, and keep going right back to the personal stuff? Aren't you dying to know more about how you go from riches to rags and it all turns out O.K.? Thought you would be!)

> "My family didn't understand or agree with my decision to turn down the family fortune and not follow in the family business, but in order to become the person I needed to be, I had to unearth and expose all the beliefs that didn't serve me."

Unearth, expose all the beliefs that don't serve us? WOW, this one's good.

We could use this to help us make our changes. All you have to do is stop for a second and think about what "serves you" and what doesn't "serve you."

Lack of exercise. Does it serve or not serve?

When you finish a huge greasy meal? Serve? Not serve?

How about the second night in a row of lying in bed, watching TV, and eating, eating, eating every sweet thing in the house? Serve you?

Boy, did I live in the not-serving-myself state, and did I suffer the consequences. Eating too much high-fat food, isolating, not moving, dieting, bingeing, dieting again didn't serve me, and it's not serving you.

As John was talking, I was thinking (you expected that, didn't you?) about the changes I made a long time ago, the changes that started to serve me and my life.

Exercise served me.

Eating—talk about serving your body.

These are the simple things that did serve me and did start the movement forward. Those few tiny steps have lead to things beyond my wildest dreams. Check it out, guys: I'm writing a book on food and interviewing people like John Robbins. Who would have guessed?

What isn't serving you in your life-style right now? What isn't serving you is your food choices? Take a minute and think about it. No guilt. No shame. No anger. Just a conscious inventory of the serving things and the not-so-serving things in your life.

One of the greatest parts of deciding what serves you is setting it in motion, and as you change, what serves you changes, so you can keep setting different levels of change in motion until you are where you want to be—or hopefully you'll be lucky enough never to be where you want to be, because where you want to be keeps changing, and it's just the process of growth, evolvement, learning, living. That rambled a bit, but it makes sense, doesn't it? Here's why I say that and how it's connected to the food we are eating and your food transitions: What serves me now is very different from what was right for me at 260 pounds—on every level: emotionally, physically, spiritually. You start with just the low fat, then jump into the quality thing, throwing in something whole once in a while, and keep moving forward. Use everything you need from whatever stage you want.

> Step out of the denial closet whenever you want.
>
> Listen to the experts.
>
> Bear with me if you will . . . keep moving forward.

There are things I would eat three years ago that I don't want to eat anymore, but it's the changing, the process, that is hard to define and hard to grasp when you want desperately to change your life.

It's been tough talking about food and weight loss without giving out menus. Do you know how hard I fought against TV programs, audio product manufacturers, booklet and guide guys not to have a menu or daily eating plan in any of my products? You know why I didn't want to? Because it's the process of change that's the most important—not having someone tell you every minute of the day what to do.

> Eating healthier has become easier every week.
> —*Kelly, Kyle Ann, Rae, and Donna, Elgin, Illinois*

John says all you need to start is "an image of a better way." Don't start with the world; remember, you'll work your way to that. Just think YOU right now.

/₥ Do you want your health to be better? Then start creating an image of feeling better.

/₥ More energy? Do it—think about your life with more energy.

/w Lower fat? Here's an easy thought to set in motion: Just think lean. Start to think lean.

/w More joy? Then start doing things that bring you joy.

/w Excitement back in your life? What the hell, throw in a little excitement.

/w Recover from heart disease? Think unclogged. Eat unclogged.

/w Not so saturated? Forget cholesterol.

You guys can include more in your image because you have so much more information than I did.

John had an image, an image of a better way, and he started by trying to clear up what didn't feel right to him, what didn't serve him. The lifestyle his parents led wasn't right for him, and he wanted to figure out what was.

Totally different reasons, totally different images of a better way, and totally different outcomes, but results just the same: I got lean, strong, and healthy. John got more respect from the wellness community than he probably ever imagined possible. He wrote some great books that the world should read. Raised a great family and is happy with his life.

It's the imagining and taking small steps that start the process. Then once you "set the change in motion, any change," you're on your way.

Is it really so far-fetched for anyone to suggest "imagining it" first? How can you reach your goal if you don't even know what it is? Who said that? Whoever it was, just know that I've stolen it from you and am going to use it forever.

Years ago I saw a movie called *Brother Sun, Sister Moon,* a good movie; if you haven't seen it, do—rent it and enjoy. It's the story of Saint Francis of Assisi, one of the big guys in the Catholic Church. During the movie Saint Francis was trying to build a church and was running into all kinds of problems because he was a bit of a loon for his day: Ran the streets naked because the Church told him God would provide everything. Left his family fortune to go out on his own and let God provide all. AAAAAHHHHHHHHHHHH, John Robbins, isn't that what you did? Not run naked but give up the family fortune??

Are you Saint Francis reincarnated? If you are, I can't talk to you anymore, because I know the lightning bolts are gonna come down and strike me dead for even putting these things down on paper.

Bless me, Father, for I have sinned—I alluded to reincarnation and the Catholic Church in the same sentence . . . had a conversation with someone who could possibly be the modern-day Saint Francis.

> I still have a tub of margarine in my refrigerator since July. It is a symbol of what I have learned to do without while eating, eating, eating better foods.
>
> —*Gail, Stoughton, Massachusetts*

The reason for bringing up *Brother Sun, Sister Moon* at all is the one-stone-at-a-time principle that Saint Francis built his church on. Each stone with love, and one at a time.

Now you guys may be reading this and thinking: Where the hell has she been? Hasn't she ever gone to a twelve-step meeting for anything? Dependency? Enabling? Eating disorder? If she'd been living anywhere but under a rock for the last ten years, she'd have heard that one-step-at-a-time thing a million times.

I know—true, true—but two points need to be made here. Number one is that the twelve-steppers stole from Saint Francis. And number two is that if Saint Francis could build a church one stone at a time, then imagine what you can build one change at a time. Each small change sets into motion the movement forward.

Saint John Robbins said that, and he's right.

> You imagine the life you want.
>
> How you want to feel.
>
> What you want to look like.
>
> The energy level you want.
>
> Then you set one or two changes in motion.

Eliminate the saturated fat and cholesterol one change at a time; cut back on your total daily fat intake—one change at a time. Processed foods? A single stone here, too. And the next thing that happens is you "ignite the belief" in the possibility of change. John said that.

That's exactly what happened when I weighed 260 pounds and started walking and cutting back on the fat in the suburbs of Dallas, Texas.

> A belief did ignite.
>
> The belief that I could feel better.
>
> Hope.
>
> A ray of light.

There was an answer other than starvation, deprivation, and beating myself to death with the body-image sledgehammer. The belief did ignite that I could regain the control I thought was lost forever. (A couple of years into the yo-yo-dieting, losing-and-gaining-weight, hateful cycle will guarantee that you feel totally out of control and hopeless—you know what I'm talking about.)

Igniting the hope, the belief, and the understanding that the small changes make enormous differences—this is big, very, very big, and important. You see, everyone wants to know where and how they should begin. Everybody wants a menu.

The answer is in your getting the information you need. Understanding and adding to your change process things that you may never have thought about.

> Being open.
>
> Listening and applying.
>
> Failing and trying again.
>
> Getting results and taking it as far as you want it to go.

You've got some great food information. Eating—not a problem anymore. The charts and graphs are all there to back up the facts and to take to your doctor when he tells you you're out of your mind.

Stage two bonus: the emotional, spiritual (if you will), intangible concepts that have everything in the world to do with your making the changes that will dramatically affect your life—throw 'em in. What the heck—you're brilliant, capable, and open, right?

Of course the physical—which is what I've been focusing on for years because it's so easy to understand and start to make changes in: the low-fat food, the higher quality, the walking to burn off the fat that I'd stored all over my body—was a very important part of the process. But there was another source of power to change that isn't as tangible—the power I got from visualizing, seeing, igniting the changes in my life that I wanted to make. Dreaming or igniting the possibilities that I thought were long-lost—everything was beginning to be possible again.

John says:

> "Once the belief is ignited, a person shifts out of passive into active, and that is truly a beginning."

Do you see it? You make your own changes. I'm telling you: From here something happens, and you'll begin to want more.

> I hated our old kitchen. . . . About all it was good for was keeping pop in the fridge and reheating pizza in the microwave. Now I can't wait to get in there and cook food that I know will nourish me, give me energy, and help me get well.
>
> —*Kate, Pittsburg, Kansas*

How far did John go?

Was it worth it?

And the family? What happened to them?

Where are they now?

Don't you want to know?

Well, Uncle Baskin died of a heart attack. What a shame. Died from the life-style he lived? Lots of meat, lots of dairy. Typical American diet. Who's to know, but he's gone.

And Dad? Where's Dad?

"The family was very, very mad, confused, and frustrated with me when I made my decision to leave. For years we were estranged, but something very interesting has happened as a result of my decision years ago. Recently, Dad's health has degenerated."

With all due respect to John's dad, no wonder. According to all the medical reports, facts, and opinions during the last twenty years, he didn't have much of a chance eating what he'd been selling all those years. Chowing down on ice cream, meat, and the all-American life-style, his health was affected. It got to Uncle Baskin, and it got to him. Are any of us surprised by that anymore?

No, but here's what I was surprised by during my conversation with John. I was very surprised by the conclusion to John Robbins's "igniting":

"Dad was dealing with high blood pressure, obesity, and diabetes. His cholesterol was 300, he was taking twelve pills a day for high blood pressure, and he was sick, very, very sick. My father changed his life-style."

Based on your beliefs? The son passed right over that one and continued a story that touched me deeply:

"Dad is a businessman, so he respects and responds to financial success, which I've had. I refused his money when there was no reason to or understanding of why. He came to me when he was sick and incorporated my philosophy of living—changed his diet, started exercising, and the end result is his cholesterol went from 300 to 150. My father has gone from twelve pills a day to one every other day for his blood pressure, and his diabetes is under control without medication."

If you guys think I would stop here, you're nuts. I kept going. John, how does that make you feel?

"I didn't take his money when I could have without question. I would have been a rich person in things that didn't matter to me, and it would have been easy. Now I can look my dad in the face and ask him how he feels, knowing that he understands all I want to know is how he is truly feeling and what I can do to help him feel better. I am richer than I could have ever imagined."

I know this book is about food, and I know that I've strayed from the beaten path, bringing Saint Francis, igniting, ice-cream heirs into the whole thing, but let me tell you something: When this man made that statement, it set my mind a-thinking. Thinking about the end result for all the women I've seen make the smallest changes in their life-styles. Thinking about the thousands and thousands of letters I've read, the women I've met everywhere I go—their transitions and results.

> Change.
> Transition.
> Taking responsibility for our own lives.
> Moving toward health and wellness.
> Having the courage to define your own life.

That's what John did. That's what I did. That's what thousands and thousands of women can do. That's what you can do when you make your first small change toward a healthier, happier, more vital, higher-energy life by changing what you are putting in your mouth.

John Robbins is healthy. He is happy. He lives in healthy relationships. He has participated in the raising of a wonderful human being, his son, and it worked. The whole damn thing turned out O.K.

There is so much more to this whole issue than how much protein we need or what a complex carb is, and we are only in stage two. What magic awaits us in stage three? Who's to know? These are the intangible but very real discussions, considerations, things that you can apply to your process of change.

Imagine what you want.

Ignite the belief.

Make a change here and there.

And see what happens in your life.

If you are interested in reading more of what John has to say, try these:

Diet for a New America

May All Be Fed

If you would like to know more about Earth Save, John Robbins's organization, contact:

Earth Save

706 Frederick Street

Santa Cruz, CA 95062

(408) 423-4069

Earth Save educates and supports people in making healthier, earth-friendly food choices. The Healthy School Lunch Program offering low-fat, high-fiber, plant-based options in Santa Cruz public schools is now available to communities everywhere through the recently published Healthy School Lunch Program handbook.

The Earth Save order line for John's books and for the Healthy School Lunch Program handbook is (800) DNA-DOIT.

To find out more about Youth for Environmental Safety, contact

YES!

706 Frederick Street

Santa Cruz, CA 95062

(408) 425-6518

YES! is a powerful youth-run organization that inspires and empowers young people to take action for a healthier world. They tour the country speaking to high school assemblies and offering workshops, training, and summer camps.

Thank you, John.

STAGE 2 RECIPES

BREAKFAST

Apple Fritters   Great Morning Cereal

SOUPS

Zucchini and Spinach Soup   Broccoli Soup
Bean and Cabbage Stew

SNACKS

Granola   Oatmeal Fruit Cookies
Granola II

SALADS

Black Bean Salad   Complete Protein Tabouleh

SAUCES

Soy-Ginger Sauce   Broccoli Sauce

SIDE DISHES

Pasta and Beans

Sweet-and-Sour Lentil Casserole

Brown Rice Pilaf

Millet and Vegetable Casserole

Lentil and Bulgur Pilaf

Curried Vegetables

Spicy String Bean and Tomato Sauce

MAIN DISHES

Bean and Corn Burritos

Vegetable Lo Mein

Chinese Stir-fry Vegetables

Lemon Chicken and Bulgur

Spaghetti and Eggplant Sauce

Soba Noodles with Snow Peas

Chick-pea Sauce and Rigatoni

White Beans and Fusilli

Lentil Sauce, Vegetables, and Rice

Cauliflower–Chick-pea Sauce with
   Shells

DESSERTS

Brown Rice Pudding

STAPLES

Polenta

Brown Rice

BREAKFAST

Apple Fritters

3 medium apples, peeled, cored, and cut into ¼-inch rounds	¼ tsp salt
	¼ tsp ground cinnamon
1 c whole wheat flour	1 large egg
1 tsp baking powder	1 c apple juice
	1 Tbsp vegetable oil

1. Dry apples with paper towel and set aside. Apples need to be dry or batter will not stick.
2. Mix flour, baking powder, salt, and cinnamon in a bowl.
3. In a separate bowl, beat egg, juice, and 1¼ teaspoons of vegetable oil. Mix wet and dry ingredients together until there are no lumps.
4. In a nonstick pan, heat ½ teaspoon of oil. Dip apples in batter and let excess drip off. Sauté slices a few at a time. Cook until golden, turn, and brown the other side. Continue until all apples are done. Drain on paper towels.

 Top with cinnamon and sugar, honey, or maple syrup. Easy!

Serving size	7 oz	Total fat	6 g	
Servings per recipe	4	Saturated fat	1 g	
Calories	254			

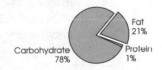

Fat 21%
Carbohydrate 78%
Protein 1%

Great Morning Cereal

4 c water	1 c steel-cut oats
1 tsp salt	1 tsp cinnamon
1 c oatmeal	

1. Boil water and salt in a large pot. When water is boiling, slowly add oatmeal, oats, and cinnamon. Mix well.
2. Lower heat and maintain a slow, rolling boil. Cook for 10 minutes, stirring frequently.

Option
Plain thick hot oatmeal cereal with a touch of cinnamon. Ready to sweeten.

I make this the night before or first thing in morning before I wake up the kids. Leave simple and sweet or dress up with jams, fruit, sugars, nutmeg, dried fruit, or syrups.

Serving size	10 oz	Total fat	4 g
Servings per recipe	4	Saturated fat	1 g
Calories	231		

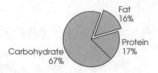

Fat 16% / Protein 17% / Carbohydrate 67%

SOUPS

Zucchini and Spinach Soup

½ Tbsp olive oil
1½–2 c onions, coarsely chopped
5 c vegetable or chicken stock (or canned broth)
3 lbs. small zucchini, or 12 medium, cut in ½-inch rounds

1 10-oz package frozen chopped spinach, or 1 lb fresh spinach with stem removed and chopped
2 lemons, juiced
1 tsp salt, or to taste
½ tsp black pepper, or to taste

1. In a soup pot, heat oil over medium heat, add onions, and cook for 10 minutes, until tender.
2. Add broth and bring to a boil. Add zucchini and return to a boil. Cook for 15 minutes, uncovered.
3. Add frozen spinach, reduce heat to low, and cook until the spinach breaks up.
4. Blend with a hand blender until smooth, but keep the spinach visible, or put in blender or food processor.
5. Before serving, add lemon juice and season with salt and pepper.

 A Braun hand mixer works great. You can blend while it is still cooking in the pot.

Serving size	19 oz	Total fat	2 g
Servings per recipe	6	Saturated fat	0 g
Calories	85		

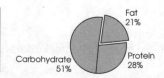

Fat 21% / Protein 28% / Carbohydrate 51%

Bean and Cabbage Stew

1 Tbsp vegetable oil	2½ c vegetable broth
1 large onion, chopped	4 c cabbage chunks
3 medium potatoes, peeled and cut into 1-inch cubes	1 c frozen peas
	1 can Great Northern beans
3 medium carrots, sliced	1½ tsp salt, or to taste
½ tsp caraway seeds	½ tsp black pepper

1. Heat oil in a large skillet. Add onion, potatoes, and carrots. Cook until lightly browned, about 10 minutes.
2. Add caraway seeds and sauté for 1 more minute. Add broth and cook until carrots are almost tender, about 7 to 10 minutes.
3. Add cabbage and peas and cook for 10 minutes, covered. Add beans, salt, and pepper, and cook 5 more minutes, uncovered.
4. Check vegetables and seasonings, and serve.

Option
Add salt and pepper on top after serving.

 Wonderful the next day. Freezes great. Can be used as a main course or can serve 6 as a side dish.

Serving size	20 oz	Total fat	4 g	
Servings per recipe	4	Saturated fat	0 g	
Calories	313			

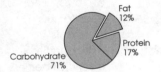

Fat 12%
Protein 17%
Carbohydrate 71%

Broccoli Soup

1 large onion, diced	2 lbs broccoli, cut into pieces
14 cloves garlic, crushed	2 Tbsp fresh dill
2 tsp canola oil	½ tsp nutmeg
8 c water	1 tsp salt
2 large baking potatoes, peeled and cut into small pieces	½ tsp pepper

1. In a soup pot, sauté the onion and garlic in the oil for 5 minutes, until browned.
2. Add the water along with the potatoes and boil for 15 minutes, until the potatoes are tender.
3. Add the broccoli and continue boiling for 5 minutes.
4. Blend three-fourths of the soup until creamy. Return to the soup pot. Add the spices, heat through, and serve.

Fabulous summer soup—add a squeeze of lemon for a little extra zest!

Serving size	13 oz	Total fat	2 g	
Servings per recipe	8	Saturated fat	0 g	
Calories	113			

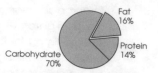

Fat 16%
Protein 14%
Carbohydrate 70%

SNACKS

Granola

⅓ c chopped assorted nuts (walnuts, almonds, filberts) or favorite nuts
1 c currants
½ c dry cherries
½ c dry cranberries
2 c apple juice

3 c puffed rice (3 oz)
3 c puffed millet (3 oz)
1 c brown rice flakes (2 oz)
2 c wheat flakes (2 oz)
½ c rice bran

2½ tsp ground cinnamon
½ tsp grated nutmeg
2 tsp allspice
1 tsp salt
⅓ c barley malt
⅓ c maple syrup
⅓ c rice syrup
2 tsp vanilla extract
½ c applesauce

1. Heat oven to 325°.
2. Roast nuts in oven for 15 minutes.
3. Plump fruits in apple juice over low heat. Cook for 10 to 15 minutes. Drain and cool.
4. In a large bowl, mix rice, millet, rice flakes, wheat flakes, and bran. Add plumped fruit and nuts and all other ingredients. Mix until all ingredients are well integrated.
5. Spread mixture on 2 cookie sheets and bake for 30 minutes, stirring a few times so that everything gets crispy. Turn oven off and allow to sit in oven for 1 hour, then cool. Keep in an airtight container until ready to use.

 Sweet, fruity, and crunchy. Terrific snack or breakfast food. Not a fast recipe but worth the effort.

Serving size	4 oz	Total fat	5 g
Servings per recipe	10	Saturated fat	0 g
Calories	224		

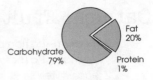

Fat 20%
Carbohydrate 79%
Protein 1%

Granola II

6 Tbsp almonds
½ c sesame seeds
1½ Tbsp vanilla extract
½ Tbsp salt
1 c hot apple juice
¾ c maple syrup
¼ c low-fat soy flour (or whole wheat flour)

¼ c whole wheat flour
7 c rolled oat flakes
1 c pitted and chopped dates
2 c raisins

1. Chop in a food processor or blender: nuts, sesame seeds, vanilla extract, salt, apple juice and maple syrup. Blend until the nuts are small bits and the mixture has thickened a little.
2. In a separate bowl, combine flours and oat flakes.
3. Pour ingredients from processor over dry ingredients. Add dates and raisins, and combine well, until evenly mixed and moist.
4. Spread a thin layer of mixture over 2 large cookie sheets. Bake in 325° oven for 30 minutes. After 15 minutes, move lower cookie sheet up and upper cookie sheet down.
5. Turn off oven and allow granola to dry for 2 to 3 hours, until totally cooled. Enjoy for breakfast or as a snack. Keep in an airtight container or bag to store.

 Top with yogurt, non-fat ice cream, and non-fat hot fudge for a sweet treat.

Serving size	6 oz	Total fat	10 g
Servings per recipe	10	Saturated fat	1 g
Calories	477		

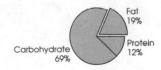

Fat 19%
Carbohydrate 69%
Protein 12%

Oatmeal Fruit Cookies

2 medium-size ripe bananas (to make 1 c mashed)	1½ c rolled oats
2 egg whites	½ c raisins
1 c pitted and chopped dates	

1. Preheat oven to 350°.
2. Mash bananas, leaving some chunks. Add egg whites and dates, and mix to make sure dates are separated and well coated.
3. Mix in rolled oats and raisins. Set aside for 10 minutes. Wipe a cookie sheet with a little oil. Place teaspoonful of dough on cookie sheet, and flatten with the back of a spoon.
4. Bake for 20 to 25 minutes, until the edges are lightly browned. Cool and remove from pan. Store well covered in refrigerator or freezer.

 Moist, sweet, chewy cookie. Easy, easy, easy—get the kids to help! Double recipe and freeze for later.

Serving size	1 oz	Total fat	trace	
Servings per recipe	24	Saturated fat	0 g	
Calories	60			

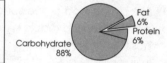

Fat 6%
Protein 6%
Carbohydrate 88%

SALADS

Black Bean Salad

2 cans black beans
½ red pepper, chopped fine
½ yellow or green pepper,
   chopped fine
1 lime, juiced
½ red onion, chopped fine
½ bunch cilantro, leaves
   removed from stems and
   chopped
½ bunch flat-leaf parsley,
   leaves removed from stems
   and chopped

1½ tsp olive oil
2 Tbsp white vinegar
4 Tbsp water
¼ tsp garlic powder
¼ tsp turmeric
½ tsp oregano
1 tsp chile habañero sauce
   (or Tabasco)
   salt and pepper to taste

1. Rinse black beans well and drain off liquid.
2. Mix all ingredients together well, cover, and chill.

 Quick and easy. Leave out the parsley or cilantro if you hate it. Heap on tacos, burritos, salads—use as a dip or enjoy it by itself.

Serving size	7 oz	Total fat	2 g
Servings per recipe	6	Saturated fat	0 g
Calories	180		

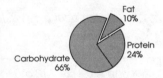

Fat 10%
Protein 24%
Carbohydrate 66%

Complete Protein Tabouleh

2 c bulgur wheat
4 c boiling water

Dressing:
3 Tbsp olive oil
2½ Tbsp distilled white vinegar
½ c lemon juice, or more to taste
pinch of sugar
1 tsp salt, or to taste
½ tsp black pepper, or to taste

1 small bunch scallions (5 or 6), chopped into rounds
5–6 large cloves garlic, pressed
2 cans chick-peas, drained and rinsed
1 bunch fresh parsley, chopped
2 large ripe tomatoes, chopped

1. Place bulgur in bowl and cover with boiling water. Cover and let stand for 15 minutes.
2. Pour bulgur through strainer and drain for 5 to 10 minutes.
3. Meanwhile, prepare dressing. Whisk together all the dressing ingredients until thoroughly mixed.
4. Put bulgur, dressing, and remaining ingredients in a large bowl and mix well. Let stand for about 1 hour before serving.

Options
Prepare this dish a day in advance and leave overnight in the refrigerator. Serve cool or at room temperature.

 It doesn't get any easier than this!

Serving size	12 oz	Total fat	7 g
Servings per recipe	8	Saturated fat	1 g
Calories	333		

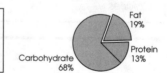

SAUCES

Soy-Ginger Sauce

½ c soy sauce
½ c water
1 Tbsp dry sherry
1 Tbsp grated ginger
½ c chopped scallions
2 cloves garlic, finely chopped

2 tsp sesame oil
2 tsp chinese vinegar or red
wine vinegar
2 tsp sugar
4 c cooked brown rice

1. Mix all ingredients together and let stand for 30 minutes.

 Easy! Wonderful! Tart, sweet, salty sauce. Spoon over veggies, salads, pasta, potatoes, and stir-fry.

Serving size	10 oz	Total fat	4 g	
Servings per recipe	4	Saturated fat	1 g	
Calories	279			

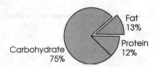

Fat 13%
Protein 12%
Carbohydrate 75%

Broccoli Sauce

1 head fresh garlic
2 tsp vegetable oil, preferably
canola
1 head fresh broccoli
1½ lb pasta (small shells or
radiatore are best; also
delicious with filled pasta
such as tortellini.)

1½ tsp salt
½ tsp pepper
freshly grated Parmesan
cheese (optional)
water for steaming

1. Preheat oven to 350°.
2. Peel all the garlic and arrange in one layer in a small ovenproof dish. Coat with oil and bake for 40 minutes, until all the garlic is golden brown. (Or buy already roasted garlic if you ever see it, already peeled and crushed.)
3. To prepare the broccoli, separate the large stems from the florets. Peel the tough skin from the stems and discard. Steam the stems for 10 minutes, until almost tender. Add the florets to the steamer and cook 5 minutes, until they are bright green and just tender. Do not overcook.

4. Do not rinse the broccoli and do not discard water from steamer.

5. Prepare pasta according to package directions. If serving immediately, do not rinse the pasta.

6. When the garlic is ready, combine the garlic and broccoli in a blender or food processor with a steel knife. Run the processor about 20 seconds, until coarsely chopped. Add 1 cup water from steamer, salt, and pepper. Process until smooth. Serve hot over pasta. If desired, top with grated Parmesan cheese.

Options
Add dill and lemon juice or add Italian seasoning and Parmesan cheese.

 Love the garlic in this pasta dish!

Serving size	15 oz	Total fat	4 g
Servings per recipe	6	Saturated fat	0 g
Calories	391		

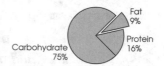

Fat 9%
Protein 16%
Carbohydrate 75%

SIDE DISHES

Pasta and Beans

1 Tbsp olive oil
2 c chopped onions
6 cloves garlic, minced
1 celery stalk, sliced
2 tsp basil
1 28-oz can tomatoes with juice
7 c vegetable broth
¼ tsp sage
¼ tsp crushed red pepper flakes

1 bay leaf
2 14-oz cans pinto beans, rinsed and drained
2 tsp salt, or to taste
½ tsp black pepper, or to taste
2 c small macaroni or spaghetti (broken into pieces)
¼ c chopped fresh parsley

1. Heat oil in a large soup pot over medium heat. Add onions and garlic, and sauté until onions are lightly browned.

2. Add celery and basil, and cook 2 more minutes.

3. Add tomatoes, broth, sage, red pepper, and bay leaf. Cook for 30 minutes, uncovered.

4. Remove bay leaf and add beans, salt, and pepper. Cook another 15 minutes.

5. In the meantime, cook pasta according to package directions, until done but still firm. Drain pasta and add to soup pot. Add parsley, season to taste, and bring to a boil.

6. Remove from the heat and serve.

 Freeze the leftovers for a quick and easy meal.

Serving size	18 oz	Total fat	3 g
Servings per recipe	8	Saturated fat	0 g
Calories	238		

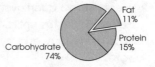

Fat 11%
Protein 15%
Carbohydrate 74%

Sweet-and-Sour Lentil Casserole

1 c dry lentils
¼ c soy sauce
3 Tbsp honey
⅓ c white vinegar
1 tsp grated fresh ginger
2 oz fine egg noodles
1 Tbsp dark sesame oil
2 Tbsp water

1 clove garlic, chopped
1 large carrot, thinly sliced
1 small pepper, chopped
4 bunches scallions, thinly sliced into rounds
salt or extra soy sauce to taste

1. Wash lentils in several bowls of water until clean: make sure to remove all stones. Place lentils in pot, cover with water. Cook in covered pot until lentils are tender but still firm.

2. Mix soy sauce, honey, vinegar, and ginger, and set aside. Cook noodles according to package directions and drain.

3. Heat sesame oil and water, and sauté garlic and carrot for 3 to 5 minutes, until carrots are almost tender. Add pepper and scallions, and cook until scallions are barely wilted, about 2 minutes.

4. Add cooked lentils and soy mixture, and cook for 10 minutes over low heat. Add noodles and mix together until heated through. Remove from heat, check seasoning, and serve.

 Lentil casserole's a big family favorite with us!

Serving size	15 oz	Total fat	5 g
Servings per recipe	2	Saturated fat	1 g
Calories	579		

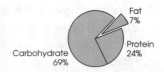

Fat 7%
Protein 24%
Carbohydrate 69%

Brown Rice Pilaf

1 Tbsp olive oil	½ tsp thyme
2 medium onions, chopped	1½ c brown rice, uncooked
6 cloves garlic, minced	5¾ c boiling chicken broth
10 oz mushrooms, sliced	1 tsp salt, or to taste
(canned or fresh)	½ tsp black pepper, or to taste

1. Preheat oven to 350°.
2. Heat oil in a 3-quart ovenproof casserole on medium heat. Sauté onions and garlic for 10 minutes, until onions are transparent.
3. Add mushrooms and thyme. Raise heat and sauté mushrooms until liquid evaporates.
4. Add rice and mix until rice turns opaque.
5. Add broth, salt, and pepper. Cover casserole tightly and cook in oven for 1 hour. Check to see if all the liquid is absorbed.
6. Fluff with a fork and serve.

 Fabulous as a stuffing!

Serving size	13 oz	Total fat	4 g	
Servings per recipe	6	Saturated fat	1 g	
Calories	230			

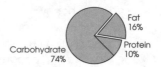

Millet and Vegetable Casserole

1 Tbsp olive oil	2 tomatoes, peeled and
1 medium onion, finely	chopped
chopped	1 c millet
4 cloves garlic, minced	2 c boiling vegetable broth
1 stalk celery, sliced	2 tsp fresh ginger, minced
1 medium green pepper, cut	1½ tsp curry powder
into strips	1½ tsp salt, or to taste
2 carrots, thinly sliced	½ tsp black pepper
2 small zucchini, cut in half	
and sliced into ½-inch slices	

1. Heat oil in a large frying pan. Add onion, garlic, celery, green pepper, carrots, zucchini, tomatoes, and ginger. Sauté the vegetables for 5 minutes, stirring often.
2. Meanwhile, wash the millet thoroughly, changing water often, and let drain for 10 minutes.

3. In a dry skillet over medium heat, toast the millet lightly, stirring constantly.
4. To the vegetables, add millet, broth, curry, salt, and pepper. Mix all ingredients well. Cover pan and simmer for 10 to 15 minutes, until the liquid is absorbed.
5. Adjust seasoning and serve.

 Try this one—you'll be surprised.

Serving size	14 oz	Total fat	6 g
Servings per recipe	4	Saturated fat	1 g
Calories	281		

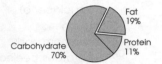

Fat 19%
Protein 11%
Carbohydrate 70%

Lentil and Bulgur Pilaf

½ lb lentils, washed and picked over
5½ c water
4 cloves garlic, minced
1 bay leaf
1 tsp ground cumin
1 c bulgur

¼ tsp cayenne pepper
1½ tsp salt, or to taste
½ tsp black pepper
2 c thinly sliced onions
1 Tbsp olive oil
2 Tbsp fresh parsley

1. Soak lentils in water for 1 hour in a large casserole. Add garlic, bay leaf, and cumin, bring to a boil, and cook for 20 to 30 minutes, or until lentils are just tender.
2. Add bulgur, cayenne, salt, and pepper, stir, and cover pan. Remove from the heat and let stand for 30 minutes, until the bulgur has absorbed the liquid and becomes tender.
3. Meanwhile, sauté onions in skillet with oil over low heat, until lightly brown. Transfer bulgur to a serving platter, spread onions and parsley on top, and serve.

 Love, love, love those lentils!

Serving size	18 oz	Total fat	5 g
Servings per recipe	4	Saturated fat	1 g
Calories	387		

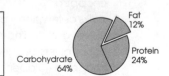

Fat 12%
Protein 24%
Carbohydrate 64%

Curried Vegetables

2 medium onions, sliced thin	3 c water
1 Tbsp olive oil	4 c 1-inch pieces of cauliflower
5 cloves garlic	2 c green beans
2 tsp minced ginger root	(fresh or frozen)
1 tsp minced hot chili pepper	1 c chopped ripe tomatoes
(fresh jalapeño)	½ lemon, juiced
1 tsp turmeric	2 tsp salt, or to taste
4 cardamom pods	
2 lb potatoes, peeled and cut	
into ½-inch cubes	

1. Sauté onions in oil for 10 minutes until soft.
2. Add garlic, salt, and all the spices, and sauté for 5 minutes.
3. Add potatoes and water, cover, and cook over moderate heat for 20 minutes.
4. Add cauliflower and green beans, stir well, cover, and cook over low heat for 30 minutes.
5. Add tomatoes and lemon. Stir, and remove from heat.

 Spice this up with capers or jalapeños—it's even better the next day.

Serving size	12 oz	Total fat	2 g	
Servings per recipe	6	Saturated fat	0 g	
Calories	157			

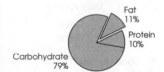

Fat 11%
Protein 10%
Carbohydrate 79%

Spicy String Bean and Tomato Sauce

2 Tbsp olive oil	1½ lb string beans, trimmed,
2 medium carrots, finely	washed, and cut into
chopped	1½-inch pieces (can use
2 stalks celery, finely chopped	frozen)
6 cloves garlic, minced	2 Tbsp chopped capers
2 hot peppers, seeded and	1½ tsp salt, or to taste
chopped (jalapeños)	½ tsp black pepper
1 27-oz can plum tomatoes,	¼ c chopped fresh parsley
chopped	

1. Heat oil in a large saucepan. Add carrots, celery, garlic, and hot peppers. Sauté for 10 minutes, until vegetables begin to golden. Add tomatoes and continue cooking until sauce begins to thicken, about 15 minutes.
2. Add all other ingredients except parsley and cook, covered, until string beans are

tender, about 20 minutes. Check to make sure there is enough liquid; if not add enough water to have sauce for pasta.

3. When beans are ready, turn off the heat, and add parsley.

Options
Serve over spaghetti cooked according to package directions. Great also with rice or just plain.

 Salty, spicy, Italian-tasting.

Serving size	11 oz	Total fat	2 g
Servings per recipe	6	Saturated fat	0 g
Calories	103		

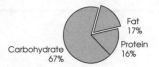

Fat 17%
Protein 16%
Carbohydrate 67%

MAIN DISHES

Bean and Corn Burritos

1 c dry red kidney beans or 2 c canned kidney beans	1 jalapeño pepper, seeded and minced
2 c frozen corn, cooked	1 tsp basil
2 tsp canola oil	½ tsp oregano
1 medium onion, chopped	2 Tbsp cilantro, chopped
2 cloves garlic, chopped	1 lb corn tortillas
½ red pepper, chopped	1 tsp salt, or to taste
½ green pepper, chopped	1 tsp sugar

1. Pick over beans, soak them overnight, and discard liquid. Wash and cook, drain, and reserve liquid. If using canned beans, drain and rinse them.
2. Cook corn and blend half into a creamy sauce with a blender, hand blender, or food processor.
3. Heat oil in a pan and sauté onion and garlic for 3 minutes. Add peppers, basil, and oregano, and continue cooking for 5 minutes.
4. Partially mash beans and add to pan. Cook for 2 minutes. Add whole and creamed corn and cilantro. Mix all ingredients together. Add salt and sugar, and check consistency, making sure it is soft and easy to use as a filling. Set aside.
5. Heat tortillas on a hot griddle, 2 or 3 at a time, until they become flexible. Fill them with a few spoonfuls of the filling. Roll up tortilla around the filling.

6. Set aside in a warming pan until all are done. Heat in the oven and serve with salsa. Keep covered to keep tortillas moist.

 Mexican heaven!

Serving size	12 oz	Total fat	6 g
Servings per recipe	4	Saturated fat	1 g
Calories	527		

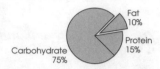

Vegetable Lo Mein

1 Tbsp dark sesame oil
¼ c vegetable broth
3 cloves garlic, chopped
4 c diagonally sliced broccoli
1 medium onion, sliced
2 stalks celery, cut into diagonal slices
1 c sliced mushrooms
1 8-oz can sliced bamboo shoots

1¼ c cooked frozen peas
3 Tbsp chopped cilantro
½ lb vermicelli
Soy-Ginger Sauce (see recipe)
Salt or extra soy sauce to taste

1. Heat oil and vegetable broth in a pan. Add garlic and sauté for 3 minutes. Add broccoli and onion, and cook for 3 minutes. Add celery, and cook for 3 minutes. Add extra vegetable broth if pan gets dry—½ cup at a time.
2. Add mushrooms and bamboo shoots, and cook for 3 minutes. Add peas and cilantro, and remove from heat.
3. Cook the vermicelli according to the package directions and drain.
4. Add the Soy-Ginger Sauce to the vegetables and heat through. Serve over noodles with salt or extra soy sauce to taste.

 Slice, chop, sauté. Done!

Serving size	13 oz	Total fat	5 g
Servings per recipe	4	Saturated fat	1 g
Calories	217		

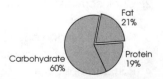

Chinese Stir-fry Vegetables

2 Tbsp cornstarch
Soy-Ginger Sauce (see recipe)
2 Tbsp dark sesame oil
2 medium onions, cut into ¼-inch slices
3 carrots, cut on the diagonal into slices; and then slices cut into matchsticks
1 head broccoli, stem peeled, sliced, and cut, and florets cut small

12 black Chinese mushrooms, soaked for 20 minutes in hot water, stems removed, and cut into ¼-inch strips
2 medium red peppers, cut into ¼-inch strips
4 c cooked brown rice

1. Add cornstarch to Soy-Ginger Sauce and stir until smooth. Set aside.
2. Heat oil in a heavy pan. Sauté onions for 5 minutes. Add carrots and broccoli, and cook for 10 minutes. Add mushrooms and peppers, and cook for 3 minutes.
3. Stir the Soy-Ginger Sauce to make sure the cornstarch is evenly mixed. Add to the vegetables and bring to a boil. Cook for 3 minutes, until slightly thickened and all vegetables are coated with sauce.
4. Serve with the brown rice.

 Look for dried Chinese mushrooms in the Asian section of the store.

Serving size	13 oz	Total fat	7 g
Servings per recipe	5	Saturated fat	1 g
Calories	317		

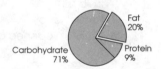

Fat 20%
Protein 9%
Carbohydrate 71%

Lemon Chicken and Bulgur

1 tsp canola oil
2½ lbs whole chicken, skinned and cut into serving pieces
2 tsp salt, or to taste
½ tsp black pepper, or to taste
3 medium onions, chopped (to make 1½–2 cups)
4 cloves garlic, minced

1¾ c bulgur
½ tsp ground cardamom
½ tsp ground coriander
½ tsp ground cumin
2 lemon rinds, grated
2½ lemons, juiced
3½ c boiling chicken broth

1. Preheat oven to 350°.

2. In a large skillet, heat oil and sauté chicken pieces until golden. Add salt and pepper and place into an ovenproof dish.
3. Add onion and garlic to skillet and cook until onions are soft but not brown.
4. Add bulgur and sauté until lightly browned. Add spices, lemon rinds, and lemon juice. Mix well and spoon over chicken.
5. Bring broth to a boil, pour over everything, and cover dish.
6. Bake for 1 hour. Chicken should be tender and bulgur soft.

 Light and lemony.

Serving size	16 oz	Total fat	11 g
Servings per recipe	4	Saturated fat	3 g
Calories	481		

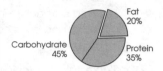

Fat 20%
Protein 35%
Carbohydrate 45%

Spaghetti and Eggplant Sauce

1 Tbsp olive oil
1 large onion, chopped
4 cloves garlic, minced
1 tsp basil
1 tsp oregano
3 lb (48-oz) canned plum tomatoes

2 lb eggplant, cut into ½-inch cubes
olive oil spray
3 tsp salt, or to taste
½ tsp black pepper
1 lb spaghetti

1. Heat oil in a large saucepan over medium-high heat. Add onion and garlic, and cook until soft.
2. Add herbs and cook for 2 minutes. Add tomatoes with juice and stir to break up the tomatoes. Cook for 15 minutes, until thick.
3. Preheat oven to 400°.
4. Spread out half of the eggplant on a large cookie sheet and spray with oil (not too much, just enough to lightly coat the eggplant). Bake the eggplant for 10 minutes in the upper portion of the oven, then bake for 10 minutes in the lower portion of the oven. The eggplant should be golden brown. Repeat with the remaining eggplant.
5. Stir the eggplant into the sauce and season with salt and pepper to taste. Cook for 20 to 25 minutes.
6. Cook the spaghetti according to package directions and serve with the sauce.

Rich, zesty, tangy red sauce. Pour over pasta, rice, potatoes, toasted bread.

Serving size	29 oz	Total fat	6 g
Servings per recipe	4	Saturated fat	1 g
Calories	595		

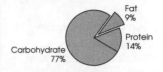

Soba Noodles with Snow Peas

½ lb soba noodles
1 Tbsp dark sesame oil
1 large onion, sliced
1 large carrot, sliced thin

2 c snow peas
Soy-Ginger Sauce (see recipe)
soy sauce or salt to taste

1. Break noodles in half and cook according to package directions. Drain.
2. Heat sesame oil in a pan. Add onion and carrot and sauté for 3 minutes. Add snow peas and cook 5 more minutes. All vegetables should be cooked but not raw.
3. Add Soy-Ginger Sauce to the vegetables and heat for 2 minutes. Pour the vegetables and sauce over the noodles and check for seasoning.

 Got extra veggies in the fridge? Throw some in to change this into a whole different meal.

Serving size	6 oz	Total fat	4 g
Servings per recipe	4	Saturated fat	1 g
Calories	267		

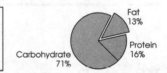

Chick-pea Sauce and Rigatoni

2 cans chick-peas, rinsed and
  drained
1 c vegetable broth
1 Tbsp olive oil
1½ c thinly sliced onions
1½ Tbsp minced garlic
1 16-oz can crushed
  tomatoes

1 tsp crushed rosemary
¼ c chopped fresh parsley
1½ tsp salt, or to taste
½ tsp black pepper
1 lb cooked pasta (small
  shape) or regular spaghetti

1. In a food processor or blender, puree half of the chick-peas with ½ cup of vegetable broth. Set aside.
2. Heat the oil in a large saucepan. Sauté the onions and garlic until lightly
   browned, about 5 to 7 minutes.
3. Add the tomatoes, rosemary, chick-peas, chick-pea puree, and ½ cup of vegetable broth. Cook, stirring well, for 15 minutes, or until the whole chick-peas are
   soft.
4. Add the parsley, salt, and pepper. Serve over rigatoni cooked according to package directions.

  An extra can of tomatoes makes this even zestier.

Serving size	15 oz	Total fat	5 g
Servings per recipe	6	Saturated fat	1 g
Calories	442		

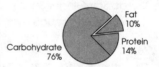

Fat 10%
Protein 14%
Carbohydrate 76%

White Beans and Fusilli

1 Tbsp olive oil
6 cloves garlic, minced
1 small onion, finely chopped
1 head escarole, chopped
2 c cooked white beans or
  canned
1½ tsp dried rosemary

2 c vegetable broth
2 tsp salt, or to taste
½ tsp black pepper
1 lb fusilli pasta
2 Tbsp finely chopped flat-leaf
  parsley
1 lb fusilli pasta

1. Boil water for pasta. Meanwhile, warm oil in a sauté pan over medium heat. Add
   garlic, onion, and escarole, and cook, stirring frequently, for 5 to 10 minutes, until
   the escarole is wilted.

2. Add the beans and rosemary, and sauté for 1 minute. If you use canned beans, rinse before cooking.
3. Add the vegetable broth, salt, and pepper, and simmer for 5 minutes. Taste, and adjust the seasoning. Cover and set aside.
4. Cook the fusilli according to package directions. Drain.
5. Toss the pasta and warm beans together. Garnish with parsley.

 Yummy mild pasta and bean dish.

Serving size	*17 oz*	*Total fat*	*6 g*	
Servings per recipe	*4*	*Saturated fat*	*1 g*	
Calories	*621*			

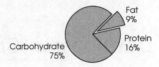

Fat 9%
Protein 16%
Carbohydrate 75%

Lentil Sauce, Vegetables, and Rice

1½ c brown lentils, washed and picked over
1 qt water
1 bay leaf
3 stalks celery, sliced
2 medium carrots, sliced
1 bunch scallions, sliced
2½ c canned crushed tomatoes
½ lb zucchini, cut in half and sliced
1 tsp ground coriander
1½ tsp ground cumin
⅛ tsp cayenne pepper
1½ tsp salt, or to taste
½ tsp black pepper
1 Tbsp olive oil
1 large onion, sliced
4 large cloves garlic, minced
¼ c chopped fresh cilantro
1 lemon, juiced
2 c brown rice

1. Place the clean lentils in a large pot and cover with water. Soak for 1 hour. Add the bay leaf and bring to a boil. Cover pot. Cook for 20 minutes, or until the lentils are just tender. Take out the bay leaf.
2. Add the celery, carrots, scallions, tomatoes, zucchini, spices, salt, and pepper. Cook for 15 minutes or less, until the vegetables are just tender.
3. Meanwhile, heat the oil in a frying pan and sauté the onion and garlic until golden. Mix into the cooked lentils.
4. Add the cilantro and lemon juice. Serve with brown rice cooked according to the package directions.

This has all my favorites in it—you've got your bean, your grain, and your vegetable.

Serving size	22 oz	Total fat	5 g
Servings per recipe	6	Saturated fat	1 g
Calories	474		

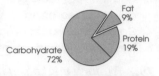

Cauliflower–Chick-pea Sauce with Shells

1 can chick-peas, rinsed and drained
1 Tbsp olive oil
4 cloves garlic, minced
⅛ tsp red pepper flakes
1 small head cauliflower, cut into small pieces
4 c chopped ripe tomatoes

1 c vegetable broth
1 Tbsp wine vinegar
1½ tsp salt, or to taste
1 tsp dried basil
2 Tbsp pitted and sliced black olives
¼ c chopped fresh parsley
1 lb small shells

1. Heat the olive oil in a pan and sauté the garlic for 2 minutes. Add the pepper flakes and cauliflower, and sauté for 2 minutes. Add the tomatoes, broth, vinegar, salt, basil, and olives. Bring to a boil and cook until the cauliflower is tender, about 5 minutes.
2. Add the chick-peas. Check the seasoning and cook 5 more minutes. Add the parsley and stir. Serve over pasta cooked according to package directions.

 Spicy, rich, and Italian. I throw it on rice, toasted bread, baked potato (plain, of course), or just eat, eat, eat it alone.

Serving size	17 oz	Total fat	5 g
Servings per recipe	6	Saturated fat	1 g
Calories	386		

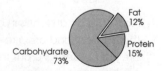

DESSERTS

Brown Rice Pudding

3 c cooked brown rice	¼ c brown sugar
6 c apple juice	¼ tsp salt
¼ c golden raisins	1 Tbsp tahini
½ c dark raisins	2 tsp vanilla extract
1½ tsp ground cinnamon	1 tsp grated lemon rind

1. Place rice, juice, raisins, cinnamon, salt, and brown sugar in a heavy-bottomed pot. Simmer on very low heat for 2½ hours, stirring occasionally. Check to make sure the rice does not get too dry. Add more juice if necessary.
2. When the rice is very soft, take 1 cup of the rice and the tahini and blend until smooth. Return to the pot and mix. Cook 15 to 20 more minutes. Add the vanilla extract and lemon rind, and pour into a serving bowl.

Options
Try with other dried fruits instead of raisins.

 Creamy, thick, rich, rice pudding—just as good for breakfast as for dessert!

Serving size	8 oz	Total fat	2 g
Servings per recipe	10	Saturated fat	0 g
Calories	196		

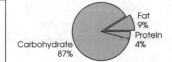

Polenta

1½ c yellow cornmeal	4 c boiling water
1 c cold water	2 Tbsp grated Parmesan
1 tsp salt	cheese (optional)

1. Mix cornmeal, water, and salt until all lumps are gone and it has a puttylike consistency.
2. Place in a pot with boiling water. Lower the heat and mix with a wire whisk. If the mixture gets too stiff, add ½ cup of cold water and continue mixing. Cook for 8 to 10 minutes. Taste for doneness.
3. Pour into a 9 by 12-inch pan and cool. Cut into squares for serving.
4. Prior to serving, heat in the oven for 10 minutes, covered, or sprinkle Parmesan cheese on top and place under a broiler until the surface starts to brown.

 Pour mushroom stew over this—outstanding!

Serving size	12 oz	Total fat	3 g	
Servings per recipe	4	Saturated fat	1 g	
Calories	180			

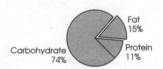

Brown Rice

2 c brown rice (short grain is best)	4 c water
	1 tsp salt

1. Wash rice in a bowl, changing the water 3 times until it rinses clean. Drain.
2. Bring water and salt to a boil, add rice, cover, and simmer for 45 minutes. Do not uncover pot. Let sit on the side for 5 to 10 minutes.

 You can always find a huge pot of this stuff! Toss, throw, combine in soups, salads, veggies, and on and on and on . . .

Serving size	11 oz	Total fat	3 g	
Servings per recipe	4	Saturated fat	1 g	
Calories	342			

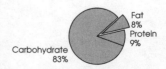

Stage *3*

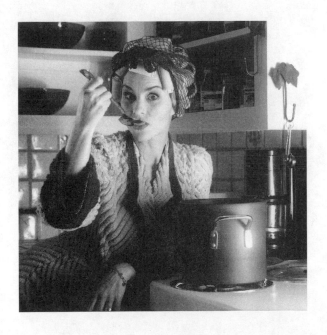

CHAPTER 13

STAGE 3

Yep, yep, yep. Who would ever have thought about the streamline inspection system, protein, calcium, Walton's mountain, or any of it. And then you gotta bear with me and go on and on. Do you think I've asked too much?

NAWWWWWWWW, it ain't over yet. We've still got stage three. And if stage two went from sticking your toe in to jumping, then stage three goes from grounded to flying. Lots of interesting connections to food. Just a tad over the edge. Consider it a personal challenge. Going further than you ever thought you'd go when we're talking about how breakfast, lunch, and dinner are connected to how you look and feel.

Blurbs. Thoughts. Connections that may have never been made. Whatever you want to call them, stage three is stage three. To be used as stage one and two are—whenever, however, and to whatever degree you want to use it.

And if it's food you want, the recipes at the end of this high-flying section may knock your socks off. I told you by the end of this book you'd be looking at seaweed wondering why anyone in their right mind would consider eating it. Arame. Amasake. Miso. Fly, fly, fly right into them with me. You've gone this far, you may as well take it to the end.

My "end" with food was the beginning of our discussion. Fat. Getting fat was the end, the club over the head, the big (pardon, pardon, pardon that one) slamming lesson for me connected to food. But the beginning took me right to things like miso, arame, and amasake. Your stage three was my stage one, and it was all connected to my cervix. Yep. Female reproductive system.

Actually it started with my and my friend Deborah's cervix. You see, when

I was nineteen, twenty, something like that, my friend Deborah told me I was out of my mind, needed to get a grip and act like an adult. I was working in an office, connecting people with jobs and jobs with people, otherwise known as the personnel business. Deb worked in the same office, different department, and the minute I met her I loved her and knew I was going to be her friend. I'm thrilled to say that twenty years later she is one of my dearest friends in the world. The heart bracelet I wear on my wrist all the time— Deb gave me that! The dedication to the woman in New Jersey in my first book—that's Deb! She loves me, I love her. Simple and wonderful, that's what our friendship has been for twenty years, and that's what it's going to be for the next however long we have together.

So this friend of mine was yelling at me years ago, trying to make me come to my senses because I had gotten a call one day in our office from my doctor telling me that I had a bad pap smear and needed further testing, blah, blah, blah. Deb had gotten the same call just a short time before and did the "right" thing—went straight to her doctor, had the freeze biopsy done, got the results, went in for surgery, and did it all without a second thought. The whole damn thing cost a couple of thousand dollars, some pain, a chip off the old cervix, and it was over—except, of course, for regular pap smears she has to get for the rest of her life, and she does, now that she is "high risk."

What Deb's cervical cancer surgery has to do with your and my transition from high-fat living to lower-fat living may be the pressing question on your mind right now, or maybe it's gone way beyond Deb's cervix to my sanity. Understandable, but you'll see soon how it all ties in beautifully.

We all know now that certain cancers are very much connected to high-fat diets, but that's not where I'm going with this. This is about going from very fat and unfit to leaner and healthier, and it did all begin with Deb's cervix.

The call came in to my office. The bad pap smear was confirmed, and I told Deb. Within minutes she'd lined up an appointment with her doctor, the best in New York, and as far as my friend was concerned, there was nothing more to think about except the results of the cryosurgery that were sure to follow.

My thoughts on the whole bad pap smear thing were very different, and in the year and a half that followed, we went through some tough, wonderful, difficult times as I asked my questions, got my answers, and made decisions that Deb and everyone else thought were completely nuts. I started looking into alternative treatments during a time when it was not cool to say you were going to an acupuncturist. Food and health—the connection was as far-fetched as you could get, completely disconnected. Vitamins and herbs were considered the imaginative nonsense of the hippie generation, and treating what was being called cancer with anything other than Western medicine was unheard of.

Family and friends consulted on the state of my sanity quite a few times during that year. My medical diagnoses changed a couple of times, depending on which lab I went to and which doctor I consulted, going from a grade 2–3 pap smear (not necessarily cancer, just some kind of funky cell stuff going on) to a grade 5, big bad trouble. I heard it all:

> You are in immediate danger of losing your life, young lady, because if this gets into your uterus, the cells go wild within all the layers of that uterus of yours, and we will never be able to stop it.

> You've probably got a really bad infection, and there's nothing to worry about.

> How dare you question me! I've got the medical degree, not you.

The scare tactics and horror stories some of the doctors used to make me "come to my senses and just have the surgery" were beyond belief.

> "Who do you think you are?"
>
> "What are you so worried about? Just have the surgery. Is it never being able to have children? There's always adoption, just as satisfying."
>
> "If you feel a hysterectomy will make you less of a woman [I swear the statement was made by more than one doctor], there are plenty of support groups that I can put you in touch with."

Still, I had some questions and wasn't completely comfortable with the options I was being offered. My concern was never whether or not I could have children—with all due respect to the two whom I love most in the world, that's not what was on my mind when I thought I might be dealing with cancer. And as for being feminine without a uterus, who cared? My concern was that the answers I was being given didn't seem to be making much sense.

More questions.

More answers.

Still I didn't listen.

Doctors joined friends and family in their concern for my sanity. And I kept reading, questioning, and not having the surgery. You want to know why I didn't have the surgery? Deb knows and understands now, but we've had the advantage of twenty years together. When I got this diagnosis, I started asking questions:

What is this I've got? . . . No answer (lots of different opinions).

Why did I get this at age twenty? . . . No answer (not even opinions on this one).

What's to prevent it from happening again? . . . No answer.

If I get this surgery, does it guarantee that this whatever-it-is won't show up somewhere else? . . . No answer.

If I have to have a radical hysterectomy, will I have to go on estrogen therapy, and if so, is it true that estrogen therapy can cause cancer? . . . No answer.

Is there any other test, alternative diagnosis, or treatment? . . . No answer.

The more questions I asked, the fewer answers I got, and the more lectures I received starting with "young lady" and ending with some horror story that was supposed to snap me into action—the action they wanted me to take.

I did have a few surgical procedures during that year and decided—after enough research done at a local library and the last cold, uninvolved, hands-off, worst-bedside-manner-on-earth experience with the hospitals and doctors—that I wasn't going to continue in a medical system that not only couldn't and wouldn't answer my questions but that didn't seem to understand the concept of healing, prevention, and including me. The uterus and cervix they were looking at every day were part of someone with a head, a mind, a heart, and a soul.

My name was Susan Powter, and I was twenty years old, scared, worried about my health. And I wanted to find out what the hell was going on and to make it better. Because I didn't want to blindly commit my body, mind, and soul to a team of physicians didn't make me insane—I thought it made me smart. So I decided in the middle of the night to leave the hospital and figure this thing out on my own.

From Deb's cervix to mine, to my hospital escape, to food makes perfect sense, wouldn't you say? Well, it does: My search for a cure lead straight to food. Holistic medicine. Vitamin therapy. Visualization—thinking about the cancer/dysplasia cells as soldiers in black and the good cells as soldiers in white. Very racist but holistic as hell. That's what I spent my time doing. Food was a big part of this process. I learned back then that what I ate was absolutely connected to what was happening inside my body. How I was feeling. Diseased, not diseased—possible connection for sure. Somehow, somewhere, but connected.

// Sugary cereals in the morning—the best way to start out the day?

// Lamb chops for dinner—the best form of protein?

// The stuff added to our food—no connection to our health at all?

These are the things I started thinking about. Basic? You have no clue. The research had been done, but it was done by doctors who were considered off-the-wall physicians by regular AMA doctors. The AMA was nowhere near acknowledging anything that was going on when it came to food and our health, which is all I was thinking about back then—health, not looking good, because I looked O.K. Food connected with disease—what are you, kidding? Saturated fat having anything to do with heart disease, cancer? What are you, out of your mind?

My father thought I was killing myself running after some herbal theory, and Deb was disgusted. Here I was, open to the concept of food and health; trying like hell to find as much information as I could about food, food, food; fighting for my dysplasia/cancer life. (A note from the author here: I say dysplasia/cancer because to this day I don't believe that I ever came close to having cancer. However, half the doctors almost insisted on using that term —perhaps the ultimate scare tactic to get me to come around to their way of thinking? Who's to know.)

Living on yogurt and cheese. Cutting back on the red meat (ahead of my time, wouldn't you say?). Granola left, right, and center. Vitamins, something totally new. In my life I'd never taken vitamins, and now I was taking what seemed like hundreds. I started working out at an exercise studio—a very hip one in New York, I might add. Lots of dancers, actors, people with big theories about life . . . and me. (The exercise and the ciggy story for those who read *Stop the Insanity!*—that's the place.)

What was really new to me and a direct result of my dysplasia/cancer experience was the introduction to the concept that what I put in my mouth affected how I felt and whether or not I was healthy. The whole vitamin/herb/alternative anything. Back then chamomile tea was my cure for everything. Taking responsibility for my health was something I'd never thought about until I found myself at a very young age worried about my health.

So I started eating better than I'd ever eaten in my life. Feeling a little better than the Average Joe who was chowing down on the burgers, fries, and shakes every day without thinking about his health, and exposing myself to people, tinctures, and concepts that were as foreign to me as protein coming from a bean was to Average Joe.

Shopping in health food stores was part of my intro to alternative. And some of the stores I walked into back then—the incense was so strong, you could puke. The women and that crunchy granola look. Forget it. Not for me now, not for me then. My thoughts on the look:

Bath, try it. What could it hurt?

Let's shave our legs and our underarms and pretend that's the way it's always been done.

How about we take our hair out of the knots and give it a wash?

Then from there came the two sick babies (my second food connection), the marriage blowing up, and my adding a hundred to my frame (my third and most powerful connection). And then . . . the *Food* book. Writing about it all and trying like hell to make some sense of it all and talk with you about it.

> The possibilities.
> The connections.

Beyond butt and thigh hatred to your heart, your cervix, your moods, your emotional, spiritual, and physical well-being . . . and food. Welcome to stage three.

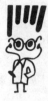

CHAPTER 14

CHEMICALS

*L*et me be the first to say that I love chemicals, certain chemicals.

> Red acrylic nails, count me in.
> Hair dye, don't ask; I live on the stuff.
> Makeup, can't live without it (a sad but true statement).

So it's not life without chemicals that you'll ever hear me talking about. But I think you know by now that I'd like to get the facts, know the truth, and make up my own mind about what I want or don't want in my life.

Suzi (you remember my wonderful friend) came into my house the other day with a box of chemicals she'd just picked up at the hardware store and a box of cereal she'd just picked up at the grocery store. She walked into my kitchen, plunked the cereal down on the counter, and proceeded to read from the carton. The yellow-and-black box contained something called TSP, a chemical used in "heavy-duty cleansers."

Suzi is usually very calm and controlled. You gotta know her to understand how out-of-range her voice got as she read the warning label on the side of the box of chemicals, then read the side of the cereal box. "I can't believe these S.O.B.'s." Suzi's not a big cusser, but this got her cussing. "Our children are eating this stuff. Babies eat this cereal. It's one of the most popular on the market." Here's where her vocal range started to compete with Whitney Houston's. "That little bunny jumps around and tells us that this stuff's fun and nutritious to eat. Read what's in this. Who 'tricks' who when it comes to our children and their health? I gotta go. I'm calling the company to find out what's going on here."

Byyyyeeee, Suzi.

Later that afternoon Suzi was sitting at the butcher block counter in my kitchen. I'm cutting veggies for tonight's soup (expect John-Boy to walk into this kitchen any moment; don't we sound like the Waltons?), and she's telling me about calling the company.

"I called the customer service representative at General Mills. I explained that I was concerned because I had seen TSP on both a cereal box label and a highly toxic industrial cleaner from my local hardware store. The customer service rep said that TSP was used as a buffering agent to control the acidic nature of some of the cereal doughs. I asked her if there had been other calls or if mine was the first. She answered that 'every once in a while' someone would call with a concern.

"She advised me to call the FDA. But you know that wouldn't satisfy me. I pushed a bit harder and she gave me the name of a vice president [if you want to call him, his number is 612-540-3760]. According to her, he was a great guy who would want to hear my concern. I wouldn't know. I was never able to get through to the man.

"Now I was getting frustrated. I looked through my resources and found a number that led me to the National Pesticide Telephone Communication Network [1-800-858-7378]. I know that TSP is not a pesticide but I gave it a shot anyway. A very accommodating gentleman searched through the computer for research on TSP. He found nothing significant. We spoke at length, and after endless questions I discovered the most profound piece of information: To this man's knowledge and all the networks he has access to, it appears that there has never been a study on the effects of combining all the chemicals and additives we ingest. TSP may be harmless in tiny amounts, but combined with dioxin residues? Or how about BHT and MSG and pesticides floating around our neighborhoods that we inhale? Combine all that with some nitrates and sulfites, and throw in a little saccharin and the three thousand different food additives we swallow? It's a miracle that we haven't blown up!"

It's a little overwhelming when you get the cold, hard facts about the chemicals that are added to our food. Maybe that's why we haven't had a look at them. Even the most seasoned Food P.I. would get a little overwhelmed and discouraged by the time he or she got through the meat, chicken, and dairy problems we've just waded through. Sure, it's a bit discouraging when you learn about the lack of policing of the food we're eating. Is everyone at the FDA asleep? Chemicals injected into, lacing the feed of the mass-produced meat we've been eating, and now cleaning agents in the kids' cereals?

It's tough, but forge ahead we must in the name of education—increasing choices and awareness, getting our butt and thighs to look the way we want them to. And at this point I think we can also include an ounce of health consciousness. What the heck, what harm can it do to give our bodies more of what they need and less of the poison?

Think about this: You can have the body of your dreams but, God forbid, what if you get sick? What good will those great upper arms do you then? So when you're talking about chemicals, let's shoot for looking good and also work toward preventing some of the things that might be connected to what we are eating in a big, big way. Let's get more info and become more aware of some of the most deadly, the already proven, the strongest things that might be causing some of the disease, contributing to the exhaustion, making our skin look bad. Who knows what reaction our bodies may have to some of this stuff. But no reaction at all? Come on. You and I know better than that, even if the manufacturers of this junk would rather go down in a ball of fire and damnation (sound like a preacher, don't I?) before they 'fess up to what's going on.

Like the TSP Suzi got so upset about. You want to know what I found when I looked into this little chemmy? It's highly alkaline; it can cause skin irritation. It's used in shampoos, cuticle softeners, bubble baths, water softeners, and cleaners. Yuuucckkkkk! Now get this one . . . It's used in incendiary bombs and tracer bullets!

Let's read the warning on the box:

 Caution, contains Trisodium Phosphate. Avoid contact with skin. In case of eye contact, flush thoroughly with water. If swallowed, give plenty of water and call a physician immediately.

Hey, Suzi—what was that number for that "great guy" at General Mills who's putting this stuff in my kids' food??

> Modern food preservation began in 1810 in France with jars and bottles sealed with wax.

What are some of the other little chemicals we've been putting in our beautiful bodies? Check out the labels of some of the foods you're eating, especially the stuff that the kids are eating. I happen to have some right here for the "do together" part of this chapter.

MSG

Sure see a lot of that MSG, don't you? Ever wondered what it is? Ever left your favorite Chinese restaurant and felt as if you were going to crawl out of your skin? Then, as fast as the feeling came on, it was over? I'd like to introduce you to Mr. MSG. Monosodium glutamate. The most widely used flavor enhancer in the world—other than salt and pepper, of course. Here are some totally different foods, all with Mr. MSG added:

Tuna Helper

INGREDIENTS: ENRICHED NOODLES (WHEAT FLOUR, EGGS, NIACIN, IRON, THIAMIN MONONITRATE, RIBOFLAVIN), CORN STARCH, PARTIALLY HYDROGENATED SOYBEAN OIL, CREAM, SALT, *CORN SYRUP, *PEAS, *ONION, *CARROTS, HYDROLYZED VEGETABLE PROTEIN (SOY, CORN, WHEAT AND YEAST), SODIUM CASEINATE, DISODIUM PHOSPHATE, MONO AND DIGLYCERIDES, SUGAR, LACTOSE, DIPOTASSIUM PHOSPHATE, MONOSODIUM GLUTAMATE, NATURAL FLAVOR, NONFAT MILK, *PARSLEY, CHICKEN, SOY LECITHIN, MODIFIED CORN STARCH, TURMERIC EXTRACT COLOR, WHEAT STARCH, SPICE. FRESHNESS PROTECTED BY BHT, SODIUM SULFITE AND BISULFITE.
*DRIED

Let's take a look at a popular just-add-tuna mix. Maybe it "helps" out that tuna, but I gotta wonder how much it's helping out my body when I check out the list of chemmies this little goodie has packed into one box.

Hydrolyzed vegetable protein—alias MSG. More to come on this chemmie.

Sodium caseinate—soluble form of milk protein. (Could this be a problem to people allergic to milk?)

Disodium phosphate—a buffer to adjust acidity. When you look this one up in the chemmie dictionary (*A Consumer's Dictionary of Food Additives* by Ruth Winter. Very scary reading, I might add!), it says "it may cause mild irritation to the skin and mucus membranes, and can cause purging." Yeah, something I want to be putting in my stomach.

Mono and diglycerides—glycerides of edible fats and oils. Is this a hidden fat?

Dipotassium phosphate—again, a buffering agent to adjust acidity. What is the acid in this mix?

Monosodium glutamate—MSG again, already.

BHT—we'll be talking about this little goodie a little later.

Sodium sulfite—oh, this is great. Also used in hair dyes, developer in photography, used to bleach straw, silk, and wool.

Bisulfite—also a member of the sulfite family of horrors that we'll be talking about shortly.

This is hardly a complete rundown of these chemmies, but I think you get the general idea about what's being put in our foods.

According to the specialists, MSG:

> Is used to make foods taste better.
>
> Removes the tinny taste from canned foods.
>
> Stimulates "tired" taste buds.

MSG is a drug that acts directly on the taste buds, altering their sensitivity.

It acts peripherally on blood vessels, the lobar esophageal sphincter, the brain, and the central nervous system.

It's a cheap way for foods to be made without using expensive ingredients.

At least 20 million people in the United States have a reaction to MSG. MSG intolerance is not an allergic reaction but a true drug effect, a reaction to a drug because it is a drug. Reactions to this drug range from mild headache and flushing of the skin to:

> Asthma
>
> Acute headaches
>
> Mood swings
>
> Irritability
>
> Depression
>
> Paranoia
>
> Migraine headaches
>
> Nausea
>
> Life-threatening heart irregularities

In large concentrations MSG is a potent nerve toxin.

Tobacco leaves have been cured with MSG for "smell and flavor enhancement." Add that to the list of five hundred-plus other things that are in the ciggies we've been smoking—HEY, I'd say this is some mighty powerful stuff that seems to be in almost everything we are eating and smoking, wouldn't you agree?

Tortilla Chips

INGREDIENTS: CORN, PARTIALLY HYDROGENATED CANOLA OIL, BUTTERMILK, SALT, TOMATO, PARTIALLY HYDROGENATED SOYBEAN OIL, CORN SYRUP SOLIDS, WHEY, ONION, GARLIC, MONOSODIUM GLUTAMATE, CHEDDAR CHEESE (MILK, CHEESE CULTURE, SALT, AND ENZYMES), SUGAR, NONFAT MILK, DEXTROSE, MALIC ACID, SODIUM CASEINATE, NATURAL AND ARTIFICIAL FLAVORS, SODIUM ACETATE, EXTRACTIVES OF ANNATTO, DISODIUM PHOSPHATE, MONO- AND DIGLYCERIDES, SPICE, CITRIC ACID, SODIUM CITRATE, DISODIUM INOSINATE, AND DISODIUM GUANYLATE. NO PRESERVATIVES.

Snack Chips Made With Popcorn

INGREDIENTS: GROUND WHOLE POPPING CORN, DEGERMED YELLOW CORN MEAL, RICE FLOUR, PARTIALLY HYDROGENATED CORN AND SOYBEAN OIL, MODIFIED CORN STARCH, SUGAR, SALT, *WHEY, NONFAT MILK, *SOUR CREAM (CULTURED CREAM, NONFAT MILK), DRIED ONION, SODIUM CASEINATE, TRISODIUM PHOSPHATE, DEXTROSE, SOY LECITHIN, ARTIFICIAL AND NATURAL FLAVOR, MONOSODIUM GLUTAMATE, PARSLEY, SODIUM CITRATE, CITRIC ACID. FRESHNESS PRESERVED BY TBHQ AND CITRIC ACID.

Beef Stew Seasoning Mix

INGREDIENTS: CORN STARCH, ONION, SALT, PAPRIKA AND OTHER SPICES, MONOSODIUM GLUTAMATE (FLAVOR ENHANCER), HYDROLYZED CORN GLUTEN, SOY PROTEIN, AND WHEAT GLUTEN, CITRIC ACID, AND CARAMEL COLOR.

Chicken Flavor Stuffing Mix

INGREDIENTS: ENRICHED WHEAT FLOUR (NIACIN, IRON, THIAMINE MONONITRATE, RIBOFLAVIN); CORN SYRUP; ONION; SALT; PARTIALLY HYDROGENATED SOYBEAN AND/OR COTTONSEED OIL; YEAST; CELERY; COOKED CHICKEN AND CHICKEN BROTH; HYDROLYZED VEGETABLE PROTEIN; SOY FLOUR; WHEY; MONOSODIUM GLUTAMATE, PARSLEY FLAKES; SPICES; FRESHNESS PRESERVED BY CALCIUM PROPIONATE, SODIUM SULFITE, BHA, TBHQ, CITRIC ACID AND PROPYL GALLATE; SUGAR; CHICKEN FAT, ONION POWDER; CARAMEL COLOR; TURMERIC; DISODIUM INOSINATE AND DISODIUM GUANYLATE (FLAVOR ENHANCERS).

Egg Noodle and Beef Sauce Mix

INGREDIENTS: ENRICHED EGG NOODLES (DURUM FLOUR WITH NIACIN, IRON [FERROUS SULFATE], THIAMINE MONONITRATE, RIBOFLAVIN, EGG YOLK), HYDROLYZED CORN, SOY AND WHEAT PROTEIN, FOOD STARCH-MODIFIED, SALT, PARTIALLY HYDROGENATED SOYBEAN AND COTTONSEED OIL WITH EMULSIFIER (MONO- AND DIGLYCERIDES), SUGAR, CHEDDAR CHEESE (MILK, CHEESE CULTURE, SALT, ENZYMES), BUTTERMILK, DEHYDRATED ONION, COLOR (CARAMEL, YELLOW 5 AND 6), CORN SYRUP SOLIDS, SOYBEAN OIL, DISODIUM PHOSPHATE, CORN STARCH, MONOSODIUM GLUTAMATE, AUTOLYZED YEAST EXTRACT, DEHYDRATED GARLIC, SPICE, SODIUM CASEINATE, CITRIC ACID, LACTIC ACID, BEEF EXTRACT, MALTODEXTRIN, DISODIUM INOSINATE, DISODIUM GUANYLATE, NATURAL FLAVOR.

BHT AND BHA

Moving on in the discussion of the common chemicals we are eating, here's one you also see all the time, BHT, and its cousin, BHA. Check it out, they're in

---

Creamy Vanilla Frosting

INGREDIENTS: SUGAR, A BLEND OF PARTIALLY HYDROGENATED SOYBEAN AND COTTONSEED OILS, WATER, CORN SYRUP, WHEAT STARCH, CONTAINS 2% OR LESS OF: MONO- AND DIGLYCERIDES, ARTIFICIAL FLAVOR, YELLOWS 5&6 AND OTHER COLOR ADDED, SALT, POLYGLYCEROL ESTERS OF FATTY ACIDS, SODIUM-STEAROYLLACTYLATE, SODIUM ACID PYROPHOSPHATE, DIACETYLATED TARTARIC ACID ESTERS OF MONO-GLYCERIDES, DISODIUM PHOSPHATE FRESHNESS PRESERVED BY POTASSIUM SORBATE AND BHT.

Corn Puffs with Sprinkles

INGREDIENTS: CORN MEAL, SUGAR, CORN SYRUP, WHEAT STARCH, PARTIALLY HYDROGENATED COTTONSEED OIL, WHOLE OAT FLOUR, SALT, ARTIFICIAL FLAVOR, TRISODIUM PHOSPHATE, VITAMIN C (SODIUM ASCORBATE), A B VITAMIN (NIACIN), IRON (A MINERAL NUTRIENT), YELLOWS 5&6 LAKE, YELLOWS 5&6, RED 40 LAKE, BLUE 1 LAKE, RED 40, BLUE 1, VITAMIN B_5 (PYRIDOXINE HYDROCHLORIDE), VITAMIN A (PALMITATE), VITAMIN B_2 (RIBOFLAVIN), VITAMIN B_1 (THIAMIN MONONITRATE), ALMOND OIL, CARNAUBA WAX, CONFECTIONERS GLAZE, A B VITAMIN (FOLIC ACID), VITAMIN D. VITAMIN E (MIXED TOCOPHEROLS) AND BHT ADDED TO PRESERVE FRESHNESS.

Chocolate Corn Puffs

INGREDIENTS: SUGAR, CORN MEAL, COCOA PROCESSED WITH ALKALI, CORN SYRUP, WHEAT STARCH, CORN FLOUR, PARTIALLY HYDROGENATED COTTONSEED AND SOYBEAN OIL, SALT, FRUCTOSE, BEET POWDER AND CARAMEL COLOR, DICALCIUM PHOSPHATE, BAKING SODA, ARTIFICIAL FLAVOR, TRISODIUM PHOSPHATE. FRESHNESS PRESERVED BY BHT.

Honey Graham Cereal

INGREDIENTS: CORN FLOUR, SUGAR, BROWN SUGAR, HONEY GRAHAM CRACKER CRUMBS [ENRICHED FLOUR (FLOUR, NIACIN, REDUCED IRON, THIAMINE MONONITRATE, RIBOFLAVIN), CORN SYRUP, GRAHAM FLOUR, PARTIALLY HYDROGENATED VEGETABLE SHORTENING (SOYBEAN AND/OR COTTONSEED AND/OR PEANUT OIL), LEAVENING (SODIUM BICARBONATE), SALT, WHEY, HONEY], PARTIALLY HYDROGENATED COTTONSEED OIL, CRISP RICE (RICE, SUGAR, SALT, BARLEY MALT), OAT FLOUR, RICE FLOUR, ROLLED OATS, SALT, HONEY, ARTIFICIAL FLAVOR, SODIUM ASCORBATE (A VITAMIN C SOURCE), NIACINAMIDE*, REDUCED IRON, VITAMIN A PALMITATE, ZINC OXIDE (A SOURCE OF ZINC), CALCIUM PANTOTHENATE*, PYRIDOXINE HYDROCHLORIDE*, VITAMIN D, BHT (A PRESERVATIVE), THIAMINE MONONITRATE*, RIBOFLAVIN*, FOLIC ACID*, VITAMIN B12.
*ONE OF THE B VITAMINS.

Frozen Ready to Bake Pie Crust

INGREDIENTS: FLOUR, LARD (WITH BHA, BHT PROPYL GALLATE AND CITRIC ACID ADDED AS PRESERVATIVES), WATER, CORN SYRUP, SALT, WHEY, BAKING SODA, SODIUM BISULFITE (DOUGH CONDITIONER), ARTIFICIAL COLOR (YELLOW 5, YELLOW 6).

Some of the highest concentrations of BHT can be found in chewing gum and dry active yeast. And those aren't the only places they are hiding. You can find them in lots of processed foods like potato chips and oils and, get this one, food-packaging materials.

Don't think for a second that this chemmy is used as a food additive alone. Only 5 percent of this little baby is used in our food. The other 95 percent of the BHT produced is used in rubber and plastics as an antioxidant, and it's also found in liquid petroleum products like gasoline and motor oil.

I'm having a little trouble with this one. Flavor enhancers I can understand, but eating the same stuff that's in motor oil? That's harder to swallow—pardon, pardon, pardon that pun, please. But detectives we will be and detect we must—the reason for what seems to be craziness (eating drugs and toxic chemicals and not believing that there are any side effects or disease connected to it). What does it do for motor oil, and what does it do for our food?

Check out some of these facts reported by the Burton Goldberg Group:

"Many consumers eat nearly 20 milligrams or more of BHA or BHT daily."

"Babies beginning to eat solid foods are estimated to eat as much as 8 milligrams per day."

BHA in pregnant mice caused brain enzyme changes in offspring, including a 50 percent decrease in the brain activity that transmits nerve impulses. BHA and BHT "affect animals' sleep, levels of aggression, and weight." Both may "affect the normal sequence of neurological development in young animals." Possible side effects? How about

> Elevated cholesterol levels
> Allergic reactions
> Liver damage
> Kidney damage
> Infertility
> Sterility

Behavioral problems

Loss of vitamin D

Weakened immune system

Increased susceptibility to cancer-causing substances

A little scary, wouldn't you say, for chemmies that the FDA boys have approved as food additives but are "still reviewing" as of April 1994 when I gave them a call? Oh, and by the way, our brothers and sisters across the ocean in England prohibit BHT as a food additive. Might we say they are just a little more "enlightened"?

The oldest food trademark in the United States (1868) belongs to Underwood Deviled Ham.

SULFITES

Onward chemmy soldiers . . .

Have you ever had a glass of wine and felt as if your head was coming off? How about eating at some of the fast-food restaurants and getting a headache from hell? Sulfites? Remember a couple of years ago when "20/20" and a bunch of other news shows did the sulfite thing? Warning signs needed in restaurants that use sulfites. People with asthma need to be aware. Babies, pregnant women. And then it died down. The sulfite fuss died down, but the use didn't.

Go into the kitchen of most restaurants and ask them to show you the "stuff" they dip the lettuce in. I swear. Liquid that can make lettuce look fresh for months. How do you think everything at the salad bar looks as though it's just been picked? Sulfites. Yeah. Or look into the processing of the wine you're drinking and check out the sulfites, otherwise known as:

Sulfur dioxide

Sodium sulfite

Sodium bisulfite

Potassium bisulfite

Sodium metabisulfite

Potassium metabisulfite

What for? Hey, if you want color retained in dried fruits and fresh veggies—sulfites. And if those black spots in shrimp annoy you (or you don't want the people buying your product to see them)—sulfites.

In 1990 the FDA banned sulfite use on fresh potatoes, but the National Coalition of Fresh Potato Processors joined forces with some other potato companies and got the ban overthrown on a legal technicality. Makes me feel safe!

In the late 1980's at least four people died as a result of eating sulfite-treated potatoes in restaurants. Yet in 1990 sulfites are still used by commercial potato processors who provide "ready-for-frying" peeled potatoes to our restaurants.

Consumer awareness and new FDA actions slowed the number of reported adverse reactions from 1990 to 1992—but remember, the only way FDA gets this information is from voluntary consumer and physician reports!

In 1989 it was estimated that eighty thousand to one hundred thousand Americans were sensitive to sulfites.

In 1990 the FDA estimated one million Americans may be sulfite sensitive.

Asthmatics are the most at risk. Most of the reactions and reported deaths occur among asthmatics, 5 percent to 15 percent of whom are sulfite-sensitive.

Possible side effects range from diarrhea, hives, abdominal cramps, and chest tightness to elevated pulse rates, lightheadedness, and lowered blood pressure, just to name a few.

And where can you find this wonderful stuff? A 1990 pamphlet from the American Academy of Allergy and Immunology tells us it's mainly in

> Canned foods
> Frozen foods
> Dehydrated foods (for example, dried fruits)
> Processed grain foods (such as cookies and crackers)
> Shrimp
> Beer
> Wine
> Wine coolers
> . . . and the list goes on.

And what do Davey and his friends at the ol' FDA have to say about sulfites? In 1986 they banned the use of sulfites on fruits and vegetables that were sold or served raw. The same year they ruled that sulfites used as preservatives must be listed on labels no matter what amount but that sulfites used in food processing, and not as a preservative in the final food, have to be listed only if "present at levels" of 10 ppm (that's science talk for parts per million) or higher. In 1990 they extended their regulations to include standardized foods.

While they do require it to be identified on products, they don't require a warning label. But get this: They prohibit using it on important sources of thiamin (vitamin B1) because it destroys it. Does that tell you anything?

DIOXIN

If sulfites aren't enough of a headache, here's a chemical in our foods that you may not be as familiar with. Consider this one of the behind-the-scenes guys. When you think dioxin, think milk carton, microwave dinner packaging, fruit juice container. Think white, think bleaching. Then think about this:

/ⁿ/ According to Dr. Diane Courtney, dioxin is by far the most toxic chemical known to man.

/ⁿ/ Congressman Ted Weiss, chairing hearings on dioxin in 1992, said that "dioxin is unsafe at any dose."

/ⁿ/ Dioxin has been found to be toxic to lab animals at every level tested.

/ⁿ/ Dr. Arnold Schecter of the State University of New York said that according to their studies, "the fatty tissue of the average American contains about 7.2 parts per trillion of TCDD dioxin." This is a big problem for most of us but particularly for nursing mothers.

/ⁿ/ John Harte, in his book *Toxics A to Z*, reported that "the FDA estimates that for every one million average milk drinkers in the U.S., five will get cancer as a result of dioxin in milk containers."

One of the really big suppliers of dioxin in the standard American diet, which is beginning to look more like a lab test result than lunch, is milk. It's that five-out-of-a-million argument popping up again. I don't know about you, but if my child or someone I loved dearly was one of those five and died because of the deadly chemical in a milk carton, I'd be some kind of angry.

So what's the solution—glass bottles, cartons without dioxin, even if it's just some kind of acknowledgment of the poison we are talking about and movement toward a result? That's all we are talking about here.

NITRITES, NITRATES

Some of these chemicals may be new to you, but I'll bet there's one that you've heard something about over the years. Nitrites, nitrates? Have a clue what they are? They've got something to do with hot dogs and bacon, and they were big news a couple of years back, but who knows what's happened since then and who's thought about them since?

Well they're back. Actually, they didn't go anywhere. Sodium nitrite and sodium nitrate, to be exact, are used to preserve meats. Takes that meaty red color and keeps it meaty and red. They are a bit of a flavor enhancer and can be considered botulism stoppers. That's what they are used for. And side effects? Any?

They've been blamed for causing headaches and hives in some people and, more important, they've been connected to human cancer and birth defects by some sources. Frances Moore Lappé stated in her wonderful book, *Diet for a Small Planet,* that

> "even if nitrites themselves are not shown to cause cancer, nitrosamines may be formed from the nitrites either in cooking or in the digestive process, and nitrosamines have been linked to cancer."

In the 1970's our FDA buddies banned sodium nitrate from most processed meats and lowered the permitted levels of sodium nitrites, but they still don't require a warning label.

> I could actually care less at this point whether I ever eat another egg yolk or piece of bacon.   —*Betsy, Los Angeles, California*

It doesn't take a rocket scientist to figure out that the long-term effects of some of these deadly agents should have been considered *before* (the operative word here) they were sprayed on, injected into, or poured over our food. It also doesn't take a great mind to blow apart the old "it's only minuscule amounts" arguments given by the companies that are doing the adding. Think about the other side to the "minuscule amount" theory. How about adding up every small amount of all of these chemicals and telling me it isn't connected to how we are feeling?

Doesn't it make sense that if it says on the label of some of these chemicals, "Warning: causes skin irritation, could cause blindness, keep away from children," and has that skull and crossbones we all grew up knowing means don't go near it, we shouldn't be eating the stuff, even in "minuscule amounts"?

There's a new application necessary, a different interviewing technique required immediately over at the FDA. (ANOTHER VILLAGE PEOPLE HIT!). DAVID . . . (as you can see, I'm not too happy with him after reading about the chemicals) here's Interviewing 101 for your FDA staff. For every applicant who walks in the door, hold up some weed killer and ask: "Would you suggest that your two-year-old eat this, even in minuscule amounts?" If that person says yes—no job! Nothing complicated about it, is there?

We Americans consume 150 pounds of food additives per year. Yo! This has no effect? None whatsoever? Doesn't have a thing to do with how we are feeling and doesn't affect our bodies, our health, at all??

All right. Let's say for a moment—or, if you want to be like the FDA, for thirty years—that it doesn't.

That's cool.

But if you, like me when I found out about this stuff, are a little confused and want to know what you can do about those 150 pounds of food additives, the five to ten pounds of enriched vitamins, flavors, preservatives, and colored dyes that we take in a year, you may want to contact organizations, read, learn more, and make different decisions about what kind of chemicals you and your family are eating. Who knows if there are consequences connected to eating poison—are you willing to gamble on it? That's really the only question.

PESTICIDE/CHEMICAL RESOURCES

EPA (Environmental Protection Agency)   (415) 744-1510

FDA (Food & Drug Administration)   (301) 443-3170

National Coalition Against Misuse of Pesticides   (202) 543-5450

National Pesticide Tele-Communication Network   (800) 858-7378

CHAPTER 15

FOOD AND RECOVERY

*A*ddicted to drugs and alcohol? Can food help? Does what you eat have anything to do with whether or not you can get sober, stay sober and be healthy again? Come on. What next? From portion control to recovery.

When you mention food, recovery, addiction, healing, any of this stuff to most medical people, what you get back is one of those stares that lets you know they think you're a loon and have no chance of credibility now that you've let on you even think there's a connection between what you eat and something like recovery from addiction.

To say that the connection hasn't been made yet is an understatement. We're having a hard enough time figuring out that what we put in our mouths has anything to do with heart disease, cancer, and obesity. To ask most people to stretch as far as food and recovery is unreasonable. But I'm not talking to most people, I'm talking to you—and you are more than capable of entertaining the idea.

Here's where all this came from. After I changed my life and started to feel healthy and alive again, I started thinking (one of the wonderful side effects of getting well) about all the people who weren't getting this basic information about changing what they were eating, adding a little exercise, oxygen, and strength in their lives, and giving their bodies some basic things that could make such an enormous difference.

The obese, of course, were my focus—after all, look where I'd just come from. The unfit and overfat folks who wanted to look and feel better.

The sick folks of the world. People suffering from degenerative diseases. Anything we can do to make their daily lives a little easier?

The kids whacking out. The young people who were having a hard time sitting still, concentrating, functioning in this world. What if they were eating something other than sugar once in a while and got physically well? Could it do any harm to include some high-volume, low-fat, quality food and some exercise, and see what happens?

People dealing with depression? Since we know for sure that what we eat and drink, and anything else we ingest, affects our moods, was there anything we could add to an effective treatment program to make their lives easier?

Then there's addiction, something I'm all too familiar with. Isn't there anything we can do for the millions of people living their lives in the hell of addiction?

You're dying to know what that "something I'm all too familiar with" means, aren't you? Well, I'll tell you. Addiction is all over my family. It's all over most of our families, because it's all over our society.

Nicotine is a drug, and millions of us are addicted to it.

Caffeine is a big-time drug, and a morning doesn't go by when I don't have a cup of it.

Ever thought about all those chemmies in your morning cup o' coffee? The insecticides, pesticides, fungicides, defoliants, and fertilizers used to grow that little bean before it was ground up . . . the list is in the hundreds. Don't you think some of those little goodies might just be passed on to you? And how about the chemicals used to process that little bean into your morning fix?

Now, mind you, I've gone from the chemically processed to the organically grown. Gone from three heaping cups to one small cup a day, but bottom line: I'm addicted, because caffeine is a drug, and I take it in daily.

A simple goatherd in Ethiopia discovered the coffee bean in 850.

Then there's alcohol. Alcoholism—it's everywhere you look in my family. Forget about soil; our family tree was germinated in alcohol, and like most families with this disease running through its veins, all you gotta do is look back and you can find a few people in each generation who had a problem with the bottle. A nice, steady pattern that most people living in alcoholic homes who ever looked past the nose on their face know about. The experts, however, are still arguing about whether alcoholism is a genetic disease. Guys, visit with any of us who've lived with it for a day or two, we'll show you a pattern that can't be denied. But they argue on . . .

Millions of people are affected by this disease, and like so many other diseases in our society, we have spent so long talking about it, throwing the theories around, that nobody's addressing some of the practical, daily, easy-to-solve issues such as eating, breathing, and moving (pardon me, had to plug my own system) that can help anyone who's dealing with it. So what better place to talk about it than in this *Food* book? Logical place, don't you think? When you bought this book, did you figure you'd end up talking about alcoholism? Maybe not, but you gotta admit that this is very, very stage-three stuff, an interesting discussion for sure, one that I hope and pray will reach anyone who needs it.

Does what you eat have anything to do with alcoholism? How about recovery? Could the food you are or aren't eating help in any way?

"The power of nutritious food and vitamin and mineral supplements to promote healing and health in recovering alcoholics is supported both by research and clinical experience. . . . The research solidly links diet to mental as well as physical health, and the ever growing evidence points clearly to the connection that what we eat directly influences how we think and feel."

Get 'em, girls. That's straight from the fabulous book *Eating Right to Live Sober* by Katherine Ketcham and L. Ann Mueller, M.D.

"There is such a thing as a permanent end to the craving for alcohol. You can rebuild your physical as well as your emotional health."

That's a mouthful out of the mouth of Joan Larson, whose book *Seven Weeks to Sobriety* is a book and a half. Sounds right to me. This how-you-think-and-feel tagging right along with how-you-look just about says it all as far as I'm concerned. Wellness—the whole picture, here we are again!

See how we've all evolved during the three stages of this book? We started out just caring about the size of our thighs, and now it's also about how we think and feel!!! I'm so impressed with us all that I can't stand it!!! We know that eating saturated fat, cholesterol, and the old sedentary life-style can lead to disease. And it's clear that eliminating a few of the damaging things and including some of the healing things—strength; oxygen; whole, high-quality fuel; etc.—can greatly reduce the chances of and even eliminate some of these diseases. Just ask Dean Ornish about reversing heart disease.

Then why doesn't it make sense that nutrition and life-style can help with the disease of alcoholism?

It does.

It makes perfect sense.

FACT TIME:

There's only one thing that cures alcoholism, and that's not taking it in. Not drinking. Abstinence. We are not talking about the road to abstinence or whether or not to stop drinking. Getting to the point where you choose sobriety over addiction is a completely different book. We're talking about staying stopped once you choose sobriety; recovering from the physical damages that drinking causes; rebuilding a strong physical foundation to do the work of healing (common sense again raises its consistent little head, no matter what); rebuilding physically as well as doing the emotional work necessary to recover. Joan Larson says,

"Recovery is possible. Alcoholism is not a character defect. It's not a sign of weak will. It is a devastating physical disease that damages both mind and body. An enormous number of well-controlled scientific studies by distinguished researchers the world over have shown that alcohol undermines physical health and mental stability by destroying the vital nutritions responsible for their maintenance. Additional studies have shown that alcoholism can be conquered by undoing this damage."

"Aiding recovery by creating a strong physical foundation. Can it hurt?" Can anyone in his right mind deny that being healthy and strong can help you deal with recovery, that it's important and should be considered? Can anybody argue with the fact that including all the therapies, the emotional support along with the physical along with abstinence, would do more good than focusing only on half of them? If someone does, run like hell, because he's got a lot of catching up to do before he can effectively advise you.

"Eating the right foods in the right amounts and avoiding those foods that upset the body's chemistry and weaken the mental and physical health" [is what Katherine and Ann say makes a big difference]. "Most alcoholics have no idea that their diet can contribute to relapse. The most common mistake they make is to load up on sweets. For alcoholics sweets can actually be deadly, weakening sobriety to the point where the alcoholic is no longer able to fight the urge to drink."

Personal story here. As I mentioned earlier, alcoholism is all over our family, so I'm all too familiar with A.A. meetings, adult children of everything, codependent, enabling, the whole thing. I've been there from the time I was eleven years old. It was during one of my very first experiences with A.A. that I noticed something interesting. The meeting, in an old church basement, had lots of people you'd never expect to be there. Funny how when you reach out for help, you're always surprised at how many other "normal" people suffer from the same problem.

So there I was in a room filled with recovering alcoholics who were drinking lots of coffee, eating lots of sugary sweet things, and smoking lots and lots of cigarettes. Even at eleven I thought that was odd—so many people talking about one problem while they were creating a couple more. But what does an eleven-year-old know? So I concentrated on what was being said and tried like hell to be a good support person and do what I could to help solve the problem, but not enable or be the codependent supporter of this thing that was affecting our whole family.

That was then. Now, of course, you've got every kind of twelve-step program available under the sun. Political correctness like you've never. Today you'll find

> The Non-Smoking Group.
>
> The Recovery from Caffeine Group.
>
> The Gay Men Group.
>
> The Straight Men Who Accept and Love Gay Men Group.
>
> The Jewish Christian Group.
>
> The Feminist Group.
>
> The Housewives and Proud to Be Group.
>
> The Large Ladies and Glad to Be Group.

But in the days before this political correctness and a twelve-step group for every problem imaginable, it seemed a little strange that nobody was talking about anything other than hanging on from day to day and sharing with each other the problem that everyone was suffering from. How about a thirteenth step, as unlucky as it may be? What about how you are living? What you are eating? The physical health that you're in? Doesn't it make any difference at all? I swear, that's what I was thinking years and years ago sitting in my first of many twelve-step programs.

A food book author in the making, you might ask? Possibly, but back then all I knew was that I was a confused kid trying to deal with a family issue that was causing havoc in the home and craziness in my head. So I stopped thinking about it until a few years later: my cervix, the sick babies, then the extra 133, then the *Food* book and research done on all kinds of food connections . . . and there it was again. The question about alcoholism, addiction, nutrition—but this time there was an answer.

"A great majority of alcoholics suffer from varying degrees of both malnutrition and unstable blood sugar chemistry. Recovery from alcoholism must involve every aspect of the alcoholic's mental and physical being. Abstinence, body healing, and counseling."

Sounds like a good plan to me. Why the hell not? It makes sense that doing all that would make it a whole heck of a lot easier to fight alcoholism or drug addiction.

I must ask: Aren't they the same thing? Why do we separate alcoholism and drug addiction?

> Alcohol is an addictive drug.
>
> Crack is an addictive drug.
>
> Alcohol ruins lives.
>
> Crack ruins lives.
>
> Living with both is hell for everyone involved.

What's the difference? Doesn't this stuff do damage? Is it possible that blood sugar balances or imbalances are involved? A sick body that needs repair? Damage done that must be undone, including the mind and the body in recovery? Is it that simple? Is there something more we can do for people going through the process of recovery that may give them something to work with, to help them make it?

If it would help to treat the physical as well as everything else, why haven't you heard about it? Who's doing it, and how can you get the information you need if you are searching for it? Glad you asked, because we've got the answers right here.

There are some wonderful programs for working with addiction, working with abstinence, counseling, and the nutritional approach, and their results are staggering. We'll talk about them, but first . . . you're probably thinking, "What's she talking about, wonderful programs? We know it's called A.A., and she hasn't been very respectful toward a program that's helped millions of people."

Give me a minute with this one. Before every person reading this who's been through A.A.—and has the almost religious fervor that goes hand-in-hand with having been through addiction and been helped by the program—picks up his or her pen and starts slashing at me, will you do me a favor and listen to me before you defend?

A.A. is a wonderful program and has helped a lot of people. However, it's not the only answer for everyone. That's the statement that usually sets all A.A. people off. The truth is that the recovery rate in the traditional A.A. program is 15 percent to 25 percent. So not everyone who desperately needs it is being helped.

As Joan Larson says so beautifully:

"Alcoholics Anonymous does not provide treatment. It is a support group, a fellowship through which an alcoholic can become and remain abstinent with the help of other members."

Which is great, but it's not all there is. We have a monopoly thing going on with a treatment program, and it's just as dangerous as any other monopoly. When most hospitals, institutions, detention centers, and other facilities use only one program because it's considered to be the only answer, it's a problem—because it's not the only answer, it doesn't work for everyone, and there is more to recovering from addiction than the twelve steps. Where's the body in all the discussion? Hasn't half the treatment been left out? Isn't it even a consideration?

Maybe you're open to the thought that your body—healthy or unhealthy, repaired or broken—has something to do with recovery, no matter what your sponsor says. You're dealing with the problem, or thinking about dealing with the problem of alcoholism, and you want info. You've got it, but first let's wipe out a few myths so that we can get on with helpful hints, try to clear up all the muck around this issue, and help you get some answers, shall we?

Physical addiction or a sign of a weak will? Shame, guilt, can't control yourself? Baloney. All a load of crap.

"In times past, alcoholism has been seen as a weakness of will—alcoholics, it was assumed, have the same appetite for alcohol as other people, but they lacked the willpower to stop drinking. Research conducted in the last twenty years strongly indicates, however, that alcoholics have the same willpower as everyone else, but their appetite is somehow different; and this appetite for alcohol is determined by a weakness in the physical makeup of the drinker. In other words alcoholics don't abuse alcohol—alcohol abuses them."

"Alcoholism is not a character defect. It is not a sign of a weak will. It is a devastating physical disease that damages both mind and body."

Here it is, the root of the controversy. Is alcoholism a disease, or isn't it? Is it a matter of willpower or not? An emotional or physical issue? Who knows and who cares is what I have to say about it. How's that?

When it comes to recovery—recovery is recovery, and the process seems to have the same basic elements, no matter what it is you're trying to recover from. First you gotta not want to do it anymore, really not want to do it, and be ready to face and clean up the mess that addiction leaves in its trail. Then you gotta abstain. No way around that one. You can't do what you're addicted to anymore.

Support groups are always good to help with that.

Emotional help is important.

Therapy can be really beneficial.

Understanding and education, big important factors in recovery, for sure.

Facing yourself and your addiction seems to be important.

And the physical? Pretty much ignored when it comes to treatment centers around the country.

A.A. and nutritional connection? None.

State hospitals and nutrition? It ain't happening.

Jails and nutrition? Forget about it.

Juvenile detention centers? No chance in hell.

When you find out how many people are suffering from the same thing, it's a little crazy that we haven't looked into the physical connection. If you thought for a minute that you were the only one with the problem, have a look at this:

According to the Seventh Special Report to the U.S. Congress on Alcohol and Health released January 22, 1990:

- 10.5 million American adults show signs of alcoholism or alcohol dependence.

- 7.2 million show signs of "abusing alcohol" although are not yet showing signs of dependence.

- 11.2 million American adults are estimated to be alcohol dependent by 1995.

So a lot of us have a problem, and if it's help you want, then it should be help you get, and there's no reason for the physical to be ignored any longer.

Back in the days of the old basement meetings with my family, nobody knew that the foods we ate had anything to do with anything. There was no connection made between eating the sugar, sucking down the coffee, or nutritionally correcting the deficiencies that drinking causes. They never talked about working with the disease on any other level but giving your power to something other than you, and hoping like hell one day at a time that you had the control and support you needed to make it. Fair enough. Did a lot of good for a lot of people, but it also left a whole lot of people without a place to go. There's a whole lot of people who didn't make it.

After twenty years of living around and with the disease of alcoholism, I'll tell you what I've learned. Just like heart disease, it's a quiet disease. Changes start to take place in your body early on that you don't know are happening. Eating the saturated fat and cholesterol, smoking, and a sedentary life-style are some of the things that set your arteries up for rotting. Drinking sets the alcoholic's body up for cellular changes and nutritional deficiencies, "laying down the groundwork for the massive damage that occurs later." (*Eating Right to Live Sober* by Katherine Ketcham and L. Ann Mueller, M.D.)

Alcohol creates changes in our cells. We're not talking about the damage done if you're the lying-in-the-gutter kind of skid row wino we've all associated with the disease. We're talking about a respectable mother and wife living in a nice house and drinking socially with her friends. That's who's setting herself up for disaster. Cellular changing city is what's going on all over the place.

You, like the rest of your tennis partners (how stereotypical and WASPy can I be? You'll have to pardon my stereotyping, but that's what I grew up with and that's what I was sitting in A.A. meetings with. It's a personal thing I can't seem to shake, even twenty-five years later, so throw me an emotional bone, will ya?) may just be having a few drinks after the game. The problem is that your drinks affect you differently from the way theirs affect them. You're not a bad person.

"She wasn't a weak person, one of the strongest I knew, with more discipline and willpower than anyone I'd ever met, but her drinks affected her differently than her friends' drinks did. It's during this early stage of the disease that she didn't even know there was anything wrong with her. No symptoms. This disease takes time. The shame, the guilt, the disease—it all built slowly until it was such a mess, with so many people involved, that it took a face-down-in-the-gutter experience to have a look at what was going on and make her see that it had to end."

The pain and suffering that go on during the course of this horrendous disease cannot be described. Anyone growing up in an alcoholic home or dealing with the disease, or living with trying to hide the disease, knows exactly what I'm talking about when I say it takes years for all those exposed to it to sort it all out.

Like heart disease, alcoholism doesn't come easy. You gotta work at it. Constantly poisoning your cells. And like heart disease, it's socially acceptable, of course!!! I mean, it's not as if you're putting a needle in your arm, eating that butter, drinking that drink, are you?

"If she'd gone in for a checkup, no doctor in the world would have seen the early stages of this disease—not then, 'cause they didn't know about malnutrition and alcoholism, and they still don't. Blood sugar and alcoholism. No clue. Very, very few doctors even considering it. Forget about including it in treatment."

While the groundwork is being done, you don't feel sick, you aren't craving the stuff, you're not drinking any more than anyone else. Hey, think about heart disease. You keep eating the steak, put the butter on the potatoes, have a few cigarettes, don't have time to exercise—laying that pavement—and bammo! You wake up one day with heart disease. How'd that happen? Why you? And what can you do about it?

Think about this. You drink the alcohol. Your body doesn't deal with it the same way the bodies of people who aren't alcoholics do. You're an alcoholic. Your cells are being damaged; your brilliant machine adapts by adjusting to the presence of what for you is poison. Everything is affected by this stuff. Alcohol and acetaldehyde, the poisonous by-product of alcohol, screw up the electrical and chemical signals in this brain of ours (have we become one during the reading of this book?).

Your liver? Forget about it. There's something in your liver called mitochondria, tiny little things within each cell that help release energy from food. If it's an alcoholic you're looking at, even in the paving stages of this disease:

"The liver mitochondria are noticeably altered: While normal mitochondria are round with clearly defined outer walls and inner structures, in alcoholics the walls stretch, becoming enlarged and misshapen, and the inner structures are visibly distorted." (*Eating Right to Live Sober* by Katherine Ketcham and L. Ann Mueller, M.D.)

Do you know what the cellular change means? It means that you can drink more and more. And anyone who has sat next to this beast of a disease will tell you that's exactly what starts happening before you know it. It may take years, but you can bet that if you're looking at a drinking problem, you're looking at your alcohol intake increasing. It never decreases.

Textbook. This disease never gets better and doesn't go away. It always gets worse. Varying degrees of worse but always worse.

Next stage. Unable to stop once you get started? Drinking more than you planned? Drinking differently than others do? And knowing it. Not admitting it, but in your soul knowing that your drinking is different.

You see those commercials—"Hey, bartender, just one more—" and you get that cold feeling inside whenever the truth hits you upside your head. Have a glass of wine with your friends and start to notice that you're three to one on them. Watching people who just have a few sips of their wine and leave the rest—knowing you'd never do that.

One hangover too many, and getting more and more severe. Wondering if you acted like an idiot and discreetly checking what happened the night before when you were out with your friends?

Knowing it isn't funny anymore. Glimpses of the truth and not being able to face it because you're afraid. If you are an alcoholic and you're drinking at all, damage is being done. And it ain't pretty what's happening physically.

> "Alcoholism does not do its damage cleanly, nor does it concentrate its attack in one easy-to-reach part of the body. Instead it requires a messy, complex clean-up job that takes time, patience, and a considerable amount of effort for the healing to be complete." (*Eating Right to Live Sober* by Katherine Ketcham and L. Ann Mueller, M.D.)

Bad news for anyone suffering from this disease? No. Because at last we are finally talking about healing. Not white-knuckle sobriety, the old dry drunk, the craving that never ends, and the dread that so many alcoholics live in from day to day, hoping that they won't lose the whatever they are supposed to hang on to. There's more to recovery than just living with it and fighting against it emotionally.

Consider the concept of nutritional support another life vest in the rough waters of recovery. (Is that too corny? Just what I felt while I was typing this, but I had to throw it in.)

> "To counteract the damage caused by years of drinking, the alcoholic must strengthen his defenses, making himself as strong as possible. An essential part of this building and maintaining body strength is good nutrition." (*Eating Right to Live Sober* by Katherine Ketcham and L. Ann Mueller, M.D.)

That's all we are talking about here.

> "Most alcoholics don't realize that alcohol, in addition to its direct poisonous effects on organs such as the liver, heart, brain, and stomach, works indirectly as a sort of nutritional vacuum cleaner sucking up vit-

amins and minerals and leaving the body with numerous deficiencies."
(*Eating Right to Live Sober* by Katherine Ketcham and L. Ann Mueller,
M.D.)

Don't you think that being a walking nutritional deficiency has got to make
the emotional, spiritual, and recovery work that faces anyone dealing with
this monster more difficult? Come on, everyone, let's get off our twelve-step
high horse and consider something that could help millions of people who
are suffering.

What is this stuff that we all grow up thinking is the fun at the party? The
relaxation at the end of a hard day. One of the big keys to the "good life," for
sure. Do you want to know more about it?

Alcohol is considered a food. Did you know that? It's a food because it has
calories. Every ounce of this stuff gives your body about 70 calories. Small
amount of food, lots of calories. But the problem with this alcohol-as-fuel theory is that it's missing something—any nutritional value at all. It's not something you want to be using as food, as many late-stage alcoholics tend to do.
Forget about eating nutritionally when most of your calories are coming from
a bottle. When you're addicted to something, your first thought isn't a good
high-quality, low-fat meal. Whatever you're addicted to tends to override just
about anything after a while. Haven't we seen enough movies-of-the-week
to know that by now?

It's still fuel, though, and quick-absorbing energy at that. Your body
doesn't have to work too hard to digest this stuff, and very quickly and efficiently your cells have the fuel they need, but there's a catch.

"Cells . . . need continual and careful maintenance if they are to stay
healthy and carry on their normal everyday functions, but they won't get
any help from alcohol, which provides only energy. Without the proper
nutrition, damaged cell parts cannot be replaced, new cell materials cannot be created, and the cells cannot build or replenish tissues and organs. If the cells are continually denied nutrients for too long, if they are
denied even just one nutrient, they will weaken, become sick, and eventually die." (*Eating Right to Live Sober* by Katherine Ketcham and L. Ann
Mueller, M.D.)

Weaken the foundation by taking in poison—alcohol.
Weaken the foundation by clogging it all up—saturated fat.
Weaken the foundation by not getting oxygen to every cell and muscle in
your body—unfit.
What, what, what are we talking about here? Seems to me we are talking

about the same thing, just different symptoms (diseases) of the same problem: overloading our bodies with stuff that damages and not giving our bodies the stuff we must have. When we don't, there's trouble. Different kinds of trouble, for sure, but trouble all the same. Screwing up the system that works pretty damn well in all kinds of ways—and who doesn't do it? We all do things that screw up our bodies, and we probably always will. It's your life and your body. What we are talking about here are some of the big issues surrounding health in this country today.

Getting the information.

Finding out about the options.

Making them make a little sense and opening it all up for discussion.

Here's a thought: how about working with your body and supporting it more than screwing it up are really what this is all about. Just knowing enough to know that there is a nutritional connection is a huge start for most of us. I mean, think about this: If "alcohol can produce changes in the digestive system that lead to interference in the absorption and use of nutrients in the body," (*Eating Right to Live Sober* by Katherine Ketcham and L. Ann Mueller, M.D.), and it can, then wouldn't you think that it can be interfering with the whole system? The important stuff going on inside your body that keeps it all balanced and functioning properly?

I'm not a doctor, nutritionist, or recovery expert. I'm just someone who has lived with this problem for more of my thirty-six years than I want to think about. When three out of five members of the family are hit with the same problem, and every relative for as far back as you look has dealt with it, please don't tell me that there isn't a physical, genetic connection going on. When I see people I love struggling with recovery and can clearly see a mood change after a huge bowl of ice cream, don't tell me what you eat doesn't affect you.

This book is about food, not about addiction. My goal in bringing this up at all is to open up discussion about the possibility of food being connected to alcoholism. And if you have experienced that cold, scary feeling of truth when you hear the commercials, watch other people drink normally, feel the horrendous shame when you're too hung over to go to your kids' school play, I want to say that the best books I've ever read about this disease are the following:

 Eating Right to Live Sober by Katherine Ketcham and L. Ann Mueller, M.D.

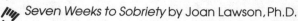 *Seven Weeks to Sobriety* by Joan Lawson, Ph.D.

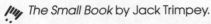 *The Small Book* by Jack Trimpey.

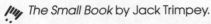 *Many Roads, One Journey* by Charlotte Kasl.

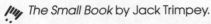 *The Truth About Addiction and Recovery* by Stanton Peele, Ph.D., and Archie Brodsky with Mary Arnold.

I'll tell ya what I really believe.

"If she had had this information, she might have been healed, not just sober. Life would have been so very much easier for the people who loved her. I would have understood more about the physical turmoil that she lived in daily, even with the strength and courage that she had in not drinking for the last fifteen years of her life. . . . We may have had a chance to have her in our lives, but nobody told her or us."

If you're interested in additional information:

RECOVERY RESOURCE LIST

Rational Recovery Systems
Jack Trimpey, LCSW
Box 100
Lotus, CA 95651
(916) 621-4374

Save Ourselves or Secular Sobriety
 (SOS)
James Christopher
P.O. Box 5
Buffalo, NY 14215-0005
(716) 834-2921

Women for Sobriety and Men for
 Sobriety
P.O. Box 618
Quakertown, PA 18951
(215) 536-8026

Alcoholics Anonymous
P. O. Box 454
Grand Central Station
New York, NY 10017
(212) 686-1100

OTHER USEFUL
PHONE NUMBERS

Adcare Hospital Helpline
1 (800) 252-6465

Alcohol and Drug Helpline
1 (800) 821-4357
1 (801) 272-4357 (in Utah)

CHAPTER 16
SEXUALITY AND NUTRITION

$\mathcal{S}ex$ and diet. Sex and health. Sex and self-esteem. Sex and the way you look and feel. Wow. Talk about a big subject and one that I've got to spend some time on because I've been in the middle of this discussion more times than you can imagine. You see, when I weighed 260 pounds, my sex life wasn't so great. Forget about the fact that I hated the way I looked naked. Let's talk here. Even if you have the self-esteem of a completely functional, well-loved, worked-through-all-the-issues-in-therapy, totally clear, loves-her-self-more-than-anybody kind of person, you still can't say that 260 and naked is a pretty picture—'cause it ain't, I promise you.

Naked and 260—doesn't scream romping around in bed full of confidence, at least it didn't in my life. Naked at 260—we're not talking feeling very sexy. Naked and 260—there were not a lot of body parts that I could look at with-out running for cover, forget about sharing the view with anybody else.

Now this would be the time for anyone who believes that how we look shouldn't have an effect on us at all, and that what other people think about us means absolutely nothing, never will, and never should, and that it's only the surfacey, insecure, unintelligent folks of the world who would let some-thing like a hundred-plus-pound weight gain affect their sex life to put this book down and not read this chapter, because I'm about to tell everyone reading this about the reality of what it did to my sex life.

It very much affected my sex life. It didn't look or feel sexy to me. The flab, the fat, the jiggly stuff all over my body wasn't my idea of good-looking. But I always hate getting caught up in the self-esteem issue. It's a never-ending argument about whether or not sexy should mean certain body images, skinny, the media's idea of what's sexy, what men want, what women have the right to have, blah, blah, blah.

First, you'll never hear me talking skinny. We're talking fit and strong and a healthy percent of body fat here. Second, I couldn't care less what men say they want or don't want in a woman. And third, this isn't about and never has been about what the media think looks good. It's always been about being well, being healthy, taking your body and making it as lean, as strong, and as healthy as YOU want it to be. That's what I'm talking about.

And finally, finally, I found someone who was talking the same language as I was when it came to sex and wellness. This guy and his book—I loved it. Dr. Morton Walker, *Sexual Nutrition*. Check it out, because it's full of great information about sexuality and wellness.

So those who are about to give up on this food book because they are convinced that I'm a surfacey, stereotyping person who's contributing to the image of the waif or nothing and that I am totally unhealthy and screwed up when it comes to a healthy body image and sexuality—calm down. I am surfacey, but I'm not contributing to any stereotype of a skinny, waify woman or "no sex life for you, babe." I am very much contributing to and promoting wellness when it comes to your living up to and having the wonderful advantage of a healthy sex life and a healthy body. The two go hand in hand no matter what you look like.

You see, I have something on my side in this little discussion. If you are well and healthy, you will be lean and strong.

You can't be fat and healthy.

You can be fat and flexible.

You can be fat and strong.

You can be fat and have good cardio endurance.

But you can't be fat and healthy, because fat isn't healthy and nobody can argue with that one.

So even though we are not talking skinny, we are talking a healthy percentage of body fat, strong, and well. See how one feeds the other?

Does your sexual appetite, (pardon that pun) have anything to do with what you eat? How can it not be connected to your diet is the better question. Of course it is. But let's let the doctor explain. After all, he's the expert. (Aren't you dying to know what his sex life is like? Imagine the burden of being a sex expert. You'd have to be really, really good in bed. I mean, how could you not?)

"Sexual dysfunction is a degeneration of body parts. It can encompass a number of different organs or systems including the mind, nerves, genitals, endocrine glands, or blood vessels. Diet-related problems with sexuality that commence in [your] twenties or thirties and steadily increase [into your] forties and fifties and later ages are often tied to overeating, improper selection of foods, and lack of exercise."

Here it is again, that slow-building damage thing that we are seeing over and over again, laying the groundwork for heart disease, cancer, alcoholism, laying the pavement for disaster, and now sex. It's the common thread in each of these areas. Diet and exercise. Diet and exercise. Diet and exercise. Connection number two.

Whether you call it unintelligent decision-making or just not getting the information about what's killing us and what isn't, we are all talking about the same basic things. And it's the same answer to most of the problems that I think Doc Morton puts so well. (Of course, he's talking about sexuality because that's probably all he ever talks about. Imagine being at a cocktail party and saying you're a sex expert for a living—talk about igniting everyone's curiosity.)

"To be a homeostatic lover you need to focus on achieving and maintaining good health along with giving and receiving sexual fulfillment. At a high level of wellness you function at your greatest potential."

Love this!! Wellness. High level of. Functioning at your greatest potential. See, the same thing we've been talking about all along, but this time it's connected to how many times a day, week, or month you may get that wonderful feeling when you look at the person you love and lock the bedroom door for a few short minutes of pleasure before the phone rings, the kids need you, the boss starts demanding, the bills need paying. Remember when nothing was as important as being with the person you love? When you were dying to make love with him or her? Isn't that the greatest feeling in the world?

That spark. That tingling inside. That physical release when you finally make love. I may have to take a cold shower in the middle of writing this chapter. Hey, maybe I'll just turn the computer off and give the husband a call. The kids are in camp, and he's working on his music. Must have been that great breakfast I ate this morning that's feeding this sexual frenzy 'cause, boy oh boy, is what we eat connected directly to our sex drive, and what we are not getting is directly connected to our lack of it.

"The results of a national survey conducted by the U.S. Department of Agriculture indicated that out of 7,500 average American families, only half had diets that met the Recommended Dietary Allowances for calories, protein, iron, calcium, magnesium, vitamin A, thiamin (vitamin B1), riboflavin (vitamin B2), and vitamin C. Industrialized peoples consume too many refined, processed, canned, frozen, precooked, or ready-to-serve items in place of fresh, whole foods. They drink an overabundance of soft drinks, alcoholic beverages, coffee, tea, and water polluted with toxic heavy metals. The price that is paid for such faulty food habits is low-level health."

You can't argue with the man when it comes to that very well said statement. If you've made it this far in this book, then you know there is very much a connection between what you are putting in your mouth and the way you look and feel.

But if you're like me, you may never have thought about the way you feel—as in sexually stimulated when you look at the one you love, that tingly feeling that may have been missing in your life for a while without your really giving much thought to where it's gone.

No time—sure that contributes to the lack of lovemaking. Stress—absolutely affects everything. Married or together for a long time and you think the flame just naturally dies—probably true. I've never been married long enough to test that theory. But what about the flame inside you?

Your spark. Your sexual appetite. Your desire for sex. Did you ever think it could be decreased or increased just by what you put into your body (don't even think about that pun—I know you did!!—I'm being mature and responsible and letting it pass). The doctor has an opinion on that one:

"Although health authorities do not agree on the precise role diet plays in sexual dysfunction [surprise, surprise, health authorities not agreeing; unusual, isn't it?], they generally do agree that diet is a major factor in many serious degenerative diseases. In the United States alone, the incidence of degenerative disease has reached more than one-half of the adult population, a staggering 125 million people. High-level wellness does not mean simply that you are not sick. It means that you are trim, eat properly, enjoy sexual relations, regularly exercise, sleep soundly, do not smoke, and do not drink to excess. You have learned to relax deeply and completely, and you know how to counterbalance stress."

I must say that all these years that I've been out there talking wellness, I left out the "enjoy sexual relations regularly" part. Sure, sex is different now from when I was 260, and finally I can get away from the argument that it's only about my self-esteem improving directly along with my body image—because it's about more than that, according to the good doctor, and I've got story after story to back that up.

You think I'm gonna spend the next few pages telling you sexually explicit stories, don't you? Well, I'll be very explicit about coming back to life sexually and what happened to me as I got well, but if it's some great sex stories you're looking for, then forget it, because not much was going on sexually as I was changing my body. Sure, I got energy as soon as I started to eat, breathe, move, and get well, but it wasn't as if weeks into it I was on the sexual hunt. When I say energy I mean just enough to get through the day. Forget about any activity other than getting the laundry done and the kids to bed, that was it.

Lacking a sex drive? Your sex drive in the gutter? Don't you think it may have something to do with not having the energy you need to do the basics? The experts can argue about this till they're blue in the face, but I can tell you right now that it does. It did for me. Getting well: The stronger I got, the more body fat I burned off, the more energy that came back into my life. Slowly the sexual energy that had been in a deep coma started to come back. It wasn't connected to a man or to my lousy self-esteem because I couldn't be with a man even if I had been looking good, because there wasn't a man in sight. After what I'd just been through with my ex-husband, the last thing on earth I was interested in was going out with a man.

That's not what ignited me. I just ignited. Who knew then what happened? I just know that I began thinking about lovemaking, romantic connections, sex—and it just happened, came back from the dead. Now I know it was all a part of getting well, healing, giving my body what it needed to live—and living was what it was doing.

Sexual thoughts, dreams, desires started flooding back into my life, and I was thrilled. It took me a while to know what to do with them, because it had been a while and things had changed. I was a divorced single mom, whereas before I was just a young, selfish (selfish goes with youth, they say; don't ask me who "they" are) girlfriend of Nic's. Talk about a big sexual turnaround, an adjustment, and some new things that needed to be considered.

I needed to set boundaries. I needed to formulate rules, and to think about a whole lot before I talked about dating any man. But that didn't stop my body from feeling or my mind from thinking about sex, and it was great to have it back in my life. Apparently this wellness thing includes everything about how we feel and think, how we look, the condition of our bodies.

> Every 120 days, every red blood cell in your body dies and is reborn, replaced.
> It's replaced or reborn from what you put in your mouth. The food we eat builds
> cells, feeds and nourishes our bodies, and is the most direct interaction we have
> with our planet.
>
> —*Dr. Marc Micozzi*

What a concept. We are what we live. The better we live, the better we are.
The worse we live, the more destruction we live with. Whether it's a heart
that doesn't work too well anymore because its not getting enough blood and
oxygen, or a sex life that isn't happening because you aren't getting enough
blood and oxygen into your body, what's the difference?

"Sexual responsiveness and sexuality require a healthy internal signal-
ing system of nerves, brain, gonads; [thought that was a made-up word
until I read this book; I swear, I couldn't believe it was real], endocrine
glands, blood vessels, and other parts. The fact is that sexual desire
along with the ability to fulfill sexual desire is greatly affected by physical health."

Damn. I knew it. It had to do with something more than the pictures in the
magazines that were supposedly brainwashing me. I never believed that theory. Please. When my body is strong, healthy, and looking the way I want it
to look, I don't walk around pining for the body of someone who's skinnier
than me. Now I have seen some backsides that I'd pay good money to own.
And hair, don't ask. When I see a full curly head of the stuff . . . I can't wait
for the day when hair transplants are better than those plug things. I'll be the
first in line when you can buy Cindy Crawford's mane. But that's not because
I'm brainwashed about body image or about what someone else thinks is at-
tractive. It's because she's got great hair and I don't, that's all. I still love myself, I just like her hair better. What's the problem with that?
The doctor's view is something that makes just a bit more sense to me.

"My premise is that a healthy body enjoys greater sexuality than does an
unhealthy body. Sexy has in many ways come to mean healthy, and
health is brought about in large measure by the quality of what is consumed."

Good point, but why do these guys talk like that? Well said, you have to
admit, but heavy, very heavy. Pardon me for interrupting . . .

"Today being sexy means for both men and women being well nour-
ished, fit, and trim, being active and vital."

When you think about it, sex is pretty physical. When you're in the middle of some good lovemaking, you are pretty much using your whole body,
unless your religion teaches you that moving is wrong. (Sorry. Grew up sur-
rounded by the old-missionary-position Catholic jokes; had to put that in
there.)

> When you think sex, think strong muscles.
> Healthy heart rate—sex.

Did you know that when you have an orgasm, your heart rate can elevate
anywhere between 140 to 180 beats per minute? When you think about the
fact that 70 beats per minute is normal, that's what you call an elevated heart
rate. Now stay that way for thirty minutes or more, and you'd be . . . dead.
But bring it down a bit and jump on a stationary bike, and you'd be aerobic.
I'll let the doctor explain what else happens during sex:

"The genital muscles of both partners go through a patterned series of
contractions. All the muscles of their bodies react much like the genitals
by contracting involuntarily."

Sounds good to me and doesn't sound as if we can argue with the fact that
sex is a very physical thing and that having a healthy, well-nourished, strong
body can't do anything but make it better.

> Stamina.
> Endurance.
> Healthy blood flow.
> Oxygen pumping.
> Muscles contracting left, right, and center.

Let's start to include more of this stuff into our discussions of sex, and less
about self-esteem, loving ourselves, and all the other stuff that's been talked
about ad nauseam.

And until the experts agree, let's get down to some facts about what may
be affecting your sex life and a few things that you may never have thought
about:

"To help protect yourself against or control ailments involving the sex organs, authorities recommend a diet that is low in fats (especially saturated fats), cholesterol, salt, sugar, and other refined or concentrated foods and high in fresh fruits, fresh vegetables, and protein from plant sources."

Well, I'll be damned. Doesn't it amaze you how many problems are connected to just a few little things in our average American diet? How can so few things do so much damage? This high-cholesterol level that we have by taking in so much saturated fat is causing a hell of a lot of problems. How about that enormous sugar intake that we are living (or dying) on? Or the un-food—the frozen, instant stuff that after processing gives us very little value for our money? How about whole food instead—something off a tree once in a while. Something that grows from the ground that hasn't been processed to the point of needing enrichment.

Seems we keep bumping up against the wall of good, solid, basic food rules when it comes to talking about a whole lot of symptoms.

> The biblical rules of food.
> The basics of good health.
> The 1, 2, 3 of getting rid of a whole lot of problems.

Call them whatever you want, but you can't get away from the facts when they are as clear as daylight.

You remember when I was talking about the clarity and the monks? What starts to happen when you heal the body, get healthy? Slowly my body came back to life and everything with it, including sex.

When you talk to the sex experts about what to look out for, you hear the same old thing:

"A diet too high in protein, putting strain on the liver."

Heard that before, connected to a lot of problems?

"Elevated blood sugar levels. The nerves, brain, and gonads depend on blood sugar in the form of glucose. When the glucose serum level drops too low, the organs and systems utilized for sex are weakened."

Here's the difference between eating tons of sugar and having a bowl of brown rice. Instant, quick, no nutritional value, or a whole lot of value that gives your body what it needs to function—sexually function, if you will.

You won't believe what else the good doctor suggests.

"Chewing your food."

True. Can you believe it? Taking us right back to stage one in a big, big way.

"Chewing your food thoroughly is the first step in proper digestion and also brings out the full flavor of whole unrefined natural foods."

Stress—talk about the basics of good health. These things go hand in hand with avoiding the things that are killing us.

"Use meditation or other relaxation techniques. Deep-breathing exercises. Plenty of exercise. Collective actions smooth the metabolism of what you eat to keep your blood sugar normally elevated in accordance with your sexual requirements."

Summing up the sexual 1, 2, 3's: We are talking your sexual health being directly connected with your physical health. And when it's health and food we are talking about, it seems that we always end up at the same few points.

> Fat.
> Cholesterol.
> Sugar.
> Refined foods.
> Chemicals.
> Cut back on.

Seems to be the same ending to a hundred different stories.

> Heart disease.
> Obesity.
> Sexual dysfunction.
> Cancer.
> Recovery.

And some good suggestions:

Increasing whole foods.

Getting the nutrients that your body needs to live and thrive on.

Exercise.

Stress reduction.

A healthy body, healthy gonads.

"Sex can be supreme, but it requires work." Dr. Morton Walker.

"Life can be supreme, but you gotta be well." Susan Powter.

CHAPTER 17

BEAUTY AND FOOD

I know you've tried the old cucumber-on-the-eyes trick at least once in your life. And after a long night, which of you hasn't steeped the tea, sucked down the caffeine, and put the tea bags over your swollen eyes for just a few minutes, wondering if it really works? Now that you know where all the fat and cholesterol are in your eggs (the yolks) and it's egg whites or nothing for you—egg whites will be working overtime in your home. Egg whites cooking in everything you ever used to prepare with whole eggs, and egg whites all over your face for the stiffest facial in the land—can those things harden, or what?

Ah, but there is more to the food-and-beauty connection than meets the cucumber over the eye. Sure, we're talking big information compared to what's in the monthly tips column of your favorite fashion magazine. We're talking beauty from the inside. Internal. Beauty and food as in what you eat and what you look like.

If ever there was an argument to be made to the believers that food and lifestyle don't have much to do with how you look, seems to me all you'd need to do is look at people who have been living the standard burgers-and-fries, drinking-lots-of-coffee, all-stressed-out, had-a-little-too-much-to-drink-and-smoke kind of life, and then check out those who've been eating right, exercising, not smoking, maybe meditating once in a while, and generally taking good care of themselves.

Come on. You've seen that ragged-looking guy or gal and turned to a friend and whispered, "He/she looks like he's been dragged home by the back of the horse" (or is this the first time you've heard that stupid expression?). I know you've met people who, during the course of conversation, mention that they are forty, while you've been thinking the whole time that they look ninety-eight . . . I'm not talking ugly, I'm talking haggard, old, unhealthy looking, which pretty much means ugly, doesn't it?

Here's where the road crosses in this beauty and food discussion. There's a big, heated debate over one thing—the definition of beauty. What does beautiful mean? Who defines the standard? What is healthy or unhealthy in trying to live up to beautiful? How far will we go? And so on and on and on and on . . . It's as never-ending and long-winded as the "what defines a healthy body image?" issue, and as far as I'm concerned, just as easy to clear up. We'd better clear it up now so we can get on with an uninterrupted Beauty Hour with Susan Powter, Food P.I.

Nobody defines beauty.

Beautiful means every human being under the sun.

No matter how hard you and I may try, we will not look like Sophia Loren, Elizabeth Taylor, Catherine Deneuve, Racquel Welch, Katharine Hepburn . . . it just doesn't happen. Some people are astoundingly beautiful. You know it when you see them. Some people are very, very good-looking. Some people have a look that's unique, fresh, appealing, striking; others physically miss the mark. Some people are ugly—what's the matter with saying that? Just like some people have magnificent bodies—they just do.

> What's magnificent or beautiful?
>
> What makes you gasp for air when you see it?
>
> What rocks your boat?

I don't know, but I do know it when I see what I think is beautiful—whether it's a nice face or great arms or beautiful bone structure or great hair or perfect skin.

I've got a little statement to make and an explanation to follow that's gonna clear up all the muck in the beautiful-or-not-beautiful argument once and for all. Beauty, just like a healthy body, is attainable by anyone. Making your body beautiful and healthy means taking what you were born with—whether your legs are long or short or you don't have any—and making it as lean, as strong, and as healthy as you want it to be.

And the same thing applies to your face. Whether it looks like it's been chiseled from stone or it's kind of crumpled looking, making it as radiantly healthy looking as you want it to be—that's beautiful. And that has a hell of a lot to do with how you live, what you're eating.

Our friend Doctor John McDougall said something in one of our conversations that fascinated me. (Yeah, just one thing!!! Do you like that? The man has amazed me with his information since I started reading everything I could get my hands on ten years ago—you know what I mean?)

"The American diet makes us ugly. It makes us pimply, pussy, swollen, gray, greasy, diseased, and ugly."

Gag me for just a moment, wouldn't you, doc??? Big statement. But when you spend a second thinking about it, isn't it true?

I haven't lied to you yet, and I'm not starting now. But if I were to suggest for a second that looking fresh, clean, or anything close to that ever crossed my mind when I thought about changing my body, then you could chalk me up as the biggest liar ever, because it didn't. It was the heart attack or at least the loss-of-consciousness kind of response that I wanted desperately to happen the minute someone who'd been mean to me, refused to date me, or made me feel bad about my life saw me minus 100-plus big ones. A gasp for air was more like what I expected, not comments like . . .

"You look so much younger than your age."
"Your skin looks so pretty."
"You glow with energy and health!!!"

. . . not even a thought!!!!

But you know what happened? Nobody had a heart attack when he saw me after many years (although there were some wonderful moments of sweet revenge and there still are). Instead, it's the "healthy," "glowy," "you look good" comments that I hear all the time. And in my newfound maturity, these comments have started to mean quite a bit to me. (Not to say that I'd rather have them over a good pain in the chest for a couple of people still on my newly revised, mature revenge list, but it's nice to hear "You look healthy" or "You glow with energy." Who'd have thunk it back then?)

> I feel so great. Even though I really feel I'm eating more, it doesn't leave me feeling tired, stuffed, greasy, or bloated.
>
> —*Avery, Sherman, Texas*

Since beauty is more than skin deep (did I just change a very famous, very old expression to suit my needs, or did I get it right?), then let's start with skin.

Nothing simple about it. Your skin makes up about 15 percent of your body weight. (Glad I didn't know that during the old diet days—there were times when I would have considered being skinned alive to drop 15 pounds). Did you also know your skin takes up about one third of your body's circulation?

Back to the haggard-looking guys and gals of the world—whenever I've run into them, it was the condition of their skin that usually left a lasting impression on me, and anyone who knows you have pounds and pounds of skin and still says that how it ends up looking has nothing to do with the food you eat is out of his mind.

Hear this:

"The health of the epidermis, dermis, sebum, fatty layer, and connective tissues depends on the quality of nutrients they receive from the bloodstream."

At least that's what Aveline Kushi has to say about it. Just like the old sex organs—pardon the personal reference, but can you blame me? We keep hearing the same thing over and over again. The quality of the nutrients you put in seems to have a lot to do with a lot of things.

"Nutrients provided by food are absorbed into the bloodstream and supplied to the cells of the skin."

Take a guess at which foods may be not so good for your skin. What do you think? High-fat foods—they seem to be doing not too well all around.

"Eating too many foods high in cholesterol and saturated fat contributes to hardening of the skin and can give it a tight, dry, and weatherbeaten look."

That's a more polite way of saying "haggard" and "dragged home by the back of a horse."

And guess what else can age you quicker than a cheating husband (there it is, Country Western hit number 4 or 5, at least, from this *Food* book)? The drinking, the smoking, the stress—sure, right along with the nasty saturated fat and cholesterol. Look at what some of the experts have said.

ALCOHOL

"Inhibits the body's ability to use certain nutrients, especially zinc, potassium, and magnesium, and alters the rate of absorption of calcium, folic acid, vitamins B6 and B12, and thiamin."

—The Canyon Ranch Health and Fitness Program

"Use of alcohol seriously depletes the body's magnesium supply. Since our usual daily intake of magnesium is low, drinking alcohol as a regular habit can lead to serious problems."

—*Maggie's Woman's Book* by Maggie Lettvin

"All types of alcohol encourage internal dehydration, leach much-needed moisture from the dermis, and destroy the B-complex vitamins.

Skin tissue consists of 20 percent water and, as alcohol leads to dehydration, it should be avoided by those whose skin is the slightest bit dry or sensitive.

Alcohol also dilates the fragile blood vessels in the face, encouraging the tiny capillaries to expand and burst.

Skin rashes are often triggered by the additives or chemical colorants routinely added to wine and liqueur drinks, and virtually all wine contains sulphur dioxide which is also known to cause skin blotchiness."

—*Save Your Skin with Vital Oils* by Liz Earle

SMOKING

"Slows the circulation of blood to your skin, releases clouds of dry, dirty smoke into your face, and makes you purse your lips and squint on a regular basis . . . Smoking regularly can age the skin up to ten years."

—The Canyon Ranch Health and Fitness Program

"Smokers suffer from chronic respiratory diseases. Smoking diminishes the supply of oxygen to the body."

—*Every Woman's Health* by D. S. Thompson, M.D.

STRESS

"The most common instigator of skin boils, eruptions, etc." [yuucckk!]

—*Nutrition Almanac* by Lavon Dunne

"Nothing shows up faster on the face than the tension and stress that quickly builds up during a busy working day.

The muscles in our faces and necks can soon become hardened into a fixed expression, and our brows become knotted together into an irreversible form."

—*Save Your Skin with Vital Oils* by Liz Earle

And even though nobody has proven conclusively or pinpointed exactly how a healthy lifestyle affects the aging process, makes skin look better, and helps you look healthier and more beautiful, all you have to do is look at people who are living a good healthy lifestyle and people who aren't—or ask me, because losing my weight, increasing my awareness of foods, and changing what I ate absolutely changed my complexion and added a shine to my eyes (as Ivory commercial as that sounds, it's true).

If it's a glow you're looking for, check out some of the good glow foods:

• •

Good Skin Food Chart

Vitamin	Best Sources	Effects
A	carrots, winter squash, rutabaga, yellow or orange vegetables, broccoli, kale, dark green leafy vegetables	keeps skin elastic; prevents dryness, wrinkling, unnatural aging
B2	whole grain, beans, leafy green vegetables	protects eyes, skin, mucous membranes
B3 (Niacin)	whole grains, beans, leafy vegetables, shitake mushrooms, seeds and nuts, fish and seafood	promotes healthy circulation keeping adequate supply of oxygen and nutrients to skin, hair, nails
B5	whole grains, broccoli, cabbage, green vegetables, cauliflower, corn, sunflower seeds, unrefined vegetable oil	anti-stress vitamin, helpful in reduction of skin inflammations
B6	whole grain, brown rice, buckwheat flour, beans, carrots, cabbage, sunflower seeds, fresh fish	valuable in functioning of skin, nerves, hormone production
B9 (Folic acid)	whole grains, green leafy vegetables, tempeh	aids in red blood cell formation, body's utilization of fats

continued

C	broccoli, mustard greens, kale, parsley, watercress, turnip greens, cabbage, leafy greens, strawberries, cantaloupe, cherries, apricots, fresh seasonal fruits	cooperates with protein in the formation of collagen and elastin, both essential for soft well-toned skin
D	sunlight, fish liver oils	promotes calcium absorption essential in formation of bones and teeth
E	green leafy vegetables, whole grains, soybeans, beans	keeps skin healthy and youthful by slowing the aging of cells resulting from the interaction of oxygen with other chemicals in the body

Adapted from: *Diet for Natural Beauty,* by Aveline Kushi

• •

You don't need to spend a fortune once you know the glow foods. Just go to your cupboard.

What you put in affects what you look like on the outside, but so does what you put on.

Yogurt: can be applied externally as a deep cleanser for the skin.

Mustard oil: a natural skin cleanser. It drains toxins from the pores and is very healing.

Olive oil: very good when applied to the skin.

Chidee (liquid from yogurt after draining through cheese cloth): mixed with ground sandalwood, almond oil, and garbanzo flour to make a paste, then massaged into the face until cheeks are red to soften the complexion.

Cucumber and papaya skins: beneficial as a facial rub.

Milk: rub your hands with milk for several minutes, wash them in warm water, then soak them in milk for several minutes. Rinse with clear water.

Potatoes: make a paste from ground potatoes and use it for burns.
—from *Foods for Health and Healing* by Yogi Bahjan

Oil-based cleansers (for dry skin): jojoba oil, almond oil, and peach kernel oil are useful for removing all types of makeup and will gently dissolve dirt and grime.

Skin tonic: chamomile floral water, made by infusing a chamomile tea bag in a jug of freshly boiled bottled water. Leave in for a few minutes while the herbal infusion steeps before removing the bag and bottling the fluid.

Skin exfoliation: finely ground oatmeal mixed with yogurt or milk, or ground almonds made into a paste with a few drops of water.

Moisturizers: avocado oil is extremely nourishing. Wheat-germ oil is the richest of all plant oils and has the highest vitamin E content.
> —from *Save Your Skin with Vital Oils* by Liz Earle

Essential oils for skin:

Normal skin: avocado, grape, lemon, peach, wheat germ, jasmine, lavender, aloe, and chamomile

Dry skin: avocado, carrot, melon, aloe, wheat germ, sunflower, jojoba, figs, almonds, and olive oil

Oily skin: cabbage, lemon, strawberry, and pear

Blemished skin: grape, cabbage, juniper, and bergamot

Mature skin: aloe, apple, banana, wheat germ, and jojoba
> —from *Natural Organic Hair and Skin Care* by Aubrey Hampton

Beautiful means taking what you've been given and making it glow, making it fresh, and making it as healthy as possible. Just like fitness, beauty is for everyone.

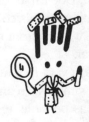

CHAPTER EIGHTEEN
BEAR WITH ME

I couldn't leave this book without introducing you to Dr. David Lapan, cardiologist extraordinaire, nice guy like you couldn't imagine, and one of the most interesting connections in my life.

In order to understand what I'm talking about, you've got to go back with me a couple of years. Once upon a time there was a doctor (and there still is, because the guy's not dead)—Dr. David Lapan. He happened to own and operate the fitness facility where I was teaching (which has one of the catchiest names I've ever heard in the old fitness business—FIT, which stands for the Fitness Institute of Tucson. Cute, don't you think?).

One day five years ago, he called me up to his office to talk to him. I figured I was going to get fired, because I'd been fired from so many fitness facilities for things like teaching too much, not smiling enough, not doing what all the other aerobics teachers were doing (jumping around like lunatics and not teaching a thing other than how to count to eight and yelp).

So up to his office I went, and Jamie, the aerobics coordinator at the time, introduced me to this good-looking guy—nice face, kind eyes, nice smile—kinda young-looking to be a big-shot cardiologist who owns this great fitness facility. And instead of firing me, Doc Lapan did something that shocked me. He asked me where I was going with this concept, resisted movement, different style of teaching. What I wanted from it and what my plans were. He asked me if I wanted to be a star.

Dr. Lapan in Tucson, Arizona, a very nice man but a total stranger, was the first person I shared my goals with, my dreams, my plans of getting this information to as many women as possible against all odds. I think I talked faster than I've ever talked in my life during that however-many-minutes we had together.

At the speed of lightning, I told Dr. Lapan everything I thought about what the aerobics industry was doing: How it had to change so that fitness would be for everyone. Why there was no need for specialty classes. What we could all do to make a difference. And how he could totally change his facility, as good as it was and still is—who couldn't use a little aerobics overhaul? I went on and on and on and on, and finally, when I stopped long enough to take a breath, he looked at me and said, "Susan, you're going to make it." That everything I was saying was going to happen because "I see something special [his words, not mine] sitting in front of me."

A cardiologist, owner and operator of FIT—and a psychic? Who knew? I just knew that someone important, a doctor who understood the importance of fitness, was listening to my opinion, and while I had an ear to bend I was going for it—because it might be the last chance I got and the only ear to bend for the rest of my aerobics life.

How I ended up in Tucson is another little story that we should revisit if we are ever going to get to one of the most interesting interviews in this book—and that's a pretty big billing, because they've all been good, wouldn't you agree?

So here it is. Five years ago, when I'd first married husband number two, I ran from Dallas, the Prince, the Christmases of doing it all alone and not getting any credit, his visits with the girlfriends in the car, the house in the suburbs, the broken dreams, the extended family—ran to Tucson to begin my new life.

That's what I was doing there, working, teaching aerobics, and talking to anybody who'd listen about this concept that I had. Everywhere I went and talked slower music and movements, no more choreography, fitness for everyone, teach, teach, teach your heart out, most clubs or fitness facilities were not listening. But FIT being the open, advanced facility it was/is had hired an aerobics coordinator, Jamie, who really took a chance on me. She hired me to teach and helped me set up a few seminars, teacher workshops, and special classes. Because she thought what I was saying had some merit.

You guys can't imagine how far out she went in doing this, supporting a concept that the governing agencies of the aerobics world didn't back up. Introducing this concept to her teachers and clients at FIT—and she had bosses she had to answer to, one of whom you already know, Doc Lapan.

You probably know what it's like to work for a company—fitness facilities are just like any other company I've ever worked for. You'd think because everyone runs around half-naked, in leotards, shorts, and sneakers, sweating for a living that it would be a little more laid back, but it isn't. The rules, the reasons why, the rights, the wrongs, the politics, the bull are the same in a fitness facility as in the company you work for, believe me. If you don't say the right thing, teach like everyone else—God forbid you try something different—remember there's an industry standard that we are all supposed to follow, even if that standard is way off base, that's the way it was, that's the way it is. So Jamie went out of her way and took some risks when she hired and encouraged me.

(A private moment here. I haven't seen Jamie in forever, but if you happen to be reading this, thanks Jamie. It all worked out well. I'm still doing the same thing I was doing back then, I'm just doing it in print, on video, audio, radio, and T.V. But it's the same thing, done with the same energy level and commitment.)

Jamie had a lot to do with my meeting David that day years ago. Just before one of my Saturday morning classes, Jamie came up to me and told me that one of the owners and his wife were coming to class. You can imagine what it's like to be in an important position, coordinator of aerobics for a fitness facility, and have your boss coming to the new teacher's class—the teacher you just hired who has very short hair and an unusual style, is wearing rags (I never really went for the coordinated leotard look), and teaches differently than any teacher on staff. So you can probably sympathize with Jamie when you hear that as she was telling me that the owner and his wife were coming to take my class, my response with a smile on my face was, "To hell with them, they are no more important than anyone else in this class, and if they get it, they get it, if they don't, they don't. Come on, let's get started." And right into teaching the class I went, never for a moment thinking again about the owner and his wife and whether or not they were in my class, were enjoying the class, or understood the class.

I spent the next hour and a half teaching. My only concern was all the rest of the wonderful people who were there learning, moving within their fitness levels, and getting stronger, burning some fat, and building some cardio-endurance. Fun class. Great people. Wonderful focus. We had a great workout and a great time together, and then I left.

Turns out that the owner and his wife *were* in the class. Jamie was probably sweating bullets the whole time, and it wasn't the exercise, if you know what I mean. And it was just after that I met Dr. David Lapan.

We met, we chatted, he told me he thought I was special, I loved him immediately (who's not gonna love someone who tells you you're special) and I left.

Tucson, that is.

Within months I was gone.

Back to Dallas, the Prince, the extended family, the new husband—never to see David Lapan again!!!

The Prince and I were starting what turned out to be work on the oddest arrangement ever, ex-husband and wife staying together and working through what we could never work through in our marriage, all for the sake of the children—the issues, the living arrangements, being the divorced family of all times. And that and my work were what I spent the next couple of years focusing on.

Opened a studio in Dallas.

Taught my own thing without having to explain it to anyone.

Read, listened, learned, worked my butt off.

Paid the bills, raised the boys, worked on the ex-marriage and the new one.

Busy little bee.

But don't expect it to end there with David Lapan. First, what would the point of this whole chapter be if that was it, and second, nothing in my life ends there, believe me.

My life is not that simple—there's always an ending with a bang, sometimes not such a good bang, but this ending has a big wonderful bang.

> I am probably eating a quarter of the fat compared to this time last year. . . . The most important thing is that I feel great!
>
> —*Patricia, Sterling Heights, Michigan*

Here I am years later writing a book on food, and you wouldn't believe where I've just spent the last couple of hours, just got back this minute and had the best time.

David Lapan's house. Swear. Five years later, I'm back in Tucson sitting in David Lapan's living room, interviewing him for my new book called—you know already—*Food*. I'm so excited. This is such a joy, and I'll tell you all about it.

Great house. Backyard like the garden of Eden. Cute kids. Wonderful wife—kinda liked her more than him (pardon me, David, but you're married to a bright, interesting, "works-for-the-betterment-of-woman" kind of woman, and that wins with me every time). And I must say, in one of those personal notes that I've sprinkled throughout this book, for me to be able to walk back into someone's life five years later and be proud of my accomplishments is a feeling I haven't had much in my life. God knows I've been at the other end more times than not, meeting someone and wanting to crawl into the wall.

How about that feeling when you bump into people who haven't seen you in a couple of years and you've put on about a hundred pounds—could you die??!!

And when they ask, how's Nic? And you've got to say, he's gone, he has a girlfriend, and my life is in the toilet—love that one!!!

Oh, and there's nothing in the world quite like bumping into your ex and his new girlfriend and feeling like Ten Ton Tessie while she's smiling brightly with the sweater draped over her shoulder and her youthful smile and shining eyes staring right at you—talk about wanting to disappear. . . .

But this moment, one of those wonderful WOW moments that seem to go hand-in-hand with a hell of a lot of hard work and taking responsibility for your life, sure felt good. David still had that kindness in his eyes. He looked great, and it was a pleasure sitting down talking with him—we kind of started right where we'd ended five years before, with me talking a million miles a minute trying to explain everything that had happened in the last five years, both personal and professional, and getting him caught up with where I was going with the *Food* book. Why I was interviewing him and what I wanted from this whole thing.

I think David got two words in at the first meeting, but he understood. David Lapan gets it—hey, David Lapan prophesied it.

So? What's the point? Do I expect you to be teary-eyed at this point over my reunion with David Lapan? Not really, but if you need to take a break and get a tissue, it's understandable—pretty touching story and all. But this is about so much more than our reunion, so much more than I ever dreamed it would be about when I sat down to chat with him so many years later.

We discussed heart disease because he's a cardiologist. Good start. David is pretty clear when it comes to talking about heart disease and the connection to food.

"Premature heart disease is a totally man-made disease. It is very rare that we see a patient under the age of sixty who doesn't smoke, eat a high-fat diet, live a sedentary lifestyle—all the things that contribute to this disease. It's what we are doing to ourselves, how we behave, that is causing this disease. Sure there are genetic predispositions involved, but first they're not that common, and second they're somewhat overrated, because you can't do anything about them. And if genetics are a consideration, you should concentrate even more on the things you can influence, the things that work to prevent this disease. People have this idea that it's genetics, therefore it's a fait accompli [something French that I didn't understand], that they are going to get heart disease. But the truth of the matter is that the genetic component of this disease is the smallest component. The largest [you guys take a wild guess here] is lifestyle. How people behave. Another consideration with the genetic predisposition issue and heart disease that we see over and over again is people stating their genetic predisposition, but very often, when we stop to have a look, it's the family behaviors that contribute to this disease. Everybody smokes. Everybody eats loads of beef [loads being my word, not David's], everybody is inactive. Very often it's not the genetic predisposition at all, it's the behavior pattern of the family that's the problem. Behavior. How people treat themselves."

I really like David's terminology. There was something very interesting about its coming from the mouth of a physician. It was wiser, deeper, more encompassing than the average Doctor Joe—the prophet David, perhaps?

> Yesterday I went through my fridge and every cupboard in my kitchen, bagging up every single thing that exceeded 30% fat. I had four grocery bags full of food.
> —*Jennifer, Lodi, California*

There's something more to this whole discussion, and it was up to me, Susan Powter, Food P.I., to sniff it out, dig under the rock, and drag the cat out of the bag—and that's exactly what I did. I asked Dave about it, and he told me, very clearly, just what the hell he was talking about.

How's this for the big investigative line of questioning?

"What are you talking about—'treating ourselves'?" That's exactly what I said to this very accomplished physician.

"The major contributors to heart disease [one at a time, please] are smoking, because smoking damages the arteries, setting you up for the process of atherosclerosis, and number two, the food you are eating."

What we are eating. See? *Food* book. Heart disease. Interview with David, the cardiologist—they all tie together eventually. And you know all too well at this point that if you are talking food and heart disease, you are talking about saturated fat. Even though you already had the scoop on saturated fat and cholesterol as early on as stage one, it's good to hear it from the doctor. Throw the cardiologist a bone, let him explain. The quick saturated fat review, by Dave Lapan.

"You eat saturated fat. With very few exceptions—coconut oil, palm oil, chocolate—saturated fat comes from animals, period. It is converted in the liver, as a breakdown product, into cholesterol."

Now, David made it very clear that there's nothing wrong with cholesterol. And who doesn't know that after reading this book? Your body must have it. Yeah, yeah, yeah, cells and all, and your body manufactures all that you need. So let me guess . . . it's not the cholesterol that's bad, it's the saturated fat that's being converted into cholesterol on top of what your body is manufacturing for its needs, because your body is brilliant . . . right? Right!

"High cholesterol is a major component of heart disease. So often I hear people saying 'I'm sticking to a low-cholesterol diet and having only four eggs a week' or 'I'm buying only lean red meat, low-fat cheese, trimming all the fat off that piece of meat.' Many times what I see is people eating reduced-fat versions of the highest-fat foods but still eating incredibly high amounts of saturated fat because of the foods they choose. We are being lied to. Packaging lies. Complicating the issues to create confusion. That's why I like your message so much, Susan [instant love for David Lapan], because you are uncomplicating the issue. Let's talk about what we can control, focus on, and the things that we can change. Then let's have a look at how we treat ourselves."

Fine, David, anything you say is O.K. with me since you love my message and all, but first let's connect obesity and heart disease. The way we look and the way we feel. What we eat and the fat that's all over our bodies, so that we can get down to the issues we are really interested in . . . smaller underarms, no more stomach hang, and those lean thighs and butt.

"Weight is an independent risk factor for heart disease."

So, you see? There it is . . . jumping right into the weight issue while still staying with the interview with the cardiologist—amazing, isn't it? See why I got the job? (Who else do you know could take this thing, twist and turn it around the way I just did, and make it come right back to the point?) So let's mix heart disease, weight, lifestyle, and food together for a moment—don't worry, it will all work out O.K.—and talk about David's real passion, which is going to surprise the hell out of you, I promise.

Weight being an independent risk factor. Food being connected with weight—i.e., saturated fat, too much fat, sedentary lifestyles being connected to heart disease and obesity and a million other things. What we eat being connected to everything. That's it. That's the connection, plain and simple, and one you are already very familiar with—but how about something new added to this equation (that is, if you could ever come close to calling what I just threw out on the table an equation of any kind), the mind/body connection? Yep. Dave's passion.

If you think this man is good when it comes to our hearts, you wouldn't believe how wonderful he is when he starts talking about something that really interests him. (Not to suggest for a second that your heart doesn't—could you imagine going to a specialist and knowing that his real interest lies somewhere else?) But someone as smart as Dave has to have a few interests, and the more we got into it, the brighter his eyes got, the more info I got, the more this chapter changed, and the more excited I got, because this is some good stuff that is really gonna make a difference in changing your lifestyle—talk about something to think about.

Here it is.

THE MIND/BODY CONNECTION AND WHAT THE HELL IT HAS TO DO WITH YOUR LIFE.

"The body is an intelligent machine."

WOW, kind of out there for a physician.

"The body is born in a healthy state—you have to work hard to screw it up."

A doctor said screw it up—have you ever?

"Think about it. When bacteria is introduced into the body, your immune system recognizes it and kicks it out. Viruses, tumors, excess cholesterol—your body responds intelligently and does what it has to do to solve the problem. When you eat, your body releases the acids necessary to digest, assimilate, distribute—it's a very intelligent machine. If you stop for a moment and look at disease, where it starts, how it happens, you'll very often see a loss of intelligence. It's almost a physical expression of what's going on in your mind."

If you thought the intelligent machine statement was out there, how about this physical expression stuff? But listen, because it gets better and makes a whole lot of sense.

"When people behave unintelligently—as in smoking, drinking, eating high-fat diets, not practicing safe sex . . ."

HOLD ON HERE . . . I may be able to twist and turn, weaving a web of a story with the best of them, but how do you go from lean thighs to heart disease to safe sex and have it all make any sense?

I'm doing my usual thinking while my interviewee is talking and it dawns on me . . . Dave's talking about people giving up control, not thinking about consequences, not understanding connections between what we do and how we end up living or dying.

". . . it's almost as if some people give up the control in their lives [swear he said it just as I was thinking it—we probably knew each other in another life, throw that into the pile of stuff we are talking about here] by choosing not to think, not take responsibility, blaming everyone and everything for our problems. Living the incredible victim act. Victim of genetics, victim of my parents, adult child of whatever, my boss is, my kids are—and it's this loss of control, lack of responsibility, sense of being a victim that many times leads to disease and looking and feeling horrible."

There it is.

What do you think? We're not just talking disease here—how about the same line of thinking directly connected to the way your body looks right now, as you're reading this? What do you think? Does the way you look and feel now, with or without disease—God forbid, knock wood—have anything to do with not taking responsibility for your life? Not acting intelligently?

Living the victim?

Quite a concept. I had to stop for a moment and think, because there is a lot of truth in it for me and my life. During the breakup of my marriage, I absolutely felt and acted like the victim. My ex-husband's rules were different from mine. Our lifestyles were dramatically different during the separation and after the divorce. He had the credit, he had the girlfriend, he had the 28-inch waist, he had the advantage in every way, and what did I do? Jumped right into the victim thing. You want blame? I blamed him for everything (even though he deserved it). Victim City, that's where I lived and what happened in my life as a result of what I was thinking and feeling.

What happened in my life? I started acting unintelligently. Shoving loads of high-fat food into my mouth. Not very smart if it's obesity you want to avoid.

Stopped moving. There's something that's gonna lead you right into looking and feeling horrible.

Started isolating—not a good thing if you want to stay sane. Stopped doing anything for me, forgot about books, music, beauty, growth—all the things that interested me, out the window. And look what happened.

ONE HUNDRED AND THIRTY-THREE POUNDS LATER, EVERY ACHE AND PAIN IN THE BOOK, EXHAUSTION, LITHIUM, ANGER, PAIN, STRESS . . .

Disease? If I'd continued down that path it would have been right around the corner. Never thought about the lack of intelligence that was involved in the process until now. Never, ever, thought about the taking-responsibility part of the process until I'd finished my therapy session with David, my guru at this point.

Taking responsibility is exactly how I began to change my life. The Prince was gone and never coming back, no matter what I did.

It wasn't the Prince who shoved the food into my mouth at 2 A.M. every morning, it was me.

The decisions I made daily were what got me to where I was, and where I was was absolutely unacceptable. It hurt too bad to live feeling and looking the way I did. So step-by-step, I started making different decisions. More intelligent decisions, if you will, now that we have this wonderful insight.

You know the first decision I made. Eliminate everything white and creamy, cut back on the fat, forget about the quality. Don't you think that was intelligent compared to how I'd been eating?

See it? See where it all connects in this book?

Next intelligent decision was to start moving. Couldn't do much, but I could walk. You can easily see that this "intelligent" thing has nothing to do with I.Q. Let's not pretend for a second that what I was doing had anything to do with passing a big test. We're talking intelligent as in things-that-are-going-to-get-you-what-you-want-as-opposed-to-things-that-are-taking-you-further-and-further-from-the-life-you-want-to-lead kind of intelligence.

Common sense and the truth—that's what I call it. This is it. This is the process that gave me back my life, my control, my choices, and eventually rocketed me out of the victim role and into the leader-of-my-own-life role. I'm dying, this is so big!!!

What David said he's seeing over and over again is:

"The quality of people's lives is, much of the time, directly connected to how much responsibility they take, whether you are talking about heart disease or being overfat and unfit. If you don't take responsibility, you will be a victim. You will not have control, and your life will not be yours."

Can't argue with that, it just makes too much sense. But Davey, I've got some good questions for you:

> How do we do that?
> Where do we start?
> Mantras?
> Affirmations?
> Disciplinary action?
> What, what, what do we do?

I know for me it was the basic, easy steps of cutting back on fat and moving that made the physical differences and helped make me 133 pounds leaner. And as I've said everywhere I get the chance, and over and over again, where the hell is the fat going to come from if you don't eat it?

Despite the many advances of modern science, all the major cereals (wheat, barley, oats, rice, etc.) had been cultivated by 3000 BC, and not a single new major crop has been introduced since then.

But Dave, what else can we do to make it happen? Not be victims of our unintelligent choices, get back the control and choices in our lives, and look and feel and live the way we want to.

What David said next knocked me for a big loop. (Don't you love this interviewing stuff? You ask these wonderful people a question and you get an answer that knocks you out—love it, love it, love it.)

"First it has to become a reality, dawn on you, be real that your life is in your control. It's that moment of consciousness that is the most powerful. Susan, something had to change you."

Dave, something did change me, and that something was anger. I was angry that the ex's life was so different from mine. Angry that his waist was different from mine. Anger, David, anger.

"You say it was anger that kept you going. Anger because the diet industry starved you, the fitness industry humiliated you, your ex-husband walked out on you, but that anger could just as easily have turned into something self-destructive. You could have killed someone [not that I didn't think about it after the first visit with the girlfriend in the car, but as many of you already know, I was stuck between the chair and the window with binoculars in my hand, so I couldn't kill anyone!!]. It wasn't anger that saved you, it was the consciousness that you had to take responsibility and make some changes in your life. It was that moment that saved you."

Hold on a minute, I thought I was talking to a cardiologist—this ain't no cardiologist, this man's my life teacher; we're going to India together. He's the smartest man on earth. He's right. This stuff makes the kind of sense that hits you in your soul and forces you to take a deep breath.

So what's a writer to do? Here we are talking food, heart disease, saturated fat, and now moments of consciousness. I'm always finding myself here and am always faced with the same old same old—do we talk about it, do it, does it make any sense? You guys are brilliant—I figured this is right. This is important.

Dave's got a point, and if making changes in your life-style and changing the way you look and feel are something you're interested in doing—or why did you buy this book?—then we really have to have a little chat about our belief systems. Yours, mine, and Dave's (the sequel to the movie, you're thinking?). Like the food you're eating, your belief system has to be looked at, thought about, and maybe changed a bit, so that making some of the physical changes that will change your life are possible, easier, more understandable . . . whatever.

O.K., Dave, belief systems—what do we do with them?

"Take a look at your belief systems and see if you are trapped in your self-imposed limitations of life, health, disease. When I think something isn't possible, when I hear that voice inside my head that is telling me I can't do it . . ."

HOLD ON, DAVID'S HEARING VOICES . . . just like I did. I heard the beast telling me that my thighs would never be as small as the nineteen-year-old's in the front row of my aerobics class.

It was the beast that told me not to worry when I was too tired to go for my walk or when I was faced with a high-fat or low-fat food choice. But David, a cardiologist, a mature father, a husband, a professional, hears voices?

". . . sure, it's the loudest voice I hear sometimes, the voice of self-doubt. When I hear it, I think of it as the devil, and I stop to listen to what it's telling me I can't do, think about what is making me believe it's not possible, and then spend my energy thinking about what needs to be done to make it possible and I take control of it."

Haven't you heard the voice? If you listen, you'll hear it.
"Go ahead, eat the cookies."
"Stay home, don't get dressed and go to exercise class, why bother?"
"You'll never be able to accomplish this, forget about ever being the size you want, it ain't gonna happen."

> The voice of self doubt.
> The irresponsible voice.
> The victim's voice.

Just like David, me, and everyone else I've ever talked to when it comes to the voices in our heads, the tapes that run nonstop, may be the loudest voices you hear.

But stop for a second and take the time to listen, think about what the voice has been saying to you—you may be amazed at how constant and persistent and brazen it really is. I was. Then when you feel its strength and try to hear any other voice, you will be floored at the one whispering:

> "You can do this, you want to be strong and healthy, this is important to you. It was only yesterday that you made up your mind to do this, you wanted this badly . . . don't eat the fat, eat the low-fat version, improve the quality, go ahead—it's what you want."

Yeah, the whisper, the voice we should all listen to, but before you know what hit you, BAMMO, you hear the yell:

"THE CAKE TASTES BETTER. HE WAS JUST SO MEAN TO YOU . . . GO . AHEAD AND ENJOY THE CAKE . . . EEEEEEEEEEEEAT IT, DON'T BOTHER TRYING TO LOSE SOME OF THAT FAT, IT'S THERE FOREVER . . . EAT THE CANDY, IT TASTES GOOD, GO AHEAD."

That's what most of us are up against when we take a second to look at belief systems and listen to the voices in our heads.

My intelligent, what-I-wanted-in-my-life voice was a whisper—forget about my belief system, I think it was in coma. I didn't have the support, the cash—anything—to believe I could ever get healthy, well, looking good again.

One hundred plus pounds lighter!!!

You want to fuel the fire or the beast's voice?

Just try to institute a belief system about losing 100 pounds alone, in Texas without a helpful soul in sight. If it's the beast you want to hear:

"GET OUT OF HERE, IT'LL NEVER HAPPEN. HOW ARE YOU GOING TO LOSE ALL THAT WEIGHT WHEN YOU CAN'T EVEN STICK TO A DIET FOR A WEEK?"

"But I'd like to feel healthy again," the whispering voice would chime in.

"WHO ARE YOU FOOLING? HOW ARE YOU GOING TO GET STRONG WHEN YOU CAN'T EVEN WALK? NOBODY CAN RE-GAIN THAT MUCH STRENGTH. IT'S GONE, FACE IT. THIS IS IT, YOUR LIFE FROM NOW ON."

"How about a smaller size, just to look a little better?" the whisper faded.

"SMALLER THAN WHAT SIZE, 18? WHAT'S THE DIFFERENCE BETWEEN 22 AND 18? YOU'LL NEVER GET BELOW THAT, SO KEEP EATING. YOU THINK SMALLER LIKE HIS GIRLFRIEND? THAT'LL NEVER, EVER HAPPEN!"

Feel good?

Get my life back?

Regain my sanity?

Get outta here—how possible was any of that at the time? But guess what? . . . first the intelligent decisions. Then the small amount of change. Then more and more moments of clarity and consciousness, the whisper getting stronger and stronger with each intelligent decision, each no-more-victim step I made, taking more and more responsibility, and slowly but surely, the whisper got a little louder, and louder, and louder, and soon it turned into a roar. The beast's yelling got quieter and quieter. The loud moments of self-doubt and imprisonment got fewer and further between.

And things sure as hell did change, didn't they?

My beast is locked in a cage and can't get out now, at least not the high-fat monster/beast. There are still a few other beasts roaming around my head, but when I look to quiet them or tame them, it's the same approach I take as I did for the first one. David's right about this "moment of consciousness"—it does start there—the big moment when we start taking the steps to change, taking responsibility for our own lives.

Think about what's making you believe it isn't possible. Take the small, intelligent steps necessary to make it happen. Stage one, two, or three of the information you're reading—take all of it, bits and pieces of each, whatever, but make the changes, step-by-step, in what you are putting into your body. If you want to go hog wild, throw in a walk once a day—see what happens.

> I used to dive for chocolate, cheese, and sweet rolls . . . what a wonderful feeling knowing that I can turn down all those fat foods and not look back!
> —Shannon, Kamloops, British Columbia, Canada

After this wonderful interview with Dr. David Lapan, I can say without question that there were moments of consciousness all along the way in changing my life. I never paid much attention to them—scary thought, unconscious the whole time during one of the biggest changes in my life. I may have been unaware of what was going on until now, but I did start taking responsibility for my own life, going from making unintelligent to intelligent decisions to beginning a process that has made a great difference in my life.

So if I'm going to give prescriptions for eating, breathing, and moving, then I've got to get prescriptive about consciousness—no easy task, I might add. Haven't people like Gandhi been trying to do this for a long time? If you go to hell in the Catholic religion for enough lies that aren't confessed in time, can you imagine what happens when you try to get prescriptive about consciousness? I'm a little scared, but let's give it a try—after all, I'm not listening to the voice that's yelling right now in my head, "Don't bother with this; just write about low-fat foods and forget about the rest, not now, not after all this!!!"

After reading about all this stuff, you may be feeling warm, fuzzy, and connected to the big picture . . . but what happens when you're dying for that bowl of ice cream, and low fat just won't do? It's you and the refrigerator door that separate you from the whisper or the roar.

That moment when you're standing at the fridge ready to high fat yourself to death!!! What do you do then? A great concept isn't going to help much, unless you know how to apply it. So we've got to come up with a system—our own system, designed by women who have found themselves over and over again at the fridge. Let's just design our own, because it's probably gonna be the best one out there.

We've talked about eating, breathing, and moving until we are blue in the face. You've probably got that down by now, but this new thing—making different choices, taking control (what do we call it?)—has to be added to our prescription. So it should read from now on: eating, breathing, moving, and what???

My friend Suzi and I are sitting here talking about this as I type. I asked for her opinion on this subject because she's been there fighting that low-fat battle. She also works with me as a researcher, so she's been a big part of writing this book, digging up the facts, sitting in libraries for hours, and even becoming computer literate within weeks because there was no alternative—it was either learn it or get buried alive by paper work, and learn she did. Now when we talk, we talk modem to modem, fax to fax—but always heart to heart, because she's my friend. Suzi is a mom, with three of the most wonderful kids you've ever met in your life. She's a wife. Harry is her husband, a really nice guy. And she's a brilliant, wonderful woman. She also happens to be a case manager for drug-addicted mothers, so it only stands to reason that I'd ask for her opinion about control, choices, quieting the voice, whatever we choose to call it.

Step one. Therapy. Is that what we all need? Is that what you'd think Suzi the case worker is going to recommend?

Not necessary right now. "It may be too expensive, maybe you've done years already, or maybe you just don't have the time. So without the benefit or need of immediate therapy to work out all the issues, we've got to figure out why we act irresponsibly, making the victim's decisions, and aren't taking responsibility for our lives."

So what can we do? The new and improved, no-need-for-therapy-right-this-moment stage one. We've got a step one for you that doesn't require hours of spewing your guts to some expensive paid-by-the-hour person. How about starting here:

"Accept what is. Look at the truth."

The old take-your-clothes-off-in-front-of-a-mirror. Look at your body in a bathing-suit dressing room, where they always have mirror-lined walls and wonderful yellow lighting. Actually have a look this time, without anything in mind but accepting what is. Looking at your eating habits honestly. Connecting and accepting what is.

> I used to sit and eat fried fish, shrimp, and french fries with melted cheese every day when I was pregnant—even before I was pregnant. I look back and think I must have been insane. I was.
>
> —*Karla, La Palma, California*

Suzi heard something years ago, and you won't believe who she heard say it—Richard Nixon, after Watergate. When asked how he dealt with it, he said, "Never look back." That's what Nixon said, and that's what Suzi says to do. Don't look back. Forget about yesterday. Don't worry about the past, just look at and work on accepting what is right now. At that moment of decision or when evaluating the problem.

- Your body. Does it have too much fat all over it? Where do you hold most of your fat? Stomach, legs, underarms, chest? Have a look, accept what is.

- Could you use a little lean muscle mass? Where?

- How does your skin look? Refreshed? Healthy? Or do you look as if you just died and nobody's told you yet.

- Eyes. Are they full of life, love, and laughter? Come on, I know I'm pushing it, but check it all out while you're accepting what is—why not? There's nothing to worry about because this is just being honest with yourself so that you can figure out what needs to be done and get on with doing it. Remember, nobody's judging, it's just you having a look.

The great thing about Dick Nixon's never-look-back theory is that all the mistakes you've made . . . you can forget about them, never need to talk about them again, because we are not doing anything but looking forward. The high-fat confessional time, right here and right now. The moment of consciousness in the making. So you've made the wrong decision about the foods you've put into your mouth a million times—who hasn't. That doesn't mean for a moment that you can't make the right one this time. The one that will support your effort to look and feel better.

The more intelligent one.

The self-esteem building and the conscious no-victim decision.

Who hasn't screwed up more times than not?

I've made some big mistakes in my life, most of which you've already heard about, and there's more to come, I'm sure. Because the minute you stop making mistakes, the minute you are afraid of being wrong, is the minute you stop growing. (Rusty, you know her, just said that to me this week—never thought I'd use it in this chapter, but what the hell. Why not if it works, and it certainly does right here and right now.)

When you're at the fridge and you know you've been there a trillion times before and eaten the ice cream every time, don't look back—try to accept what is. You're there. Your body doesn't look or feel the way you want it to, and it's time to change it.

You feel like eating the ice cream because you're angry, frustrated, fighting with the husband, exhausted, sick of being evolved, sick of low fat—and you're standing at the moment of choice. How does not looking back help you right now?

"Think fresh moment," Suzi says. "That moment at the fridge is a fresh moment. Looking back will send you right back into habit, and we all know how powerful that can be, it can give you a reason why—I mean, after all, you've done it a million times before, it felt good for ten minutes, it didn't do much harm, did it? Or did it? How are you feeling? Did those million moments and the wrong decisions that went with them contribute to how you are feeling about your body, your life, your everything—right now?"

It's at this moment that you must look at yourself. Feel yourself. Think about what you are feeling. Think. Think. Think. Sounds really stupid, but I'm telling you, thanks to the eye-opening interview with Dr. David Lapan, I realized that it was those moments, and there were a million of them, sometimes all in one day, when I had to look at what was, stop looking back, stop with the blaming, stop with the reasons why I couldn't, and learn how to move forward. The beast's voice may be yelling for you to do what you've done a thousand times before.

EAT THE HIGH-FAT FOOD.

But those ten minutes of satisfaction are what you'd throw it all away for right now. To hell with consciousness, you'd rather be unconscious and eating a bowl of triple fudge than anything in the world right now—but wait . . .

The next question, fifteen minutes later, the next morning, the next week: What about your life, my life, our life, that we never knew we could design, we had control over, and we could overhaul?

It's your life—what do you want it to be? Talk about a question that I'd never taken the time to ask. Three hundred pounds, 400, then what? Less energy, more anger, hating the way I looked and felt more than I did standing there at 260—could that be possible?

I know—immersed in that moment of choice, most of us could care less about tomorrow, let alone a lifetime, but just spend a minute with me and let's talk. You may want to feel good right now. And that ice cream may have done the job for ten minutes a thousand times in the past. But when the suffering, the agony, the darkness, the failure, the emptiness of the decision are worse than the ten minutes of pleasure you get when you eat it, you will change the behavior.

A very big part of changing the behavior is not looking back but looking at the moment instead—two very simple steps that are very, very effective. Recently, in one of the thousands of books on food I've read, there was a wonderful reason given for our love of fat—we love high-fat foods because they feel good. They're padding. They're filling. And they do feel good for the moment.

But the end result is being overfat.

The emptiness, lack of control, fear, anger, frustration—not liking the way you look and feel and ending up with a big, pardon the pun, problem.

When the consequences of the action, the ten minutes of pleasure turn into days of suffering one too many times, you're faced with your decision standing at the fridge. It's good news, folks—great news, at a matter of fact—because you are thinking about it. Remember what David said. (Forget about the fact that Suzi and I have made it understandable. Forget about the fact that we have no degrees, and always remember that when women get together and talk, support, and network, healing begins.) The thinking about it can be the moment of consciousness that can change your life.

Yes, you may fail. Yes, you may do it a million times over. But that moment can be very, very powerful. Just the thinking. Consider it the seed planting. Think about Suzi and me standing with you during that moment.

> This is the moment.
> We are here.
> The universe opens to us right now.
> The guardian angels are cheering.

The lights are blinking (that's the stars, you know), aliens have landed, document this right now, and you are one. E.T. is home, damn it.

But guess what? You asked the questions. You took the moment. Thinking without looking back, understanding what this is, maybe making a different decision this time, creating a new consciousness. Asking different questions than you've ever asked in your life. Making your own decisions, not just falling back into self-destructive habits and regaining the control over your own life . . . it's that simple, because when you do, in that moment, you may take action.

A different action than you may have ever taken. Those moments and those small, easy, different actions do add up to more than you could have ever dreamed of. . . .

I am sick of being controlled by food.

It's time for me to move forward.

On and on and on it goes, if you are going through anything like I did standing there at 260. What you are creating during those moments is awareness, desire, a different thought process, the beginning of control, and certainly taking responsibility for your actions—just in the thinking alone, all this is happening.

> Last month's meal is this month's body.
>
> —*Dr. Marc Micozzi*

See? See how something so intangible and nutty—a moment of consciousness changing your life—can be real? Take the moment and listen to the whisper—the roar may be roaring, but listen to the whisper.

"TO WANDA, THE AVENGER . . ." Suzi just yelled that at the top of her lungs. I have no clue what the hell she's talking about, but she's definitely very excited, so I asked her to explain.

"It's from *Fried Green Tomatoes at the Whistle Stop Cafe*. It's what Idgy said every time she was about to take charge." What the hell, let's make it our own—why not steal from the best of them?

TO THE MOMENT—TAKE CHARGE. Try it. When you are standing there, use the charts and graphs, substitution lists left, right, and center. Your newfound knowledge of fats—use it. Assessment—go for it. The interviews with the experts—use the yell, do whatever you have to do. But understand that all of us fighting this battle of overfat, unfit, and hating the way we look and feel find ourselves at the fridge facing the same decision—forget about whether to eat the high fat versus the low fat, how about the decision to take responsibility, make different choices, direct our own lives, and change things? All that happens in a million moments.

The victory isn't in whether you succeed every time—it's in the process. I would have given anything to have known that when I started my process from unfit and overfat to fit and lean—to know that the moment of consciousness was the victory and the beginning of changing my life. All I knew then was that it seemed my life was full of loud, roaring beasts, never-ending decisions that were so difficult for me and seemed to be no big deal for most people.

Me standing at my fridge having a conversation with twenty people in my head about whether to grab the higher-fat version or the lower is all I knew was happening. I wish I'd known that it was those many moments of consciousness, each one moving me forward to what I'm doing today, that were the most important work I could be doing. Had no clue.

But you guys do. It ain't about what you did yesterday. Forget the massive high-fat screw-up that happened an hour ago. Now, it's about now, it's about not looking back—just looking at what is, and it's about eating, breathing, moving, and thinking. Simple but true, and I've always liked simple but true.

"The satisfaction comes from that moment of strength."

Harry just walked in. He's a certified substance abuse counselor with twenty years' experience in prevention, intervention, and treatment. Listen to what he said:

"The moment of control, of breaking the habit and creating something new."

At my worst, the lowest emotional place, the highest weight, the hardest moments of decision I faced, the satisfaction did come from knowing or beginning to believe I could make a different decision than I'd made in the past, one that could lead me in a different direction.

Maybe the ex wasn't going to get the best of me. Someday, maybe, just maybe, I could look and feel better, but today I wasn't going to pig out on high fat . . . and maybe I could look better than the Prince's girlfriend. Call me stupid, someone you don't want to grow up to be like, but that's exactly what went through my head during my moment of recognition.

"Opening your eyes to the possibilities around you. Different decisions create a different reality. Recognizing that you are trying to do something. That you're not giving up."

Seeing the growth in the realization, the new questions, listening to the whispers are so very valuable, because being alive is about growing. These are the moments of change. Here's where the motivation comes in. This is where you take the time to comfort, guide, take responsibility for your life, and this is also the time that you respect and love yourself for taking the moment. It may be just a moment, but boy, what a powerful 60 seconds it could be, if you thought about it and felt it and were in it. . . .

Making the decision to move forward, to go against the beast, to listen to the whisper is as important as eating, breathing, and moving. Being present—something new. Something valuable. Something risky, for sure, but something that will take you in a different direction than the one you've gone in before . . . and, again, I ask you to look at where you are.

> Do you like it?
> Is it comfortable?
> Is it where you want to be?

I'm tired. It's a lot to understand right now, but it's a damn good beginning. It's that simple. If you don't want to be a victim, then don't be. If you want more control in your life and want as desperately as I did to look and feel better, then take the steps, slowly, respectfully, and consciously. You'll screw up a thousand times, who doesn't? But before you know it, the unconscious will become the conscious, the whisper a roar, the victim the empowered, and your body—don't ask how good it could look.

EAT, BREATHE, MOVE, AND THINK . . .

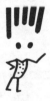

STAGE 3 RECIPES

SOUPS
....

Miso Soup   Pea Soup

SAUCES
....

Mushroom Sauce   Mochi Sauce

DRESSINGS
....

Tofu-Sesame Dressing

SALADS
....

Cold Sesame Noodles   Arame and Vegetables
Arame Salad

MAIN DISHES
• • • • • • • • • • • • • • • • •

Brown Rice, Aduki Beans, and
   Vegetables

Spicy Eggplant and Tofu

Tempeh with Apple Juice and Ginger

Soba Noodles (Buckwheat Spaghetti)
   with Yellow Pea Sauce

Millet Burger with Mochi Sauce

Vegetarian Sushi

Tofu-Rice Burgers and Arame Salad

Rice with Vegetables and Gomasio

Aduki Beans

DESSERTS
• • • • • • • • • • • •

Cherry Pudding

Date Nut Cookies

Almond Custard

Miso Soup

2	small strips kombu seaweed, washed	1	carrot, cut in pieces
1	small bunch arame seaweed, washed	1	Tbsp finely chopped ginger
4–5	dry shiitake mushrooms, washed	1	handful of collard greens, washed and cut into narrow strips
1½	qt water	2–3	Tbsp light kome miso
¼	lb soft tofu, cut into ¼-inch slices	3	scallions, cut into ¼ inch rounds: include part of the green ends

1. Place seaweeds and mushrooms in stockpot with water. Bring to a boil, then simmer for 30 to 45 minutes.
2. Let cool. Pour through a wire-mesh strainer and discard the arame. Remove the kombu and cut into 2-inch narrow strips. Remove the mushrooms, cut off the stems, and discard. Cut the mushrooms into narrow strips.
3. Return to the stockpot. Add the tofu, carrot, and ginger, and cook for 10 minutes.
4. Add the greens and cook 2 more minutes.
5. Remove some hot soup (about ½ cup) and add 2 to 3 tablespoons of light kome miso. Mix to dissolve and add back to the soup with the scallions. Keep soup warm, but don't bring to a boil.
6. Add enough water, if needed, to make 6 cups of soup. Tamari can be added if it needs more salt.

 Brothy soup—loaded with nutrients.

Serving size	18 oz	Total fat	2 g
Servings per recipe	4	Saturated fat	0 g
Calories	93		

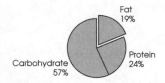

Pea Soup

1 lb dried green split peas, rinsed	2 c 1-inch strips of kale or collard greens
1 small piece kombu seaweed, 2 by 8 inches	1 small zucchini, cut into small pieces
1 small piece wakami seaweed, 2 by 8 inches	¼ c chopped red pepper
12 c water	2 Tbsp Bragg liquid aminos
1 piece parsnip, 1½ by 6 inches, coarsely chopped	3 Tbsp chick-pea miso (light miso)
3 medium carrots, sliced	1½ Tbsp mugi miso (dark miso)
1½ c chopped onions	1 Tbsp chopped dill
	2 scallions, chopped

1. Wash peas in a bowl with 3 changes of water, until the water becomes clear.
2. Wash seaweed well. Place with the peas and 8 cups of water in a large stainless pot. Bring to a boil. Control the heat to make sure the peas don't burn.
3. When the peas come to a boil, start adding the vegetables: parsnip and 1 cup of onions. Cook for 20 minutes. Add 4 more cups of water. Add carrots and cook for 10 minutes. Add remaining ½ cup of chopped onions. Cook 10 more minutes.
4. Add 2 cups of greens and continue cooking for 15 minutes. Add zucchini and pepper, and cook 5 more minutes.
5. Add 2 tablespoons bragg. Turn off the heat. Remove most of the large pieces of seaweed and discard.
6. Take one-third of the soup and blend until smooth. Return to the pot. Dissolve both misos in a little soup until smooth. Return to the pot. Add dill and scallions, and serve.

Options
If you cannot find mugi or chick-pea miso, use a light and a dark miso.

 Thick and rich—one of my favorite comfort foods.

Serving size	6 oz	Total fat	1 g	
Servings per recipe	9	Saturated fat	0 g	
Calories	101			

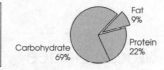

SAUCES

Mushroom Sauce

3 c vegetable stock
2 large cloves garlic, chopped
⅓ tsp thyme
10 oz mushrooms, sliced
(or 2 c fresh)
1 Tbsp light miso
1 Tbsp kuzu (acts like
cornstarch)

1 Tbsp soy sauce
2 Tbsp chopped parsley
(optional)
salt or extra soy sauce to
taste
4 c cooked brown rice

1. Heat ½ cup of stock in a pan. Sauté garlic and thyme. Add mushrooms and cook until they release liquid. Add up to another ½ cup of stock, ¼ cup at a time, to pan if it gets dry while sautéing.
2. Dissolve miso in ½ cup of stock and set aside. Dissolve kuzu in remaining stock.
3. Add the soy sauce and kuzu mixtures to the mushrooms and bring to a boil. Cook until the sauce has thickened. Add miso and parsley, and heat through. Season to taste with salt or extra soy sauce and remove from heat. Serve over rice cooked according to package directions.

 Very easy to make. Great with rice, chicken, potatoes, toasted bread.

Serving size	17 oz	Total fat	2 g
Servings per recipe	4	Saturated fat	0 g
Calories	256		

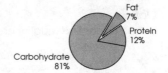

Fat 7%
Protein 12%
Carbohydrate 81%

Mochi Sauce

2 tsp canola oil
1 medium onion, chopped
1 clove garlic, chopped
1 Tbsp soy sauce, or to taste
2 tsp mirin (Oriental cooking wine)

1½ c vegetable broth (lentil broth)
¾ c shredded mochi

1. Heat oil in pan, and sauté onion and garlic 10 minutes, until soft and lightly browned.

2. Add soy sauce, mirin, broth, and mochi. Stir well and cook 3 to 4 minutes, until the mochi melts. Taste for seasoning.

 Thick, to pour over anything you love to smother with gravy.

Serving size	3 oz	Total fat	1 g
Servings per recipe	8	Saturated fat	0 g
Calories	70		

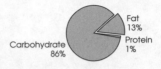

Fat 13%
Protein 1%
Carbohydrate 86%

DRESSING

Tofu-Sesame Dressing

½ lb tofu
1 Tbsp tahini (sesame butter)
1 tsp sesame oil
2 cloves garlic, sliced
3 Tbsp white vinegar
½ c vegetable stock

¼ c brown rice vinegar
¾ c soy sauce
2 Tbsp honey
1 tsp chopped ginger
¼ tsp cayenne
salt to taste

Blend all ingredients in a food processor until smooth.

 Drizzle over veggies, pasta—dip, dip, dip everything into this creamy, thick dressing.

Serving size	1 Tbsp	Total fat	.5 g
Servings per recipe	35	Saturated fat	0 g
Calories	15		

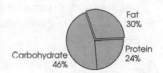

Fat 30%
Protein 24%
Carbohydrate 46%

Options

To make a low-fat pasta salad: Serve over 1½ pounds cooked pasta; 4 cups broccoli, cut into small pieces and cooked; 1 red pepper sliced into strips; 1 green pepper, sliced into strips; 1 red onion, cut into slices; 1 pound blanched frozen vegetables.

Serving size	16 oz	Total fat	5 g
Servings per recipe	6	Saturated fat	1 g
Calories	342		

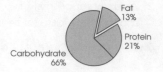

Fat 13%
Protein 21%
Carbohydrate 66%

SALADS

Cold Sesame Noodles

1 lb vermicelli
2 large stalks celery
2 large carrots
1 medium cucumber,
  seeded and sliced into
  ¼-inch pieces
1 Tbsp dark sesame oil
4 cloves garlic, chopped
1 Tbsp chopped ginger
¼ c soy sauce

Sauce:
2 tsp tahini
¾ c vegetable broth
3 Tbsp light miso
2 Tbsp honey
¼ c white wine
2 Tbsp white vinegar
⅛–¼ tsp cayenne pepper, or to
  taste
salt or soy sauce to taste

1. Cook vermicelli according to package directions and drain.
2. Cut celery and carrots into 1½- to 2-inch strips.
3. Heat oil in pan. Add garlic and ginger, and sauté for 3 minutes. Add celery, carrots, and soy sauce, and cook until crisp but not raw, about 5 minutes.
4. Mix the sauce ingredients in a bowl until well blended. Taste for spiciness and saltiness, and adjust seasoning.
5. Add cooked vegetables, cucumber, and sauces to noodles and mix until well coated.

 Salty and very creamy—try adding chopped tomatoes and onions—wonderful!

Serving size	11 oz	Total fat	5 g
Servings per recipe	6	Saturated fat	1 g
Calories	312		

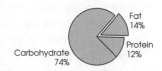

Fat 14%
Protein 12%
Carbohydrate 74%

Arame Salad

1 oz dried arame seaweed	2 tsp dry mustard powder
4 c shredded red cabbage	7 Tbsp cider vinegar
2 apples, peeled, cored, and grated	2 Tbsp honey
	3 Tbsp soy sauce
1 medium onion, sliced thin	1 tsp salt
2 cloves garlic, finely chopped	1 Tbsp fresh dill weed
1 Tbsp ginger, minced	

1. Wash arame in water until it looks clear. Drain. Mix with shredded cabbage, apples, onion, garlic, and ginger.
2. Dissolve mustard powder in vinegar and mix with remaining ingredients to make a dressing. Mix dressing and arame mixture and let sit for 1 hour so all the flavors meld.

Arame is loaded with minerals. It's a seaweed and does have a little fishy taste, which is great if you love that. But this recipe covers that taste. This will keep forever in the fridge. It's great just to mix in with other foods or on a sandwich.

Serving size	6 oz	Total fat	1 g	
Servings per recipe	8	Saturated fat	0 g	
Calories	77			

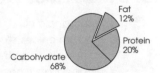

Fat 12%
Protein 20%
Carbohydrate 68%

Arame and Vegetables

2 c washed arame seaweed	2 Tbsp frozen corn
1 Tbsp dark sesame oil	¼ c ½-inch cubes of soft tofu
1 carrot, grated	1 sliced scallion
2 Tbsp diced ginger	1½ Tbsp tamari
½ large red pepper, sliced	1½ tsp mirin
2 Tbsp chopped parsley	4 c cooked brown rice

1. Soak arame for 2 minutes, drain, set aside.
2. Heat sesame oil over medium heat in a saucepan.
3. Add carrot, ginger, some pepper and some parsley. Sauté for 5 to 7 minutes.
4. Add corn, seaweed, and tofu. Continue cooking for 3 to 4 minutes. Add the remaining pepper and parsley and scallion. Stir well and cook for 2 minutes.
5. Add tamari and mirin. Stir for 2 more minutes and serve.

This is the same seaweed stuff as the arame salad, but it has a much different texture and taste. This is thick and hot and very filling. I love this with a veggie burger.

Serving size	15 oz	Total fat	6 g	
Servings per recipe	4	Saturated fat	1 g	
Calories	320			

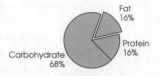

Fat 16%
Protein 16%
Carbohydrate 68%

MAIN DISHES

Brown Rice, Aduki Beans, and Vegetables

1 Tbsp canola oil
2 medium onions, sliced
2 carrots, sliced on the diagonal and then quartered
1 large parsnip, cut like the carrots
¼ lb string beans, cut in 1½-inch pieces

12 fresh mushrooms, sliced
1¾ c vegetable broth
2 Tbsp kuzu
3 Tbsp white miso
3 c cooked brown rice
1½ c cooked aduki beans

1. Heat oil in pan. Add onions and sauté for 8 minutes, until soft but not brown. Add carrots and parsnip. Cook for 5 minutes. Add string beans and mushrooms, and continue cooking for 5 minutes.
2. Mix kuzu in ¾ cup of vegetable broth until dissolved. Mix miso with remaining 1 cup vegetable broth. Combine kuzu mixture and miso mixture with vegetables. Bring to a boil and cook until thickened.
3. Serve rice, beans, and vegetables together on a plate.

Option
Use these leftovers to make soup. Add water and more soy sauce.

 Beans, rice, and veggies—what more could you want!

Serving size	15 oz	Total fat	6 g
Servings per recipe	4	Saturated fat	1 g
Calories	394		

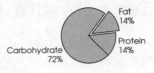

Fat 14%
Protein 14%
Carbohydrate 72%

Spicy Eggplant and Tofu

1 Tbsp canola oil
½ c ¼-inch-sliced onion
2 Tbsp garlic, chopped
1 Tbsp fresh ginger, chopped
1 large eggplant, not peeled, cut into ¼-inch slices and cut across into strips (about 6–8 cups of strips)
1 lb fresh firm tofu, cut into ½-inch cubes
12 black Chinese dry mushrooms, soaked in hot water for 20 minutes, stems removed, and cut into ½-inch strips, or dried shiitake

½ tsp salt, or to taste
¼ tsp black pepper, or to taste
¼ tsp cayenne pepper (leave out if you do not like spice)
6 Tbsp soy sauce
3 Tbsp dry sherry
2 tsp raw sugar
1 Tbsp red wine vinegar
3 Tbsp cornstarch
6 scallions, cut into small round slices ¼-inch thick
4 c cooked brown rice

1. Heat oil in a heavy skillet. Add onion, garlic, and ginger, and cook for 10 minutes. Add eggplant and continue cooking for 10 to 15 minutes, until eggplant begins to wilt.
2. Add tofu, mushrooms, salt, black pepper, and cayenne pepper.
3. Mix soy sauce, sherry, sugar, vinegar, and enough water to make 1 cup. Add to cornstarch and mix until smooth.
4. Add cornstarch mixture to eggplant. Mix well and cover. Cook on low heat for 5 minutes. Uncover and continue cooking until eggplant is tender but not mushy.
5. Turn heat off, add scallions, and serve with brown rice.

Yum, yum, yummy! Casserole in a skillet. Easy, easy. Great in cold weather.

Serving size	20 oz	Total fat	9 g
Servings per recipe	4	Saturated fat	1 g
Calories	469		

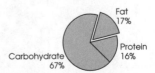

Fat 17%
Protein 16%
Carbohydrate 67%

Tempeh with Apple Juice and Ginger

2 c apple juice
2 Tbsp chopped ginger
½ lb tempeh, cut into 1½-inch
   triangles
1 Tbsp chopped garlic
¼ c lite tamari
2 tsp sesame oil
½ c 1-inch triangular-shaped
   butternut squash

½ c cut parsnip (half moons
   cut in half again to form
   triangles)
1 Tbsp umeboshi vinegar
1½ Tbsp chopped fresh parsley
4 c cooked brown rice

1. Heat apple juice in a shallow pan over medium heat. Add ginger and garlic, and lay out tempeh.
2. Add lite tamari and sesame oil. Lower heat and keep at a simmer. Liquid will cook down.
3. Add squash and parsnips. After 15 minutes, turn tempeh over to another side. Add more apple juice to the pan if necessary. Turn the tempeh every 10 minutes. Cook it for 30 to 40 minutes.
4. Add the umeboshi vinegar. Make sure the vegetables are tender. The liquid should be greatly reduced.
5. Add the parsley and serve with brown rice.

 If you've never tried tempeh, now is the time—meaty flavor and texture.

Serving size	16 oz	Total fat	9 g
Servings per recipe	4	Saturated fat	1 g
Calories	451		

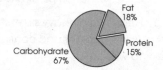

Fat 18%
Protein 15%
Carbohydrate 67%

Soba Noodles (Buckwheat Spaghetti) with Yellow Pea Sauce

½ c dry yellow split peas
1 2-inch piece kombu seaweed
1 2-inch piece wakami seaweed
1 c vegetable stock
2 cloves garlic, chopped

1 tsp oregano
1 red pepper, chopped
2 c sliced mushrooms
1 tsp salt, or to taste
2 Tbsp soy sauce
6 oz soba noodles

1. Wash the split peas and remove stones. Leave soaking until ready to cook. Wash seaweed. Place peas and seaweed in a heavy-bottomed pot with enough water to cover. Cook until peas disintegrate.
2. Keep adding water to keep the peas from boiling dry. When finished, peas should be like a sauce. Discard pieces of seaweed if they haven't disintegrated.
3. Heat ¼ cup of vegetable stock in a pan. Add garlic and oregano, and sauté for 3 minutes. Add pepper and mushrooms, and cook for 5 minutes. Add more stock, up to one cup. Add salt and continue cooking for 2 minutes. Add peas and soy sauce, and heat together. Set aside.
4. Cook noodles according to package directions. Drain and serve covered with sauce.

 Ever think you'd love seaweed? The kombu and wakami in this recipe add tons of flavor and minerals—don't worry, they don't taste fishy!

Serving size	8 oz	Total fat	5 g
Servings per recipe	4	Saturated fat	1 g
Calories	305		

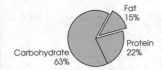

Millet Burger with Mochi Sauce

4 c water
1 Tbsp salt
2 c millet, washed and soaked for 1 hour
1 small piece kombu seaweed
1 small piece wakami seaweed
1½ c dry lentils or black beans or pinto beans, soaked overnight
1 carrot, chopped
1 parsnip, chopped
½ c chopped onion
1 c vegetable broth
2 Tbsp miso
¼ c lentil water
2 Tbsp soy sauce
1 Tbsp chopped ginger
2 cloves garlic, chopped
1 c cornmeal

1. Bring water to a boil. Add salt and millet, bring to a simmer, and cook for 20 minutes. Remove from heat and let sit for 10 minutes. Keep covered.
2. Wash seaweed and lentils. Cook lentils with seaweed until lentils are soft. Discard seaweed; drain and reserve liquid.
3. Boil vegetables in broth until soft. Mash and set aside.
4. In a separate bowl, mix millet, lentils, and mashed vegetables. Dissolve miso in ¼ cup of lentil water. Add soy sauce, ginger, and garlic. Taste for seasoning, adding more salt or soy sauce if needed.
5. Form into 2-inch flat burgers. If mixture is too dry, add more of the lentil liquid. If it is too moist, add some cornmeal.
6. Preheat oven to 350°. Place burger on a baking sheet sprayed with oil and dusted with cornmeal. Bake for 30 to 40 minutes. Serve with Mochi Sauce (see recipe).

 Eat these on a bun as a burger or just smother with Mochi Sauce.

Serving size	10 oz	Total fat	3 g
Servings per recipe	8	Saturated fat	1 g
Calories	400		

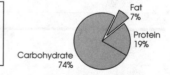

Fat 7%
Protein 19%
Carbohydrate 74%

Vegetarian Sushi

Flavoring:
- 1 Tbsp wasabi (a very hot Japanese mustard powder)
- 2 Tbsp water
- 2 Tbsp horseradish
- 2 Tbsp Grey Poupon mustard (low fat)
- 2 Tbsp umeboshi plum paste
- ½ c gomasio

- 1 roasted nori seaweed sheet
- 1 nori roller
- 1 c short-grain brown rice cooked according to directions

Vegetables:
- 3 celery stalks, cut into 1½ to 2-inch strips
- 1 lg red pepper, cut into 1½ to 2-inch strips
- 5 scallions, cut in half and into 1½ to 2-inch strips

Dipping Sauce:
- ½ c soy sauce
- 1 tsp mirin
- ½ tsp wasabi
- ¼ tsp ginger, chopped

1. Make a mixture of water and wasabi, then mix with umeboshi plum paste, horseradish, and Grey Poupon. (If the wasabi is not available, increase horseradish.)
2. Place one nori sheet in the middle of a nori roller. Place ¼ cup of cooked rice in the middle of the nori sheet and press down with wet fingers into a strip 2½ to 3 inches wide across the nori sheet. Spread a little of the wasabi-umeboshi mixture across 1 inch of this strip. Keep 1 inch clear at each end. Do not wet the seaweed.
3. Place 2 celery strips, 2 pepper strips, and 2 slices of scallions across the wasabi-umeboshi mixture and sprinkle with gomasio.
4. Wet your fingers and run them across the bottom clean strip of seaweed. Fold the top of the roll, holding on to the roll, roller, and rice, and use the heel of your hand to roll the seaweed as tightly as possible. Keep rolling until the roll has gone across the bottom and has been glued to the wetted bottom of seaweed. The roll should look like a tight cylinder. With a sharp knife, cut the roll into 1½-inch slices. Set them on end with the cut end showing.
6. Prepare the dipping sauce by mixing the ingredients together. Dip the slices in the sauce and eat.

Options
Make without flavoring and just cucumbers—a cucumber roll. Other veggies to use: cucumbers, carrots, pickled veggies, watercress, water chestnuts, bean sprouts.

 Want the best meal ever? Miso soup, sushi, and a salad with the tofu-sesame dressing.

Serving size	8 oz	Total fat	1 g
Servings per recipe	6	Saturated fat	0 g
Calories	126		

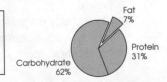

Tofu-Rice Burgers and Arame Salad

1 c vegetable broth	2 Tbsp miso
1 onion, chopped	2 c cooked brown rice
1 carrot, chopped	1 Tbsp mustard, prepared
1 celery stalk, chopped	¼ c falafel mix
½ c chopped parsnip	2 Tbsp chopped parsley
1 tsp chopped garlic	1 tsp basil
2 tsp chopped ginger	1 tsp salt, or to taste
6 oz tofu, crumbled	

1. Bring ¾ cup vegetable broth to a boil in a pot. Add onion, carrot, celery, parsnip, garlic, and ginger. Cook for 10 to 15 minutes, until all the vegetables are soft.
2. Mash tofu and vegetables in a bowl. Dissolve miso in the remaining ¼ cup vegetable broth. Add remaining ingredients and miso to the tofu and vegetable mixture. Taste for seasoning.
3. Make into 2-inch flat burgers. Spray a baking sheet with Pam and wipe off the excess or use nonstick pan. Bake the burgers in a 350° oven for 30 minutes. Serve with Mushroom Sauce and Arame Salad (see recipes).

 Never heard of falafel mix? Look for it in any health food store—while you're there look for low-fat tofu—it's high in protein and creamy just like regular tofu, but without all the fat.

Serving size	15 oz	Total fat	6 g	
Servings per recipe	6	Saturated fat	1 g	
Calories	281			

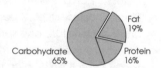

Fat 19%
Carbohydrate 65%
Protein 16%

Rice with Vegetables and Gomasio

4 c cooked brown rice	1 leek, cleaned and sliced in round, thin slices
2 oz dry shiitake mushrooms, cooked and sliced	¾ lb Chinese cabbage, finely sliced
1 Tbsp plus 1 tsp dark sesame oil	1 tsp salt
2 Tbsp tamari or regular soy sauce	2 tsp kuzu
1 Tbsp chopped garlic	½ c chopped parsley
1 medium carrot, cut in matchstick slices	1½ Tbsp gomasio

1. Wash mushrooms. Soak for 15 to 20 minutes in 3 cups of warm water. Place in a pan and cook until soft, about 20 minutes, let liquid cool. Drain and keep liquid. Remove stems and slice caps. You should have close to a cup of mushrooms.
2. Heat 1 tablespoon of oil in a sauté pan and sauté mushrooms for 5 minutes. Add rice and stir-fry with mushrooms for 5 minutes. Add tamari and heat through.
3. Heat 1 teaspoon of oil in another skillet. Sauté garlic, carrot, leek, and cabbage for 5 to 10 minutes. Add salt.
4. Mix kuzu in mushroom liquid. Pour over vegetables and bring to a boil. Cook for 2 minutes. Serve, sprinkled with parsley and gomasio, with rice.

 Never say veggies have to be boring.

Serving size	13 oz	Total fat	5 g
Servings per recipe	4	Saturated fat	1 g
Calories	646		

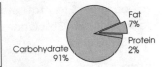

Fat 7%
Protein 2%
Carbohydrate 91%

Aduki Beans

1 c beans	4 c water
1 strip kombu seaweed	1 tsp salt, or to taste
1 strip wakami seaweed	

1. Wash beans in bowl, filling bowl a couple of times with water until the water is clean. Drain.
2. Wash pieces of seaweed under the faucet and set aside.
3. Place beans in a pot with 2 cups of water and seaweed. Bring to a boil, reduce heat, cover. Cook for 30 to 40 minutes. Uncover, add 2 more cups of water, and continue simmering for 1 hour. Ten minutes before it is finished cooking, add salt.
4. Remove large pieces of seaweed and discard.

Options
When removed from the heat, add 1 bunch of cleaned, cut-up watercress. Spice up with tamari, Bragg liquid aminos, seasoned herb salt, or jalapeños and corn.

 Perfect with Mexican food and salads.

Serving size	11 oz	Calories	172
Servings per recipe		Total fat	trace
as a main dish	2	Saturated fat	0 g
as a side dish	4		

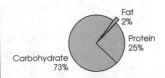

Fat 2%
Protein 25%
Carbohydrate 73%

DESSERTS

Cherry Pudding

1 qt cherry juice, less ½ cup for dissolving kuzu	5 heaping Tbsp agar flakes
½ c dried bing cherries	1 Tbsp kuzu
	1 tsp vanilla extract

1. Place juice (less ½ cup), cherries, and agar in a pan. Cook for 20 minutes.
2. Melt kuzu in ½ cup of juice and add to pot. Continue cooking until the liquid is clear, about 5 to 10 minutes. Remove from heat, stir in vanilla extract, and cool in a shallow dish. Chill. When chilled, blend until smooth and return to the refrigerator. Serve cold.

Options

The same proportions can be used with every fruit. Apple cider is great as the liquid. Use as a topping for chocolate cake or ice cream.

 I swear this reminds me of the cherry pie filling that my mom used to make. You haven't tried anything until you eat this with the Chocolate Angel Food Cake (see recipe) and non-fat ice cream!

Serving size	6 oz	Total fat	1 g	
Servings per recipe	6	Saturated fat	0 g	
Calories	120			

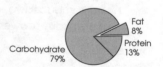

Date Nut Cookies

2 c rolled oats	¼ tsp salt
½ c chopped dates	1 tsp vanilla extract
¼ c almonds	1 tsp grated orange rind
1 c amazaki	2 Tbsp brown sugar

1. Preheat oven to 350°.
2. Cook oats in a heavy pan until they are lightly colored but not browned. Mix oats and dates together.
3. Chop almonds in a food processor, and place in a bowl. Blend oats and dates in a food processor and add to the almonds. Add remaining ingredients and mix well.

4. Spray a cookie pan lightly with Pam and wipe off excess. Place enough of the mixture to make a 1½-inch cookie. Bake for 25 minutes, cool, and keep refrigerated.

 Sweet, sweet, sweet . . . love, love, love. Make a double batch and freeze.

Serving size	1 oz	Total fat	2 g
Servings per recipe	18	Saturated fat	2 g
Calories	63		

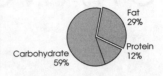

Almond Custard

2 c amazaki (set ½ cup aside to melt kuzu), original flavor	2 rounded Tbsp agar flakes
½ Tbsp kuzu	1 tsp vanilla extract
	½ tsp almond extract

1. Heat 1½ cups amazaki in a pan over medium heat. Dissolve kuzu in remaining ½ cup of amazaki.
2. Add agar flakes and melted kuzu.
3. Add vanilla and almond extracts, and stir well. Let mixture boil for 20 minutes, stirring constantly. Remove from heat and cool. When chilled, blend in blender and refrigerate.

Options
For vanilla custard, leave out the almond extract and use ½ teaspoon more vanilla extract. Can be used as a topping for fruit puddings.

 Eat on cakes, with fruit sauces, and with fresh fruit.

Serving size	1 oz	Total fat	2 g
Servings per recipe	4	Saturated fat	0 g
Calories	121		

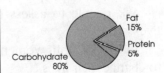

HOPE AND CHANGE

I gotta tell you something. Unscientific isn't the word for this little theory, discussion, throw-it-out-and-see-what-happens line of thinking, but boy, oh boy, would you have a hard time convincing me it's not true. So if you're looking for objectivity, don't read any further, cause it ain't in this ending.

Hope ignites change, John Robbins has already explained all this to us. But I've got a more personal view of the whole thing, and it starts with what happened to me tonight. I just left a dinner with some people, upper-middle-class and white, in a nice house in a nice section of Dallas, Texas. I'm not being a bigot when I say any of this, I'm simply including something that I think is an important part of what just happened.

In the middle of dinner, one of the men at the backyard barbecue table started a conversation with me about what I do.

· "Sell hope to people with no hope . . .

"Ask people to assess their lives who have no reason to assess their lives . . .

"Talk to fat, unfit women about changing their lives when they don't want to change their lives."

Let me make one thing clear before we go on. . . . This thirty-five plus, fat man was sitting and eating his burger, telling me that you and I have no reason to change and that what I was doing was a lost cause—can you imagine what was going through my head???

I wanna know a couple of things. Not from him, from you. Whose life isn't tough? Who doesn't have bills? I can tell you from someone who went from not having enough money to buy what I needed for my kids, waiting for an alimony check every month so I wouldn't have to call my father and ask for money (although I know I was very lucky even to have a father I could call if my pride and ego didn't get in the way), to making more money than I could ever have imagined—the battles are still the same. Whether it's the monthly rent you are struggling with or a payroll every month that includes twenty people, what's the difference? It's all money you have to come up with on the thirtieth. Is it the amount that makes it easier? I'm not sure it is.

How about the quality of your life or your relationships? Is it money that makes a difference when it comes to that? Whether it's one person or fifty you have to consider and come to terms with, does the money you make every month make a difference when you're talking about your standards, what's acceptable to you?

When you know in your heart and soul that you want to change something, anything, small or large, is that change any easier for any of us?

Here's where the unscientific part comes in. I know that it doesn't. Go ahead, call me unscientific, people have called me worse.

Change—no matter what it is you're talking about, changing is about the desire to do so. We are all equal there. Each and every one of us has the right to make changes in our lives, and we all end up in the same place trying to change it. The desire to do so.

The steps that you or I or Mr. Burger-eating-self-righteous have to go through to make a change in our lives are the same.

Knowing there needs to be a change.

Having a look at what you need to do.

Getting the information, support, steps necessary to move forward.

And then having the honesty, guts, and clarity to do it.

I have seen the other side. I was born into opportunity left, right, and center. I've seen people who had "everything," according to my friend at dinner tonight, who didn't do a thing with it. They were lacking the honesty and the guts that go hand in hand with seeing what has to be done. They lacked the courage that goes right along with taking that first step, and they had the same kind of attitude that I felt tonight—that they were better somehow than the "other" people.

Fat people.

Unfit people.

Abused people.

Unmotivated people.

And on and on and on it goes.

It would have been a whole lot easier for me to write a recipe book with a few interesting food notes here and there than it has been for me to write what you've just read. Fence sitting is a lot easier than the truth, take it from me, but that's not what makes changes. And you deserve more than that.

Information.
The truth.

Making decisions without judging is what makes the change—that's what I've tried like hell to tell you.

I believe in you.

I was the woman—unfit, unhealthy, unmotivated—Mr. Burger-eating-self-righteous was talking about. The minute I started to believe in me, ignited the hope, and had the courage to take the steps necessary to make the change, my life changed—and yours will, too.

Take what you want. Leave what you're not ready to hear or have no interest in, it's your decision. But don't ever stop questioning and getting information, and don't ever give up the hope that anything can change. The circumstances surrounding your life are just that, circumstances, and you are in charge of them . . . much better women than I am have proven that over and over again.

God bless you and be well.

Appleton, Nancy, *Lick the Sugar Habit,* Garden City, New York: Avery Publishing Group, Inc., 1988.

Bailey, Covert, *The Fit or Fat Woman,* Boston, Massachusetts: Houghton Mifflin Company, 1989.

Bailey, Covert, *The New Fit or Fat,* Boston, Massachusetts: Houghton Mifflin Company, 1991.

Balch, Phyllis and James, *Dietary Wellness. The Wellness Book of the 90's,* Greenfield, Indiana: P.A.B. Publishing, 1992.

Barnard, Neal, *Food for Life,* New York: Harmony Books, 1993.

Bieler, Henry, G. *Food Is Your Best Medicine,* New York: Ballantine Books, 1966.

Brody, Jane, *The New York Times Guide to Personal Health,* New York: Avon Books, 1983.

Bumgarner, Marlene Anne, *The Book of Whole Grains,* New York: St. Martin's Press, 1986.

Colbin, Annemarie, *Food and Healing,* New York: Ballantine Books, 1986.

Cooper, Kenneth H., *Controlling Cholesterol,* New York: Bantam Books, 1989.

Cooper, Robert K., *Health and Fitness Excellence,* Boston, Massachusetts: Houghton Mifflin Company, 1989.

Cordle-Pope, Jamie and Marine Katahn, *The T-Factor Fat Gram Counter,* New York: W.W. Norton and Company, 1991.

DeBakey, Michael E., Antonio M. Gotto, Jr., Lynne W. Scott, John P. DeForey, *The Living Heart Brand Name Shopper's Guide,* New York: Mastermedia Limited, 1993.

Duffy, William, *Sugar Blues,* Radnor, Pennsylvania: Chilton Book Company, 1976.

Dunn, Lavon, *Nutrition Almanac,* New York: McGraw Hill, 1990.

East West Journal, *Shopper's Guide to Natural Foods,* Garden City, New York: Avery Publishing Group, Inc., 1987.

Erasmus, Udo, *Fats and Oils,* Burnaby BC, Canada: Alive Books, 1993.

Feingold, Ben, *Why Your Child Is Hyperactive,* New York: Random House, 1974.

Finnegan, John, *The Facts About Fats,* Berkeley, California: Celestial Arts, 1993.

Greene, Bert, *The Grains Cookbook,* New York: Workman Publishing, 1988.

Haas, Elson, M., *Staying Healthy with Nutrition,* Berkeley, California: Celestial Arts, 1992.

Harte, John, Cheryl Holdren, Richard Schneider, Christine Shirley, *Toxics A to Z,* Berkeley, California: University of California Press, 1991.

Havala, Suzanne, *Simple, Lowfat and Vegetarian,* Baltimore, Maryland: Vegetarian Resource Group, 1994.

Hinman, Bobbie, *Burgers 'n' Fries 'n' Cinnamon Buns*, Summertown, Tennessee: The Book Publishing Company, 1993.

Holt, Tamara, *Bean Power*, New York: Dell Publishing, 1993.

Jensen, Bernard and Mark Anderson, *Empty Harvest*, Garden City, New York: Avery Publishing Group, Inc., 1990.

Jensen, Bernard, *Foods That Heal*, Garden City, New York: Avery Publishing Group, Inc., 1988.

Ketcham, Katherine and L. Ann Mueller, *Eating Right to Live Sober*, New York: Penguin Group, 1983.

Kilham, Christopher B., *The Bread and Circus Whole Food Bible*, New York: Addison-Wesley Publishing Company, Inc., 1991.

King, C.D., *What's That You're Eating*, Newport Beach, California: C.D. King Ltd., 1982.

Kushi, Avelino, *Diet for Natural Beauty*, New York: Japan Publications, 1991.

Kushi, Aveline and Wendy Esko, *The Changing Seasons Macrobiotic Cookbook*, Garden City, New York: Avery Publishing Group, Inc., 1983.

Kushi, Michio and Associates, *Crime and Diet*, New York: Japan Publications, 1987.

Lappé, Frances, *Diet for a Small Planet*, New York: Ballantine Books, 1991.

Larson, Joan Mathews, *Seven Weeks to Sobriety*, New York: Ballantine Books, 1994.

Lesser, Michael, *Fat and the Killer Disease*, Berkeley, California: Parker House, 1991.

Marcus, Alan L., *Cancer from Beef*, Baltimore, Maryland: The Johns Hopkins University Press, 1994.

Margen, Sheldon and the Editors of the University of California at Berkeley Wellness Letter, *The Wellness Encyclopedia of Food and Nutrition*, New York: Robus, 1992.

Mason, Jim and Peter Singer, *Animal Factories*, New York: Harmony Books, 1990.

McDougall, John A. *The McDougall Program*, New York: Penguin Group, 1991.

McDougall, John A., and Mary McDougall, *New McDougall Cookbook*, New York: Penguin Group, 1993.

McDougall, John A., *The McDougall Program for Maximum Weight Loss*, New York: Penguin Group, 1994.

McDougall, John A. and Mary A. McDougall, *The McDougall Plan*, Clinton, New Jersey: New Win Publishing, 1983.

Mindell, Earl R., *Food as Medicine*, New York: Simon & Schuster, 1994.

Mindell, Earl R., *Parent's Nutrition Bible*, Carson, California: Hay House Inc., 1992.

Mindell, Earl R. *Safe Eating*, New York: Warner Books, 1988.

Monk, Arlene, *Convenience Food Facts*, Minneapolis, Minnesota: DCI/Chronimed Publishing, 1991.

Murray, Michael T., *The Healing Power of Foods*, Rocklin, California: Prima Publishing, 1993.

Null, Gary, *The Complete Guide to Health and Nutrition*, New York: Dell Publishing, 1984.

Null, Gary and Steven, *Poisons in Your Body*, New York: Prentice Hall Press, 1977.

Null, Gary, *Healing Your Body Naturally*, New York: Four Walls Eight Windows, 1992.

Ornish, Dean, *Reversing Heart Disease*, New York: Ballantine Books, 1991.

Ornish, Dean, *Eat More Weigh Less*, New York: HarperCollins, 1993.

Oski, Frank, *Don't Drink Your Milk*, New York: TEACH Services, 1983.

Panati, Charles, *Panati's Browser's Book of Beginnings*, Boston, Massachusetts: Houghton Mifflin Company, 1984.

Pennington, Jean A. T. *Food Values,* New York: HarperPerennial, 1989.

Piscatella, Joseph C., *Controlling Your Fat Tooth,* New York: Workman Publishing, 1991.

Reader's Digest, *ABC'S of the Human Body,* Reader's Digest Association, 1987.

Rector-Page, Linda, *Cooking for Healthy Healing,* Griffin Printing, 1991.

Regenstein, Lewis, G., *Cleaning Up America the Poisoned,* Washington, DC: Acropolis Books, 1993.

Rifkin, Jeremy. *Beyond Beef,* New York: Penguin Books, 1993.

Robbins, John, *Diet for a New America,* Walpole, New Hampshire: Stillpoint Publishing, 1987.

Robbins, John, *May All Be Fed,* New York: William Morrow and Company, 1992.

Schwartz, George R., *In Bad Taste: The MSG Syndrome,* New York: Penguin Group, 1990.

Simmons, Maria, *Rice, the Amazing Grain,* New York: Henry Holt and Company, Inc., 1991.

Smith, Landon, *Foods for Healthy Kids,* New York: Berkeley Books, 1981.

Staten, Vince, *Can You Trust a Tomato in January?* New York: Simon & Schuster, 1993.

Steinman, David, *Diet for a Poisoned Planet,* New York: Ballantine Books, 1990.

Thompson, D.S., *Every Woman's Health: The Complete Guide to Body and Mind,* New York: Simon & Schuster, 1993.

Tracy, Lisa, *The Gradual Vegetarian,* New York: Dell Publishing, 1986.

University of California, Berkeley, ed., *The Wellness Encyclopedia: The Comprehensive Resource for Safeguarding Health and Preventing Illness,* Boston, Massachusetts: Houghton Mifflin Company, 1991.

Walker, Morton, *Sexual Nutrition,* Garden City, New York: Avery Publishing Group, Inc., 1994.

Weil, Andrew, *Natural Health, Natural Medicine,* Boston, Massachusetts: Houghton Mifflin Company, 1990.

Whitney and Hamilton, *Understanding Nutrition 4E,* New York: West Publishing Company, 1987.

Wigmore, Ann, *The Hippocrates Diet and Health Program,* Garden City, New York: Avery Publishing Group, Inc., 1984.

Winter, Ruth, *Food Additives,* New York: Crown Publishers, Inc., 1978.

Susan Powter is the star of *The Susan Powter Show,* a nationally syndicated talk show on women's issues, and of best-selling videos on health and fitness. She is the author of *Stop the Insanity!* and *The Pocket Powter.*

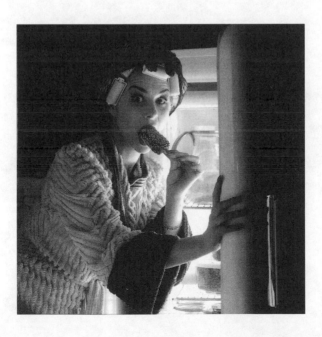

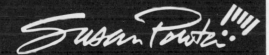
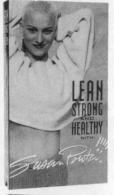
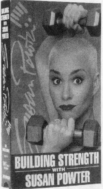
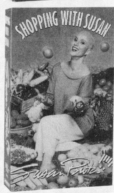
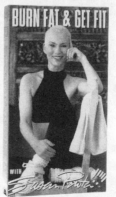

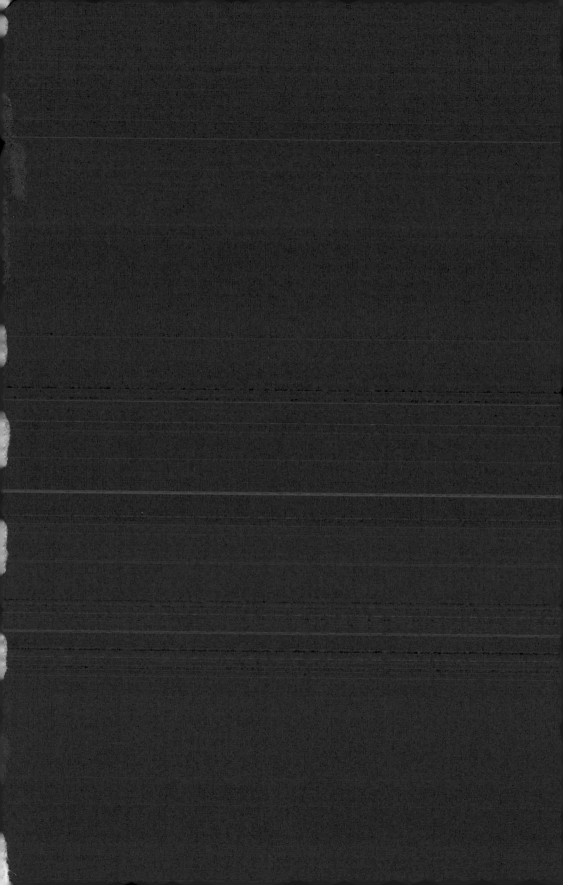